Cancer can now be CURED, not just treated

We are not accustomed to thinking about a cure for cancer. We think of remission as the only possibility. But this book is not about remission. It is about a cure. This is possible because in 1990 I discovered the true cause of cancer. The cause is a certain parasite, for which I have found evidence in every cancer case regardless of the type of cancer. So lung cancer is not caused by smoking, colon cancer is not caused by a low-roughage diet, breast cancer is not caused by a fatty diet, retinal blastoma is not caused by a rare gene, and pancreatic cancer is not caused by alcohol consumption. Although these are all contributing factors, they are not THE cause. Once the true cause was found the cure became obvious. But would it work? I set a goal of 100 cases to be cured of cancer before publishing my findings. That mark was passed in December, 1992. The discovery of the cause and cure of all cancers has stood the test of time and here it is!

You may not have time

to read this entire book first if you have cancer and are scheduled for surgery, chemotherapy or radiation treatment. You may wish to skip the first pages which describe how a parasite and a solvent cause cancer to develop. Go directly to the instructions on eliminating the parasite with herbs (Cancer Curing Recipe, page 19) or with electricity (Zapping Parasites, page 30). Using the herbal recipe along with the zapper is best. It only takes days to be cured of cancer regardless of the type you have. It does not matter how far progressed the cancer is—you can still stop it immediately.

After you have stopped the cancer, you can turn your attention to getting well (Part 2). Read the case histories to see how easy it is to stop even terminal cancers (Part 3). Learn from them to avoid mistakes.

Does this mean you can cancel your date for surgery, radiation or chemotherapy? Yes, after curing your cancer with this recipe, it cannot come back. This is not a treatment for cancer: It is a cure! But if you do not wish to make your doctor angry, you could follow her or his wishes, too. Be careful not to lose any vital anatomical parts in surgery, though, because you may need them later when you are healthy!

Remember that oncologists are kind, sensitive, compassionate people. They want the best for you. They have no way of knowing about the true cause and cure of cancer since it has not been published for them. I chose to publish it for you first so that it would come to your attention faster.

The Cure For All Cancers

Published in the United States by New Century Press
1055 Bay Blvd., Suite C, Chula Vista, CA 91911
(619) 476-7400, (800) 519-2465
www.newcenturypress.com
ISBN 1-890035-00-9 (Previously 0-9636328-2-5)
Library of Congress Card Catalog Number RC268.C96

Other books by Dr. Clark available from New Century Press:
The Cure For All Diseases - ISBN 1-890035-01-7
The Cure For HIV And AIDS - ISBN 1-890035-02-5
The Cure For All Advanced Cancers – ISBN 1-890035-16-5
Heilung ist möglich - ISBN 3-426-76152-1
The Cure For All Cancers - Japanese Translation
Heilverfahren Aller Krebsarten - ISBN 1-890035-03-3
The Cure For All Cancers – Korean Translation
The Cure For All Cancers – Italian Translation
The Cure For All Diseases – Italian Translation

30 29 28 27 26 25 24 23 22 21

Notice to the Reader:

The opinions and conclusions expressed in this book are mine, and unless expressed otherwise, mine alone. The opinions expressed herein are based on my scientific research and on specific case studies involving my clients. Be advised that every person is unique and may respond differently to the treatments described in this book. On occasion we have provided dosage recommendations where appropriate. Again, remember that we are all different and any new treatment should be applied in a cautious, common sense fashion.

The treatments outlined herein are not intended to be a replacement or substitute for other forms of conventional medical treatment. Please feel free to consult with your physician or other health care provider.

I have indicated throughout this book the existence of pollutants in food and other products. These pollutants were identified using a testing device of my invention known as the Syncrometer.™ Complete instructions for building and using this device are contained in this book. Therefore anyone can repeat the tests described and verify the data.

The Syncrometer is more accurate and versatile than the best existing testing methods. A method for determining the degree of precision is also presented. However at this point it only yields positive or negative results, it does not quantify. The chance of a false positive or a false negative is about 5%, which can be lessened by test repetition.

It is in the public interest to know when a single bottle of a single product tests positive to a serious pollutant. If one does, the safest course is to avoid all bottles of that product entirely, which is what I repeatedly advise. These recommendations should be interpreted as an intent to warn and protect the public, not to provide a statistically significant analysis. It is my fervent hope that manufacturers use the new electronic techniques in this book to make purer products than they ever have before.

Acknowledgments

I would like to express my sincere gratitude to **Frank Jerome, DDS**. for the loan of his parasite slide collection. If he had not made a slide of *Fasciolopsis buskii* in his student years and if he had not stored his slides carefully for three decades, finally to loan them to me in a generous offer, none of these discoveries would have been made. Furthermore, most of these HIV/AIDS patients could not have regained their health without his development of a new metal-free dentistry. Thanks are also due to his wife, **Linda**, for her patience and willingness to listen to new ideas. And a very special thank you is due to **Mary L. Austin, Ph.D.** now deceased, for her daily support and who, up to the age of 97, had an amazing open-mindedness. Another special thank you goes to my son, **Geoffrey**, whose suggestions, computer expertise, help with instrumentation, and editing were indispensable and very much appreciated.

In 1996, the collaboration with **Patricia Connolly Gorzen** made possible our discovery of dental toxins and better dental practices. This led directly to improved survival opportunity for many terminally ill patients. Her contribution is greatly appreciated.

Contents

i

Figures

Preface

From Time Immemorial Healthy People Have Held Sick People Hostage.

The Witch Doctor, Medicine Man and Woman, Herbalist and Clinician are all alike in this respect. They wish to keep information surrounding illness and wellness to themselves and away from the common person so that a profession of medicine can grow and become lucrative. The Herbalist did not tell which herbs could relieve colds or bring on a woman's menstrual period (birth control) for fear that the people in need would get them for themselves and not need (nor pay) the Herbalist. The modern medical profession overlooks information on prevention; it tries to make self-help and simple treatments illegal. All for the same purpose: to build and aggrandize their profession. This seems inappropriate, especially where communicable or wide-spread illness is involved. This example is taken from a text on herbology:

> This [bath] is a safe and sane procedure and will prove most beneficial to those who are obese and desire to reduce safely. In combination with the internal treatment with decoction of *Fucus*, this course is worth considerable to very stout people, and should not be sold too cheaply. It is a grave mistake to put this scientific treatment in the same class as the many advertised nostrums on the market. It is also a mistake to let your patient know what you

are using. If any do make this mistake, he will lose his client who will straight away go to a drugstore for supplies.[1]

> # I believe hostage-holding of the sick is immoral, fundamentally unethical, and needs to be stopped.

Besides the moral issue, there is a practical issue. It would benefit society much more if the sick person were quickly rescued and helped back to productivity. A healthy society benefits each of us immensely. Likewise, an ill society injures us immensely, even when it is half a planet away. With this book, I hope to give away as many secrets as I can about the cause and the cure of all cancers, letting the truth come first and "professional concerns" come last.

The human species can no longer afford to make a business out of illness. Global travel reduces our planet to the size of our backyards. In order to keep our own backyards clean, the neighbors must keep theirs clean. So it is with keeping our bodies free of viruses, bacteria and parasites. We *all* must be free of them. The concept of health as a narrow professional concern is obsolete.

This book is intended as a gift to humanity. I make a plea to the public and private sector of the medical community not to suppress this information but to disperse it regardless of embarrassment or liability from the simplicity and newness of the cure, provided only that it meets your standard of truth.

---

[1] Shook, Dr. Edward E., *Advanced Treatise in Herbology*, Trinity Center Press, 1978, p. 172.

Abstract/Summary

The human species is now heavily infested with parasites, particularly the intestinal fluke *Fasciolopsis buskii,* the sheep liver fluke *Fasciola hepatica,* the pancreatic fluke of cattle *Eurytrema pancreatica,* the human liver fluke *Clonorchis sinensis* and the common roundworm, *Ascaris.* The increase in fluke parasitism is due to the establishment of a new "biological reservoir" in cattle, fowl and household pets. The increase in *Ascaris* parasitism is probably due to harboring of household pets.

At the same time, microcontamination of the human food supply with derivatives of the petroleum industry has occurred; these include solvents, antiseptics and numerous products used directly in the food industry. In the presence of isopropyl alcohol, *F. buskii* can complete its entire life cycle in the human body, not requiring a snail as an intermediate host, as it usually does. Other solvents contributing to parasitism include benzene, methanol, xylene, and toluene which now occur as residues in our foods and pollute our body products such as toothpaste, mouthwash, lotions and cosmetics. These solvents are also contaminants of animal feed, and thus are responsible for establishing the new biological reservoir or source of infection of flukes.

Different solvents accumulate preferentially in different organs. Isopropyl alcohol accumulates in the liver, resulting in completion of the life cycle of *Fasciolopsis* in the liver. This establishes the malignant process, namely the production of the mitotic stimulant, ortho-phospho-tyrosine. Ortho-phospho-tyrosine and a variety of growth factors are produced in the human host organs, possibly for the parasites' own use, inadvertently including the human tissue in its sphere of influence. The presence of an adult fluke in the liver signals the production of ortho-phospho-tyrosine in a distant organ. This organ appears to be chosen on the basis of DNA producing bacteria present there, as well as specific carcinogens.

The difference between persons who accumulate isopropyl alcohol and those who metabolize it promptly is the presence of *aflatoxin B* in the former. The coincidence of aflatoxin B and isopropyl alcohol in the liver results in the formation of *human Chorionic Gonadotropin* (hCG). HCG becomes widespread throughout the body and is followed by ortho-phospho-tyrosine formation. Aflatoxins are contaminants of our foods and may also be produced in situ by the growing mycelia of *Aspergillus* varieties. Such mycelial growths are only seen in the presence of copper!

Vitamin C is oxidized and rendered useless in the presence of the parasite, *Ascaris*.

The killing of all parasites and their larval stages together with removal of isopropyl alcohol and carcinogens from the patients' lifestyle results in remarkable recovery, generally noticeable in less than one week. Cancer could be eradicated in a very short time by clearing our food animals and household pets of fluke parasites and by monitoring all food and feed for solvents. Stopping consumption of mycotoxins and ceasing exposure to copper, cobalt and vanadium is essential for tumor regression.

Since developmental stages of the intestinal fluke are found in blood, breast milk, the saliva, semen, and urine and can be seen directly in these body fluids using a low power microscope, it follows that this parasite can be sexually transmitted and also transmitted by kissing on the mouth and breast feeding. However, the recipient would develop cancer only if isopropyl alcohol were accumulated in his or her body.

A common bacterium species, *Clostridium*, manufactures isopropyl alcohol in the digestive tract and under dental restorations. The use of betaine as a food supplement and removal of dental fillings clear these up.

All the technical information presented here can be obtained with a device called a Syncrometer.™ The methods used are discussed in *How To Test Yourself.* A simple circuit is also described which can be built by a novice and allows anyone to reproduce my results.

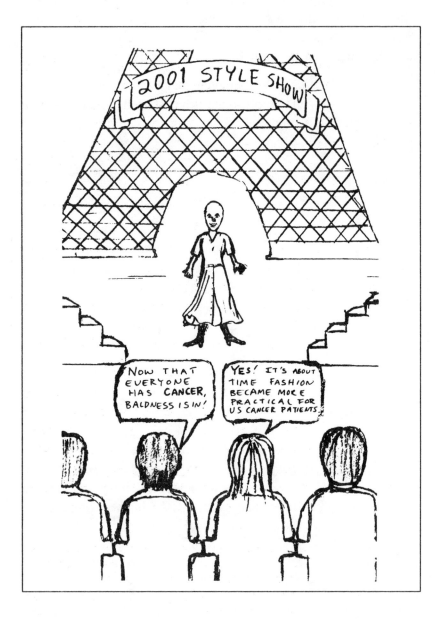

Part of the tragedy of cancer is that we now accept it as normal.

Part One: The Cause

For many years we have all believed that cancer is different from other diseases.[2] We believed that cancer behaves like a fire, in that you can't stop it once it has started. Therefore, you have to cut it out or radiate it to death or chemically destroy every cancerous cell in the body since it can never become normal again. **NOTHING COULD BE MORE WRONG!** And we have believed that cancers of different types such as leukemia or breast cancer have different causes. <u>Wrong again</u>!

> In this book you will see that all cancers are alike. They are all caused by a parasite. A single parasite! It is the *human intestinal fluke*. And if you kill this parasite, the cancer stops immediately. The tissue becomes normal again. In order to get cancer, you must have this parasite.

How can the human intestinal fluke cause cancer? This parasite typically lives in the intestine where it might do little harm, causing only colitis, Crohn's disease, or irritable bowel syndrome, or perhaps nothing at all. But if it invades a different organ, like the uterus or kidneys or liver, it does a great deal of harm. <u>If it establishes itself in the liver, it causes cancer</u>! It only establishes itself in the liver in some people. These people have *isopropyl alcohol* (often abbreviated IPA) in their bodies. All

---

[2] Cancerous cells are thought to have a special property called *malignancy*. This belief is based on scientific experiments which show that when cells are cultured in the laboratory, they become malignant in an orderly progression from initiation, through promotion, finally transformation. Transformation is irreversible. The tissue is now "malignant" and cannot be changed back. But is this really what happens in the human body?

1

cancer patients (100%) have both isopropyl alcohol and the intestinal fluke in their livers. The solvent, isopropyl alcohol, is responsible for letting the fluke establish itself in the liver. In order to get cancer, you must have <u>both</u> the parasite and isopropyl alcohol in your body.

Flukes

To understand cancer you should understand the basic facts about the human intestinal fluke. Its scientific name is *Fasciolopsis buskii*. Fluke means "flat", and flukes are one of the families of flatworms. On the next page is a photograph of the human intestinal fluke, made from a preserved and stained specimen so all the details are visible. It is as flat as a leaf. The parasite is not unknown, it has been studied since at least 1925.[3]

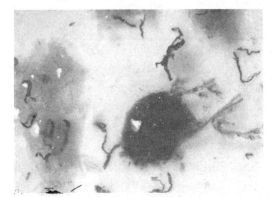

Fig. 1 Human intestinal fluke typical size

"Black hairy legs" are strings of eggs.
Fig. 2 Five flukes, in various stages of decay, expelled from bowel. They float.

---

[3] C. H. Barlow, *The Life Cycle of the Human Intestinal Fluke, Fasciolopsis buskii* (Lancaster) Am. J. Hyg. Monog. No. 4, 1925.

This Is The Cancer Causing Parasite

This parasite has stages that it must go through to keep reproducing. The first stage is the *egg*. The adult produces mil-

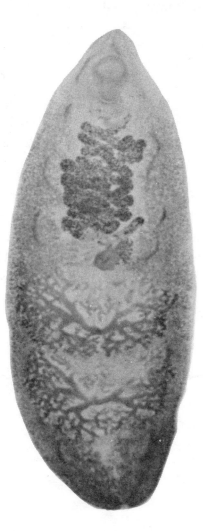

Fig. 3 Human intestinal fluke (Fasciolopsis buskii)

lions of eggs. They pass out of us with the bowel movement. The adult, though, stays tightly stuck to our intestine (or liver, causing cancer, or uterus, causing endometriosis, or thymus, causing AIDS, or kidney, causing Hodgkin's disease).

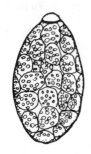

Most of us get little lesions in our intestines from time to time. These tiny sores allow the eggs, which are microscopic in size, to be pulled into the blood stream (other parasite eggs get into the blood this way too).

Size about 1/10 mm.

Fig. 4 Fasciolopsis egg

Some of these eggs actually hatch in the intestine or in the blood. The microscopic hatchlings are called *miracidia* and are the second stage. They swim about with their little swimmer-hairs. And of course, the liver whose job it is to dispose of toxins, will receive them and kill them as the blood arrives from the intestine. They have no chance to survive in normal people.

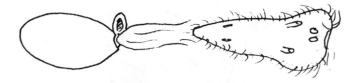

Fig. 5 Miracidia hatching

Flukes and Isopropyl Alcohol

BUT SOMETHING SPECIAL HAPPENS TO PEOPLE WHO HAVE ISOPROPYL ALCOHOL IN THEIR BODIES. The liver is unable to trap and kill these tiny fluke stages. These baby-stages are actually allowed to make their home in the liver and other tissues. It is as if the immune system has no power to kill them. The flukes begin to multiply in people with isopropyl alcohol in their bodies! The miracidia (hatchlings) start to make little balls inside themselves, called *redia*[4]. But each redia (ball) is alive! It pops itself out of the miracidia and begins to reproduce itself. 40 redia can <u>each</u> make 40 more redia! And all of this out of <u>one</u> egg!

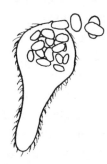

Fig. 6 Miracidia expelling "mother" redia

This parasite is laying eggs and producing millions of redia right in your body! In your cervix or lungs, wherever your cancer is growing! These redia are swept along in your blood, landing in whatever tissue lets them in. Smokers' lungs, breasts with benign lumps, prostate glands full of heavy metals are examples of tissues that give the redia their landing permits[5].

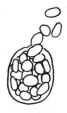

Fig. 7 "Mother" redia bearing "daughter" redia

---

[4] The Latin names are *rediae* (plural) and *redia* (singular). I have used simplified spelling, "redia", for both the singular and the plural, more like English usage.

[5] Perhaps it is the changed electrical charge or magnetic force of these damaged organs that permits further development of the fluke

Multiplying continues at a hectic pace, generation after generation. Redia are nesting in the liver and other organs. Suddenly they change their shape. They sprout a tail and can swim again. Now they are called *cercaria*[6].

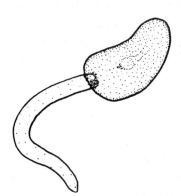

Fig. 8 Cercaria

The cercaria only need to find a place to attach. After they glue themselves to your tissue, their tails disappear and they begin to grow a "cocoon".

Now they are called *meta*cercaria. Normally, this would happen on a leaf growing near a pond, so the metacercaria develop an extremely thick shell around themselves to withstand the winter. Does the presence of the solvent isopropyl alcohol in your body dissolve this tough shell? That would remove the last barrier to the fluke completing its entire life cycle anywhere in your body!

After the shell is gone, they grow into adult flukes in your

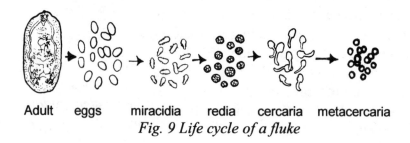

Adult   eggs   miracidia   redia   cercaria metacercaria

Fig. 9 Life cycle of a fluke

stages. Perhaps it is merely low immune surveillance. Perhaps the dying cells of a damaged organ provide food for the baby stages. Only further scientific study will reveal the truth.

[6] Again, I am simplifying the Latin *cercaria* (singular) and *cercariae* (plural) to one case.

tissue. NOT IN THE INTESTINE BUT IN YOUR LIVER! Now the cycle is complete. From egg to miracidia to redia to cercaria to metacercaria and then the adults! And all of them eating and sucking and devouring your vital body fluids.

But this is not normal for flukes. Their normal life cycle goes like this:

Stage	Normal Life Cycle
1 Egg	Expelled with bowel movement onto soil. Washed by rain into ponds.
2 Miracidia	Hatches from egg in water. Has cilia, can swim vigorously and must find intermediate snail host in one to two hours or may be too exhausted to invade.
3 Redia	Develop inside miracidia as little balls until expelled. Those are "mother" redia, and each one bears "daughter" redia for up to 8 months, all still inside the snail, and living on the fluids in the lymphatic spaces. Similarly, daughter redia are continually developing cercaria.
4 Cercaria	Have a tail, use it to exit from snail and swim to a plant. If the snail is feeding on a plant, cercaria can latch onto plant with sucker mouth and start to encyst (form a "cocoon") within minutes. Tail breaks off and swims away to dissolve.
5 Metacercaria	Two-walled cysts. The outer wall is very sticky. But as you eat the plant it is stuck to, the least pressure will break it, leaving the cyst in the mouth. The "almost unbreakable" inner cyst wall protects it from chewing, and the keratin-like coat prevents digestion by stomach juices. However when it reaches the duodenum, contact with intestinal juices dissolves away the cyst-wall and frees it. It then fastens itself to the intestinal lining and begins to develop into an adult.
6 Adult	Lives in your intestine and can produce 1000 eggs per bowel movement and live many years.

Fig. 10 Fasciolopsis' normal life cycle

As you can see, humans typically are the host for just the adult stage, and then only in the intestine. But can you imagine the havoc in your body if you did the snail's job, too?

As if these parasites were not fiendish enough, as soon as there are adults in the liver something new happens. A *growth factor*, called *ortho-phospho-tyrosine*[7] appears. A monster has been born! Growth factors make cells divide. Now YOUR cells will begin to divide too! Now you have cancer.

Now You Have Cancer

The presence of ortho-phospho-tyrosine is the beginning of your malignancy. Unless you act quickly to kill this parasite spawning machine, it will take over your body.

But first, let's sit back and think for a minute. Why is this parasite multiplying feverishly in your organs instead of living quietly in your intestine? Because having isopropyl alcohol in your body allows its development outside of the intestine. A parasite is simply doing what all living things must do: survive and reproduce. It is not the fiendish nature of this parasite that has given you cancer. It is the tragic pollution of your body with isopropyl alcohol that is at fault. And, of course, the infestation of our food animals and household pets with fluke parasites. But we will come to this later.

It is quite possible that the redia or cercaria produce the ortho-phospho-tyrosine in order to help themselves divide while reproducing. Other growth factors are produced, too. There are: epidermal growth factor (EGF), platelet derived growth factor (PDGF), insulin-like growth factor (ILGF), fibroblast growth factor (FGF). These can also be made by bacteria. But only *Fasciolopsis* makes ortho-phospho-tyrosine. These growth stimulants are not intended to make your cells multiply at all. Normally the parasite stages are developing in a pond full of snails! This parasite wasn't meant to go through its life cycle in our bodies. But since our bodies respond to ortho-phospho-

---

[7] Hunter, T., and Cooper, J.A., Ann. Rev. Biochem, 54:897, 1985. Also Yarden, Y., Ann. Rev. Biochem, 57:443, 1988.

tyrosine (and other growth factors) the same way, our cells are forced to multiply and multiply and multiply along with the fluke stages and bacteria.

Purge The Parasite, Cure The Cancer

The good news is that when the fluke and all its stages have been killed, the ortho-phospho-tyrosine disappears. In 24 hours all ortho-phospho-tyrosine is gone! Your malignancy is gone. You still have the task of repairing the damage. But your cancer cannot come back. And you have won the battle for your life.

BUT WHAT ABOUT THE BATTLE FOR YOUR HEALTH? Let us step back again into the nightmare of cancer. Why do the microscopic fluke stages choose the cervix or prostate or lung in which to settle for reproduction? Perhaps it is because this organ has developed "safety islands" for them, namely, precancerous tumors. A benign tumor has lost its immune power for you, so that it cannot catch and kill the tiny invaders. After all, there is isopropyl alcohol present, and many other toxins as well. The heavy metals copper, cobalt and vanadium are there. Often mercury and nickel are there. Lanthanide metals like yttrium and thulium are there. These are known to cause mutations. Common toxins like arsenic from household pesticides are there. PCBs and Freon are there. Fungus is even growing there and producing *patulin*, a **carcinogenic mycotoxin** (*carcinogenic* means cancer-causing; a *mycotoxin* is a toxin produced by a fungus). Is it just a coincidence that the parasite survives and reproduces itself best in your most unhealthy organs?

Clearly, you must do 3 things:

1. Kill the parasite and all its stages.
2. Stop letting isopropyl alcohol into your body.
3. Flush out the metals, common toxins, and bacteria from your body so you can get well.

We have been taught to believe that every parasite is so unique that a different drug is required to kill each one. The better drugs, such as Praziquantel™ and Levamisole™ or even Flagyl™ and Piperazine™, can each kill several worm varieties. But this is just not practical when <u>dozens of different</u> parasites are present. We have dozens of different parasites in us! It would be best to kill them all together even though only the intestinal fluke is causing cancer.

Look at the case histories. It is not unusual for someone to have a dozen (or more) parasites out of the 120 parasites I have samples of (they are listed in *The Tests*). You can assume that you, too, have a dozen different parasites. We are heavily parasitized beings! Our bodies are large enough to provide food and shelter for lots of these free loaders. If they were settled on the outside where we could see them, like lice or ticks, we would rid ourselves in a flash. Nothing is more distasteful to the imagination than hordes of biting, chewing, crawling, sucking creatures on our flesh. But what about IN our flesh? We cannot see <u>inside</u> ourselves, so we mistakenly assume that nothing is there.

Herbal Parasite Remedies

The Native American peoples knew that humans are parasitized. Other native peoples from the Arctic to Antarctic knew that we are parasitized like other animals. They had frequent purgings that included diarrhea or vomiting to rid themselves of their slimy invaders. Many cultures continued such practices right up to my own childhood. I remember being forced to swallow a spoonful of sulfur and molasses and raw onion! How dreadful it seemed. But it reduced the body's burden of worms and other parasites that we all have. **Where have we gone astray? Why have we forsaken these wise practices?** I have seen that eczema is due to roundworms. Seizures are caused by a single roundworm, *Ascaris*, getting into the brain. Schizophrenia and depression are caused by parasites in the brain. Asthma is caused by *Ascaris* in the lungs. Diabetes is caused by the pancreatic fluke of cattle, *Eurytrema*. Migraines are caused by the threadworm, *Strongyloides*. Acne rosacea is caused by a *Leishmania*. Much human heart disease is caused by dog heartworm, *Dirofilaria*. And the list goes on.

Getting rid of all these parasites would be absolutely impossible using clinical medicines that can kill only one or two parasites each. Such medicines also tend to make you quite ill. Flagyl is used for amoebas and *Giardia*; when the correct dosage is used, it can cause extreme nausea and vomiting. Quinine for malaria is quite toxic. Imagine taking 10 such drugs to kill a dozen of your parasites! Good news, perhaps, for the drug makers but not for you.

Yet three herbs can rid you of over 100 types of parasites! And without so much as a headache! Without nausea! Without any interference with any drug that you are already on! Does this sound too fantastic? Just too good to be true? They are nature's gift to us. The herbs are:

- **Black Walnut Hulls** (from the black walnut tree)
- **Wormwood** (from the *Artemisia* shrub)
- **Common Cloves** (from the clove tree)

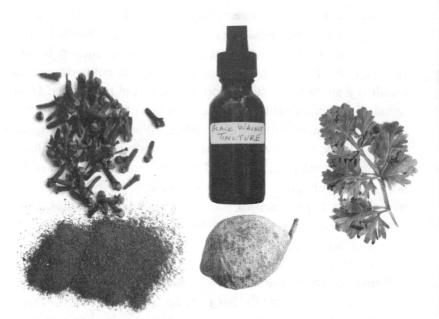

These three herbs, taken together, can cure all malignancies.
Fig. 11 Cloves, black walnut, and wormwood

These three herbs must be used <u>together</u>. Black walnut hull and wormwood kill adults and developmental stages of at least 100 parasites. Cloves kill the eggs.[8] Only if you use them together will you rid yourself of parasites. If you kill only the adults, the tiny stages and eggs will soon grow into new adults. If you kill only the eggs, the million stages already loose in

---

[8] This anti-cancer action of cloves was not discovered by me, but by a neighboring health practitioner, using a kinesiological technique she developed herself. We owe her our deepest gratitude. Not all scientific truth comes from the classically trained!

your body will soon grow into adults and make more eggs. They must be used together as a single treatment.

It is the green hull surrounding the nut of the black walnut tree that has this miraculous parasiticide. After it has turned black, it is useless. The large green balls fall to the ground early in the fall. In a week or two they will be black and decaying. Therefore, anyone wishing to make parasiticide must be careful not to let the critical time for harvesting pass. I encourage everyone to make their own parasiticides and to take back the responsibility for keeping themselves and their families free of these tiny monsters. The recipe for Black Walnut Hull Tincture Extra Strength is given in *Recipes* (page 582).

Note that it is a tincture (extracted using ethyl alcohol), not an ordinary extract (which uses water). The black walnut extract that is available from herb companies is not potent as a parasiticide. It is black, not pale green, indicating that the critical harvesting time had passed. Of course there is no time to make your own if you have fast growing or metastasizing cancer. See the chapter on *Sources*.

You will only need one 1 oz. (30 ml) bottle of the Extra Strength tincture to get started. If you have family members you will need more. While you are waiting for it to arrive, get your other two herbs ready: wormwood and cloves.

Wormwood consists of the leaves of the *Artemisia* shrub. My recommendation is that you grow it yourself if you have any space to do so. Wormwood seed is available from seed catalogs, (see *Sources*).

The amount you need to cure a cancer is very small, yet you cannot do without it. But the Food and Drug Administration (FDA) has regulated it as toxic! It is therefore unavailable in concentrated form from herb companies. The evidence for toxicity accepted by the FDA must have been hearsay. I have never seen a case of toxicity, not so much as a headache or nausea[9]. The toxic level must be much higher than is needed to kill these parasites.

This shrub is called wormwood for good reason: it kills worms! There is quite a bit of confusion over which *Artemisia* is the true wormwood. Books and nurseries can be wrong, even though they assure you they are correct! Buy *Artemisia absynthium* for your garden. Wormwood goes back to antiquity and is mentioned in the Bible.

If you grow your own, dry the leaves when they are in their prime. The leaves are greenish gray and quite bitter. Nobody would accidentally eat too much of them. Adults may put them in capsules. For a child, crumble ¼ tsp. and stir into honey. I have not done experiments to be more precise than this.

Wormwood capsules are available as a combination of *Artemisia* and other herbs (see *Sources*).

The third herb necessary to cure cancer is cloves. This is the common spice used in baking. It needs to be ground up in order to release its parasite killing properties. You can buy a can of whole cloves and grind them in a blender or grinder. Store-bought "ground cloves" <u>do not work</u>! Their parasite killing properties have evaporated long ago. Ground cloves from a health food store or herb shop may not work either! They may have been ground years ago. If an herb company were to grind cloves and fill capsules with them right away and store the capsules in closed bottles, the potency of the herb would be protected. Don't take these details for granted. You must question your source and get a satisfactory answer or grind your own (see *Sources*).

You will need about 100 capsules of cloves. To make your own, purchase size 00 (double-zero) capsules at a health food

---

[9] Of course, the FDA cannot be expected to accept experiences such as mine. We should find out what evidence they did accept.

store. (Don't try to mix cloves straight in water! It is much too strong; you may try mixing with home made yogurt or applesauce.) Size 0 capsules will also be acceptable.

You now have:

- One 30 ml bottle of pale green Black Walnut Hull Tincture Extra Strength. This is 1 ounce, or six teaspoons, enough for three weeks if you are not very ill.
- One bottle of wormwood capsules (each capsule with 200-300 mg of wormwood) or ½ cup of *Artemisia* leaves gathered from a friendly neighbor's shrub.
- One bottle of freshly ground cloves (each capsule with 400-500 mg cloves), or ¼ cup bulk powdered cloves.

These are the only essential herbs you will need to cure your cancer. They will last through the first 18 days of the Parasite Program.

Two additional items, *ornithine* and *arginine*, improve this recipe. Parasites produce a great deal of ammonia as their waste product. Ammonia is their equivalent of urine and is set free in our bodies by parasites in large amounts. Ammonia is very toxic, especially to the brain.[10] I believe this causes insomnia and other sleep problems at night and anxiety by day. By taking ornithine at bedtime, you will sleep better.[11] Arginine has similar ammonia reduction effects but must be taken in the morning because it gives alertness and energy.

Do not try to substitute drugs for herbs. **Drug parasiticides can be extremely toxic, even in the small doses needed. Nor do they kill all the stages.** Here is a clipping I saw recently:

---

[10] The brain lacks the enzyme ornithine carbamyl-transferase which is essential for making ammonia harmless by changing it into urea.

[11] I published this discovery in *Townsend Letter For Doctors*, July 1991, p 554.

Common Drugs For Parasitic Infections

Infection	Drug	Adult Dosage	Pediatric Dosage
Amebiasis			
asymptomatic	Iodoquinol	650 mg tid x 20d	30-40 mg/kg/d, 3 doses x 20d
symptomatic	Metronidazole	750 mg tid x 10d	35-50 mg/kg/d, 3 doses x 10 d
	followed by Iodoquinol	650 mg tid x 20d	30-40 mg/kg/d, 3 doses x 20d
Blastocystis	Metronidazole	750 mg tid x 10d	
	or Iodoquinol	650 mg tid x 20d	
Dientamoeba	Iodoquinol	650 mg tid x 20d	40 mg/kg/d, 3 doses x 20d
Giardia	Quinacrine HCl	100 mg tid p.c.x5d	6 mg/kg/d, 3 doses p.c.x5d
	or Metronidazole	250 mg tid x 5d	15 mg/kg/d, 3 doses x 5 d

Names & Adverse Effects of Common Drugs

Drug: **Iodoquinol**   Trade Name: **Yodoxin**.

Adverse Effects: Occ: rash, acne, slight enlargement of thyroid gland, nausea, diarrhea, cramps, anal pruritus. Rare: optic atrophy, loss of vision, peripheral neuropathy after prolonged use in high dosage (months), Iodine sensitivity.

Drug: **Metronidazole**   Trade Name: **Flagyl**

Adverse Effects: Freq: nausea, headache, dry mouth, metallic taste. Occ: vomiting, diarrhea, insomnia, weakness, stomatitis, vertigo, aparesthesia, rash, dark urine, urethral burning. Rare: seizures, encephalopathy, pseudo-membranous colitis, ataxia, leukopenia, peripheral neuropathy, pancreatitis.

Drug: **Quinacrine HCl**   Trade Name: **Atabrine**

Adverse Effects: Freq: dizziness, headache, vomiting, diarrhea. Occ: yellow staining of skin, toxic psychosis, insomnia, bizarre dreams, blood dyscrasias, urticaria, blue and black nail pigmentation, psoriasis-like rash. Rare: acute hepatic necrosis, convulsions, severe exfoliative dermatitis, ocular effects similar to those caused by chloroquine.

Fig. 12 Some clinical parasiticides

Procedure For Cure

Start by taking ornithine, 2 at bedtime on the first night you get it. You don't need to wait for the rest of the program to start on ornithine. Take 4 ornithines on the second night. Take 6 ornithines at bedtime on the third night. After this take 4 or 6 ornithines at bedtime every night till you are sleeping soundly. Then go off ornithine and see whether your sleep is as good without it. Use as needed. It is not habit forming.

Taking ornithine at bedtime may give you so much energy the next day that you don't need to take arginine in the morning. But if going off caffeine (recommended) has you dragging yourself through the morning, take one arginine upon rising and another one before lunch and supper. It can make you a bit irritable. Cut back if this happens.

Ornithine and arginine, each about 500 mg, are available in capsules, in separate bottles (see *Sources*).

There are no side-effects as you can see from the case histories.

There is no interference with any other medication. There is no need to stop any treatment that a clinical doctor or alternative therapist has started you on, provided it is solvent-free. (Over half the medications I test have traces of isopropyl alcohol, benzene or wood alcohol.)

How could you know whether a medicine is free of isopropyl alcohol contamination? Only the Syncrometer method described later (page 471) can test for isopropyl alcohol in less than a minute. If you have friends with cancer, you could become their angel by learning to use this device.

Alternatives?

Are there any substitutes for the black walnut hull, cloves or wormwood? I believe there **must be dozens** of plants that could kill the intestinal fluke.

While you are waiting for herbs, why not try all the vitamins and herbs that are presently available to you and that have been traditionally used to treat cancer? They may work by killing fluke stages, or have other value. Some of these are:

- Red clover blossoms[12] (2 capsules, 3 times a day)
- Pau D'Arco (2 capsules, 3 times a day)
- Vitamin C (10 or more grams per day)
- Laetrile (as directed by source)
- Grapes and grape juice (home-juiced, no meat in the diet)
- Echinacea (2 capsules, 3 times a day)
- Metabolic enzymes, take as directed
- The macrobiotic diet

Then, as soon as your herbs arrive, you can stop these. Or you may wish to continue them as well.[13]

---

[12] Red clover blossoms contain an inhibitor of ortho-phospho-tyrosine formation, called *genisteine* or *biochanin A*. See the *Merck Index 10th ed.*, p. 626.

[13] An excellent book listing alternative therapies is *Cancer Therapy, The Independent Consumer's Guide To Non-Toxic Treatment & Prevention*, Ralph W. Moss, Ph.D., Equinox Press, NY 1992.

Cancer Curing Recipe

Parasite Killing Program

1. **Black Walnut Hull Tincture Extra Strength** (see *Recipes*, page 582, or *Sources*):
Day 1: this is the day you begin; start the same day you receive it.
Take one drop. Put it in ½ cup of water. Sip it on an empty stomach such as before a meal.

Day 2: Take 2 drops in ½ cup water same as above.
Day 3: Take 3 drops in ½ cup water same as above.
Day 4: Take 4 drops in ½ cup water same as above.
Day 5: Take 5 drops in ½ cup water same as above.
Day 6: Take 2 tsp., all together in ½ cup water. Sip it, don't gulp it. Add sweetening and flavoring to help it go down. Or you may stir the tincture into fruit sauce. Get it down within 15 minutes. (If you are over 150 pounds, take 2½ tsp. If you are over 200 pounds, take 3 tsp.)

This dose kills any remaining stages throughout the body, including the bowel contents, a location unreachable by a smaller dose or by electric current. The alcohol in the tincture can make you slightly woozy for several minutes. Simply stay seated until you are comfortable again. You may put the tincture in lukewarm water to help evaporate some of the alcohol, but do not use hot water because that may damage its parasiticide power. Then take niacinamide 500 mg (see Sources*) to counteract the toxicity of the alcohol. You could also feel a slight nausea for a few* *minutes. Walk in the fresh air or simply rest until it passes.*

For a year: take 2 tsp. Black Walnut Hull Tincture Extra Strength once a week. This is to kill any parasite stages you pick up from your family, friends, or pets.

Family members and friends should take 2 tsp. every other week to avoid reinfecting <u>you</u>. They may be harboring a few parasite stages in their intestinal tract without having symptoms. But when these stages are transmitted to someone who has had cancer, they immediately seek out the unhealed organ to continue multiplying.

You may be wondering why you should wait for five days before taking the 2 tsp. dose. It is for your convenience only. You may have a sensitive stomach or be worried about toxicity or side effects. By the sixth day you will have convinced yourself there is no toxicity or side effect.

Going faster. *In fact, if you are convinced after the first drop of the restorative powers of Black Walnut Hull Tincture Extra Strength, take the 2 tsp. dose on the very first day.*

Going slower. *On the other hand, if you cringe at the thought of taking an herb or you are anxious about its safety, continue the drops, increasing at your own pace, until you are ready to brave the decisive 2 tsp. dose.*

Extremely ill. *Terminally ill with cancer: Take a 2 tsp. dose every hour for 5 hours; in other words, a 10 tsp. dose. Follow this the same day or next day with the Mop Up program, page 36. If this gets you out of a hospital bed, repeat the 10 tsp. dose (plus Mop Up) every other day for 2 more weeks before settling on the maintenance program once a week. Remember to include wormwood and clove* *capsules with each treatment, but increase the dose to 10 of each.*

2. **Wormwood capsules** (should contain 200-300 mg of wormwood, see *Sources*):

Day 1: Take 1 capsule before supper (with water).
Day 2: Take 1 capsule before supper.
Day 3: Take 2 capsules before supper.
Day 4: Take 2 capsules before supper.

Continue increasing in this way to day 14, whereupon you are up to seven capsules. You take the capsules all in a single dose (you may take a few at a time until they are all gone). Then you do 2 more days of 7 capsules each. After this, you take 7 capsules once a week forever, as it states in the Maintenance Parasite Program. Try not to get interrupted before the 6th day, so you know the adult intestinal flukes are dead. After this, you may proceed more slowly if you wish. Many persons with sensitive stomachs prefer to stay longer on each dose instead of increasing according to this schedule. You may choose the pace after the sixth day.

3. **Cloves**:
Fill size 00 capsules with fresh ground cloves; if this size is not available, use size 0 or 000. In a pinch, buy gelatin capsules and empty them or empty other vitamin capsules. You may be able to purchase fresh ground cloves that are already encapsulated; they should be about 500 mg. Grocery store ground cloves do not work! Either grind them yourself or see Sources.

Day 1: Take one capsule 3 times a day before meals.

Day 2: Take two capsules 3 times a day.

Days 3, 4, 5, 6, 7, 8, 9, 10: Take three capsules 3 times a day.

After day 10: Take 7 capsules all together once a week forever, as in the Maintenance Parasite Program.

Take **ornithine** at bedtime for insomnia. Even if you do not suffer from insomnia now, you may when you kill parasites. Take **arginine** in the morning and daytime.

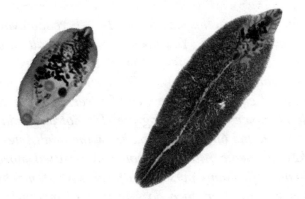

L to R: pancreatic fluke (causes diabetes); sheep liver fluke (causes "universal allergy syndrome"); and human liver fluke.
Fig. 13 Three other parasites you may be killing.

Parasite Program Handy Chart

Strike out the doses as you take them.

Day	Black Walnut Hull Tincture Extra Strength Dose	Wormwood Capsule Dose (200-300 mg)	Clove Capsule Dose (Size 0 or 00)
	drops 1 time per day, like before a meal	capsules 1 time per day, on empty stomach (before meal)	capsules 3 times per day, like at mealtime
1	1	1	1, 1, 1
2	2	1	2, 2, 2
3	3	2	3, 3, 3
4	4	2	3, 3, 3
5	5	3	3, 3, 3
6	2 tsp.	3	3, 3, 3
7	Now once a week	4	3, 3, 3
8		4	3, 3, 3
9		5	3, 3, 3
10		5	3, 3, 3
11		6	7
12		6	Now once a week
13	2 tsp.	7	
14		7	
15		7	
16		7	
17		Now once a week	
18			7

At this point you do not need to keep a strict schedule, but instead may choose any day of the week to take all the parasite program ingredients.

Continue on the Maintenance Parasite Program, indefinitely, to prevent future reinfection.

Tips on taking pills

Whenever taking capsules or pills, have a bit of bread within reach. If a pill should stick, swallow some bread. Bread pushes the pill along its way, so you are comfortable again. Never take a handful of pills together. They may clump together and give you lots of discomfort. Take them one at a time.

Maintenance Parasite Program

YOU ARE ALWAYS PICKING UP PARASITES! PARASITES ARE EVERYWHERE AROUND YOU! YOU GET THEM FROM OTHER PEOPLE, YOUR FAMILY, YOURSELF, YOUR HOME, YOUR PETS, UNDERCOOKED MEAT, AND UNDERCOOKED DAIRY PRODUCTS.

I believe the <u>main</u> source of the intestinal fluke is <u>under-cooked dairy products and meats</u>. After we are infected with it this way, we can give it to each other through blood, saliva, semen, and breast milk, which means kissing on the mouth, sex, nursing, and childbearing.

Family members nearly always have the same parasites. If one person develops cancer, the others probably have the intestinal fluke also. They should give themselves the same de-parasitizing program.

Do this once a week. You may take these at different times in the day or together:

1. **Black Walnut Hull** Tincture Extra Strength: 2 tsp. on an empty stomach, like before a meal or bedtime.
2. **Wormwood capsules**: 7 capsules (with 200-300 mg wormwood each) once a day on an empty stomach.
3. **Cloves**: 7 capsules (about 500 mg. each, or fill size 00 capsules yourself) once a day on an empty stomach.
4. Take **ornithine** at night.

	Black Walnut Hull Tincture Extra Strength Dose	Wormwood Capsule Dose (200-300 mg)	Clove Capsule Dose (Size 0 or 00)
Day	1 time per day, on empty stomach	capsules 1 time per day, on empty stomach	capsules 1 time per day, on empty stomach
1	2 tsp.	7	7
2			
3			
4			

5			
6			
7			
8	2 tsp.	7	7
9			
10			
11			
12			
13			
14			
15	2 tsp.	7	7
and so on...			

The only after-effects you may feel are due to release of bacteria and viruses from dead parasites. These should be promptly zapped (see page 30).

Children's Parasite Program

Black Walnut Tincture Extra Strength
Children follow the same parasite program as adults through day 5. On day 6, instead of 2 tsp., take the following:

Age	BWT ES	Niacinamide
Under six months	¼ tsp.	50 mg
Six months to five years	½ tsp.	50 mg
Six to ten years	1 tsp.	100 mg
Eleven to sixteen years	1½ tsp.	500 mg

The niacinamide (not niacin) is to help detoxify the alcohol in the tincture. You may crush it and put it in a spoonful of honey, if necessary. Occasionally a bit of niacin gets into the niacinamide tablet and causes a hot flush. It is harmless and soon passes.

Even though the parasite program is very beneficial to children, who tend to pick up parasites more often than adults, it should not be continued on a maintenance basis due to the alcohol content. Have children deparasitize twice a year, or whenever ill.

In case of childhood cancer, however, a much more vigorous program should be followed. Give 2 to 10 tsp. tincture as quickly as the child can take it. Follow this, several hours later with the Mop Up program, page 36.

Wormwood and Cloves

Increase dosage one day for each year. For instance a four-year old would follow the adult program until day four, then stop.

Again, it is not advisable for children to be on a maintenance dosage of wormwood and cloves. Taking them during their routine deparasitizing, or when ill, is best.

In case of childhood cancer, it is <u>not</u> necessary to use increased dosages, as with Black Walnut Tincture.

Cleanse Pets Too

Pets have many of the same parasites that we get, including *Ascaris* (common roundworm), hookworm, *Trichinella, Strongyloides,* heartworm and a variety of tapeworms. Every pet living in your home should be deparasitized (cleared of parasites) and maintained on a parasite program. Monthly trips to your vet are not sufficient.

You may not need to get rid of your pet to keep yourself free of parasites. But if you are ill it is best to board it with a friend until you are better.

Your pet is part of your family and should be kept as sweet and clean and healthy as yourself. This is not difficult to achieve. Here is the recipe:

Pet Parasite Program

1. **Parsley water**: cook a big bunch of fresh parsley in a quart of water for 3 minutes. Throw away the parsley. After cooling, you may freeze most of it in several 1 cup containers. This is a month's supply. Put 1 tsp. parsley water on the pet's food. You don't have to watch it go down. Whatever amount is eaten is satisfactory.

All dosages are based on a 10 pound (5 kilo) cat or dog. Double them for a 20 pound pet, and so forth.

Pets are so full of parasites, you must be quite careful not to deparasitize too quickly. The purpose of the parsley water is to keep the kidneys flowing well so dead parasite refuse is eliminated promptly. They get quite fond of their parsley water. Perhaps they can sense the benefit it brings them. Do this for a week before starting the Black Walnut Hull Tincture.

2. **Black Walnut Hull Tincture (regular strength):** 1 drop on the food. Don't force them to eat it. Count carefully. Treat cats only twice a week. Treat dogs daily, for instance a 30 pound dog would get 3 drops <u>per day</u> (but work up to it, increasing one drop per day). Do not use Extra Strength.

If your pet vomits or has diarrhea, you may expect to see worms. This is <u>extremely</u> infectious and hazardous. Never let a child clean up a pet mess. Begin by pouring salt and iodine[14] on the mess and letting it stand for 5 minutes before cleaning it up. Clean up outdoor messes the same way. Finally, clean your hands with diluted grain alcohol (dilute 1 part alcohol with 4 parts water). Grain alcohol is actually *ethyl* alcohol that has been made by fermenting grain. In some countries sugar cane is used to make ethyl alcohol. A common brand in the United States is Everclear. But be careful. The smaller flask sizes are polluted with solvents from the pumping and filling processes, no doubt. Choose the 750 ml or 1 liter bottle which is, evidently, bottled differently. Be careful to keep all alcohol out of sight of children; don't rely on discipline for this. Be careful not to buy isopropyl (rubbing) alcohol for this purpose.

Start the wormwood a week later.

3. **Wormwood capsules:** (200-300 mg wormwood per capsule) open a capsule and put the smallest pinch possible on their dry food. Do this for a week before starting the cloves.

4. **Cloves:** put the smallest pinch possible on their dry food. Keep all of this up as a routine so that you need not fear your pets. Also, notice how peppy and happy they become.

Go slowly so the pet can learn to eat all of it. To repeat:
- Week 1: parsley water.
- Week 2: parsley water and black walnut.
- Week 3: parsley water, black walnut, and wormwood.
- Week 4: parsley water, black walnut, wormwood, and cloves.

---

[14] "Povidone" iodine, topical antiseptic, is available in most drug stores.

Week	Parsley Water	Black Walnut Hull Tincture Dose	Wormwood Capsule Dose	Clove Capsule Dose (Size 0 or 00)
Week	teaspoons on food	drops on food, cats twice per week, dogs daily	open capsule, put smallest pinch on food	open capsule, put smallest pinch on food
1	1 or more, based on size			
2	1 or more	1		
3	1 or more	1 or more, based on size	1	
4	1 or more	1 or more	1	1
5 and onward	1 or more	1 or more	1	1

Pets should not stroll on counters or table. They should eat out of their own dishes, not yours. They should not sleep on your bed. The bedroom should be off limits to pets. Don't kiss your pets. Wash your hands after playing with your pet. NEVER, NEVER share food with your pet. Don't keep a cat box in the house; install a cat door. Wear a dust-mask when you change the cat box. If you have a sandbox for the children, buy new sand from a lumber yard and keep it covered. Don't eat in a restaurant where they sweep the carpet while you are eating (the dust has parasite eggs tracked in from outside). Never let a child crawl on the sidewalk or the floor of a public building. Wash children's hands before eating. Eat "finger" foods with a fork. If feasible, leave shoes at the door.

Solvents are just as bad for your pet as for you. Most flavored pet foods are polluted with solvents such as carbon tetrachloride, benzene, isopropyl alcohol, wood alcohol, etc. Don't buy flavored pet food.

Pets add a great deal to human lives. **Get rid of the parasites, not the pets, unless you are ill.**

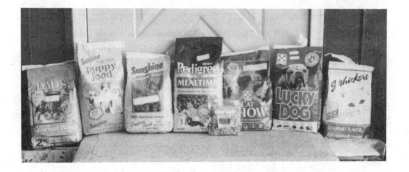

Of the collection of pet foods shown, only two were NOT polluted;
only home made food is safe.

Fig. 14 Polluted and safe pet foods

Zapping Parasites

Although the herbal parasite killing program is highly effective against parasites, you should also kill them electrically. Each method has its own areas of greatest effectiveness.

You may build a zapper (page 531) or purchase one. It is energized by a 9 volt battery. Some people can feel a minor tingling; others feel nothing. After seven minutes take 20 to 40 minutes off. During this time viruses and bacteria will emerge from dead parasites. Zap a second time. Then take another break of 20 to 40 minutes. Finally zap a third time.

You have just killed all the viruses, all the bacteria, and all the parasites including flukes that the zapper current could reach. The few remaining are stuck in gallstones, kidney stones, abscesses, or in the bowel contents. Increasing the voltage does not help. Only a 2 tsp. dose of Black Walnut Hull Tincture Extra Strength reaches them in these locations.

That is why you should use both methods.

Triple-zap once a day until you are well.

Don't wait until you have everything to begin! Start as soon as you get each item! Consider your body like a flower garden. Tiny insects are eating your leaves and petals. They are laying eggs that hatch into hungry caterpillars, spinning cocoons and emerging into new adults continually. You can't wait for anything! You must kill whatever you can as soon as you can in order to save as many petals and leaves as possible!

Tapeworm Disease

We all have tapeworm stages in our bodies, probably going back to childhood when we ate dirt. Every tumor, benign or malignant, has a tapeworm stage in the middle of it, even including warts. Growing a tumor around a tapeworm stage may be Nature's way of protecting us from it! It is not normal for these stages to hatch and develop further. Their purpose is to stay dormant. And perhaps they do little harm this way.

But I have found, using the Syncrometer, that tapeworm stages make <u>malonic acid</u>. This is a powerful inhibitor of your metabolism. It cripples your Krebs cycle, the high gear of your energy-producing machinery. Dr. Otto Warburg found, in the early decades of the 20th century, that inhibitors of the Krebs cycle caused tumors to grow.[15]

So it is very important to kill the tapeworm stages in your body—and in your tumors—even though they are responsible for the neoplasm (tumor), not the malignancy.

Cancer is a progression of developments. First, the mass is merely a benign growth, a **neoplasm**. It is instigated by a tapeworm stage. Later, the mass is invaded by the intestinal fluke causing it to become malignant.

---

[15] *The Metabolism of Tumors*, Otto Warburg, translated by Frank Dickens, M.A., Ph.D., Constable & Co., Ltd., London 1930.

Tapeworm stages do not come unaccompanied, either. They bring some very harmful bacteria and viruses with them. In sufficient numbers, they can make you feel quite ill. *Streptomyces*, a fungus-like bacterium is one of the worst. Wherever I detect *Streptomyces*, a tapeworm stage is not far away.

The herbal parasite program, taken in a very high dose kills many tapeworm stages. You simply take 8 tsp. Black Walnut Hull Tincture Extra Strength, rest for an hour, then take another 8 tsp. Black Walnut Hull Tincture Extra Strength. After each dose, take one tablet of niacinamide, 500 mg, to detoxify the alcohol. This treatment could make you woozy; do not drive a vehicle afterward. Also take 10 capsules of wormwood and 10 of cloves, slowly and carefully, to keep it all down. This treatment could save your life, if you are terminally ill.

Yet, even this very high dose parasite program is not effective against <u>all</u> tapeworms.

Tough Tapeworms

A few varieties of tapeworms, like *Echinococcus granulosis* and *Echinococcus multilocularis*, have larvae inside their larvae! And even these second generation larvae can have more larvae inside <u>them</u>. These internal larvae are <u>shielded</u> from all things that night harm them. That is undoubtedly why they are not eradicated by zapper current or the very high dose of parasite herbs. The innermost larvae are called *hydatid sand*. Testing with a Syncrometer reveals that in some persons, unfortunate enough to have these tapeworm varieties, hydatid sand is still present and alive after all these treatments. *E. granulosis* is the most common variety to survive it all. It is found the world over, infesting sheep, cattle, pigs, horses, goats, and dogs.

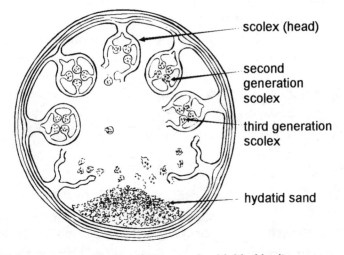

scolex (head)

second generation scolex

third generation scolex

hydatid sand

Echinococcus granulosis cysticercus is shielded by its numerous membranes but cysteine and ozonated oil penetrate them.
Fig. 15 Tough tapeworm stage

But what harm would a few left over stages of tapeworms do? With most of them dead, surely your tumors should stop growing and your health should improve. Certainly there is much less malonic acid produced. But the filamentous bacterium, *Streptomyces*, which accompanies each larva, does a great deal of harm. *Streptomyces* can spread through your body like a virus; perhaps it even hosts a virus.

Streptomyces is not merely a nuisance-invader like *Candida*. *Streptomyces* uses up your nucleic acid bases, adenine and hypoxanthine. It makes nitrites out of nitrates, leading to nitroso compounds which cause mutations. It makes a strong protease that can digest your tissues. It makes substances that stops protein manufacture by your cells. It makes ammonia out of your urea; just the opposite of what should be taking place. It has powerful immune suppressant action on T-cells. This is no ordinary bacterium although it is present in the soil everywhere.

33

Unless you kill every grain of the hydatid sand and other leftover shielded larvae, you cannot get well. But as soon as you succeed, all *Streptomyces* species disappear the same day.

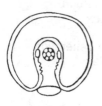 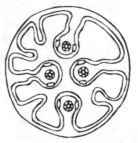 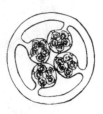

One scolex
inside cysticercus

multiple scolices
inside cysticercus

multiple scolices
inside multiple scolices
inside cysticercus

Each scolex will be turned right side-out when pressure is applied so the suckers can attach themselves to the host. But in humans the entire larva merely lodges in some organ, disturbing metabolism and spewing out bacteria.

Fig. 16 Various types of tapeworm larvae

To kill these larvae, the cyst must not be opened to let out the mischief-makers, but merely penetrated to kill the contents. Fortunately, we have found two substances that <u>can</u> penetrate a succession of membranes to kill the shielded larvae within, as well as any trapped eggs in other locations. They are **ozonated olive oil** and **L-cysteine**. We will discuss them shortly. But first, are there other parasites besides some tapeworms that can survive our treatments so far? Yes. *Ascaris*.

The Curious Case of Ascaris

If you do not get well after the herbal parasite program and the zapper treatment, you can assume you have either leftover tapeworm stages or survivor *Ascaris* eggs.

Ascaris infests animals and humans from pole to pole of this planet. It is safe to say that all dogs and cats have it and all humans have it from time to time. Domestic animals and humans each have their own variety of *Ascaris*, yet can host the other varieties, too. Horses have *Ascaris megalocephala*. Pigs have *Ascaris suum*. The human variety is *Ascaris lumbricoides*. *Ascaris* does not attach itself to you, it hardly even moves. It simply lies still in your organs absorbing nutrients and eventually filling up with eggs.

When you kill *Ascaris* worms by zapping or with the herbal recipe, they are mortally wounded. They are dying, **but the eggs inside them are not**. They were sheltered. Within a day these trapped eggs begin to leave the dying worm. Soon hordes of eggs are dispersing in your body again!

And in another 24 hours they are beginning to hatch into larvae. You can detect this as it happens with a Syncrometer and test-slides of eggs, larvae, and adults.

Of course, you are zapping and taking the herbal parasite killers. But again, these do not <u>penetrate</u> the *Ascaris* body to kill what is <u>inside</u>. It could take weeks for the dead *Ascaris* to be totally disintegrated so no more eggs are being sheltered within.

Surely, a few *Ascaris* eggs, still escaping into your body could not do much harm since the overall problem has been greatly reduced! This is not so. The eggs, even if unfertilized, may do <u>more</u> harm than the worms. *Ascaris* eggs bring three very important pathogens that spread throughout your body: *Rhizobium leguminosarum*, *Mycobacterium avium/intracellulare*, and the common cold virus, *Adenovirus*. A flood of these is responsible for night sweats and a general feeling of illness. As soon as the last *Ascaris* egg is gone, these pathogens are gone, too, and the following night becomes free of sweating. If your night sweats come back, you know *Ascaris* eggs are present again. And in 24 hours, unless you kill them, they will hatch into larvae and start the whole cycle over again.

35

It takes about three weeks for large parasites like *Ascaris* and tapeworm larvae to disintegrate completely and be cleared from your tissues. If eggs or scolices are continually released during this time, the cycle of infection cannot be broken. Fortunately, the <u>same</u> two substances that can penetrate tapeworm larvae can also penetrate *Ascaris* worms and mop up after them, whether dead or alive!

Strangle The Stragglers

Here is the three week Mop Up Program for both tapeworm larvae and trapped *Ascaris* eggs:

- ozonated olive oil, 3 tbs. taken once a day.
- L-cysteine, 500 mg, 2 capsules, three times a day.

You can easily make your own **ozonated oil**. Purchase an ozonator (see *Sources*) and a small bottle of olive oil. Pour off an inch or so. Attach an aerator to the end of your ozonator hose and drop it to the bottom of the olive oil bottle. Choose a ceramic or wood aerator, available at any pet store; the plastic varieties release benzene! The bubbles may make the oil flow over the top. In this case, pour more of it off. Turn the ozonator on before dropping the hose in the bottle. Ozonate for 20 minutes or longer. When done, cap the bottle and store in freezer until you are ready to use it. It melts quickly when needed. Would other oils work? Possibly. I have not researched them, though, since they cannot be trusted to be free of benzene (petroleum) pollution.

Measure your dose accurately. You may put it on vegetables and have it with your meal.

Ozonated oil gives you no noticeable side effects, but it should not be taken more than necessary. One could expect the ozone to jump across from oil molecules to your fat molecules, aging them too soon. Fortunately, the dose is small and may be directed at the intruders before it is directed at you.

The **cysteine** should be L-cysteine, cysteine hydrochloride, or simply free cysteine. Do not get D-cysteine or DL-cysteine which are unnatural.

Taking this supplement gives a few people side effects, perhaps due to its penetrating antiparasite property. You could have fatigue, nausea, dizziness. If you have serious side effects, reduce the dosage.

On the other hand, cysteine may make you feel better than you have in many months! The cancer sufferer is quite deficient in cysteine and suddenly supplying it could put the body into a state of euphoria. In this case, you may even double the dose!

Cysteine has other important benefits for you. It counteracts the radiation we all get from living on this planet, called "background radiation." This might even explain why supplementing animals with cysteine had the effect of lengthening their lives substantially. Cysteine is a heavy metal detoxifier, perhaps through the formation of glutathione. It is a precursor to glutathione and deserves a permanent place on your supplement list.

Nevertheless, supplementing with cysteine should not be overdone. Even if you have good side effects, reduce the dosage after three weeks to one a day. If you had bad side effects, reduce the dosage after two days to whatever you are comfortable with.

After three weeks, you can assume that all leftover *Ascaris* eggs are gone. But you can't assume this for tapeworm stages— some are still locked inside your gallstones! These can be reached with a series of ozonated oil liver cleanses (page 594).

After three weeks of Mopping Up, you may stop; do the Mop Up once a week thereafter, on days when you are doing the maintenance parasite program or the day after.

To summarize:

What you'll need for killing ALL your parasites, including tough ones, and mopping up after them:

1. Black walnut tincture, an alcohol extract of the green hull (for alcoholics, a water recipe is given).
2. Wormwood, in capsules.
3. Cloves, fresh ground, together with size 00 empty capsules.
4. Zapper.
5. Ozonator, to ozonate olive oil.
6. L-cysteine.

Optional: ornithine, arginine.

Parasites Gone, Isopropyl Alcohol Next

Now that you have killed the intestinal fluke and cured your cancer, what's next? Two tasks remain:

1. Stop getting isopropyl alcohol into your body.
2. Get rid of the heavy metals and common toxins in your body, diet and home. (This is covered in *Part Two: Getting Well Again.*) This will heal the damaged tissues and start your tumors shrinking.

Isopropyl alcohol is the antiseptic commonly used in cosmetics. Check all your cosmetics for the word "propanol" or "isopropanol" on the label. It is usually put on the label, since it is not currently suspected of causing cancer.[16] I don't know if propyl compounds like propamide, propacetamide, isopropyl gallate, or calcium propionate could be converted by the body to isopropyl alcohol, so don't take chances. Do not use anything that has "prop" in the list of ingredients. Don't give your discarded cosmetics to anybody. Don't save them. Don't have them in the house anywhere. Throw them out.

Remember, 100% of cancer patients have the solvent isopropyl alcohol accumulated in the liver and in their cancerous tissues. People without cancer do not have isopropyl alcohol in their livers. Look at the case histories. Often one spouse has cancer: you can note that she or he has isopropyl alcohol and the adult fluke in the liver. Ortho-phospho-tyrosine is present in an organ like the lung where the cancer is developing. But the other spouse does not have cancer although he or she shares the parasite. For him or her it is only in the intestine. There are no eggs or other stages anywhere. There is no solvent present!

Here is a list of common body products that may have isopropyl alcohol in them: cosmetics, shampoo, hair spray, mouthwash, mousse, body lotions, shaving supplies, and, of course, rubbing alcohol. **If in doubt, throw it out!**

---

[16] Many people use cosmetics with isopropanol in them and do not develop cancer. The isopropanol is detoxified for them by their livers. Eating moldy food with aflatoxins in it poisons the liver's ability to detoxify propanol.

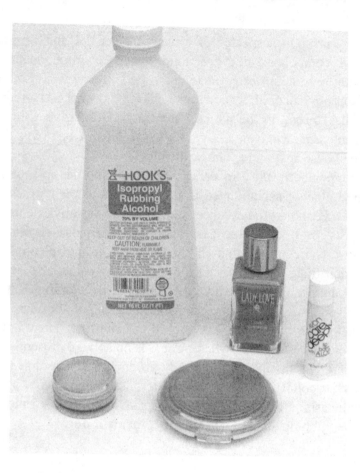

Check all labels for "isopropyl alcohol, "propanol" or
"isopropanol". Throw those products away!
Fig. 17 Some isopropyl alcohol containing products

Although body products give us our highest concentrations,
isopropyl alcohol is in our <u>food</u>, too! One primary source is flavor or color. These are extracted with <u>solvents</u>! The concentrate
extracted is called a "spice oleoresin." Naturally, the solvents

should be removed before the final product is used. But nothing can be removed completely once it is added, so there are regulations governing the amount left. Amounts are stated in "ppm", or "parts per million." 50 ppm would be like 50 drops out of a million drops, or roughly one drop per quart (or liter).

This excerpt is from the Code of Federal Regulations (CFR).

21 CFR 173.240 (4-1-94 Edition) Isopropyl Alcohol.

Isopropyl alcohol may be present in the following foods under the conditions specified:

a)   In spice oleoresins as a residue from the extraction of spice, at a level not to exceed 50 parts per million.

b)   In lemon oil as a residue in production of the oil, at a level not to exceed 6 parts per million.

c)   [Discusses its use in hops extract.]

Here is a summary of other solvents mentioned:

Solvent	Allowable residue in spice oleoresins	Paragraph in 21 CFR
Acetone	30 ppm	173.210
Ethylene dichloride	30 ppm	173.230
Methyl alcohol	50 ppm	173.250
Methylene chloride	30 ppm	173.255
Hexane	25 ppm	173.270
Trichloroethylene	30 ppm	173.290

Fig. 18 Lawful uses of solvents in food.

Another reason for isopropyl alcohol pollution (and other pollutants) in our food are the chemicals used by manufacturers to sterilize their food handling equipment.

21 CFR 178.1010 (4-1-94 Edition) Sanitizing solutions.

Sanitizing solutions may be safely used on food-processing equipment and utensils, and on other food-contact articles as specified in this section, within the following prescribed conditions:

(a) Such sanitizing solutions are used, followed by adequate draining, before contact with food. [Note rinsing or drying is not required!]

(b) The solutions consist of one of the following, to which may be added components general recognized as safe and components which are permitted by prior sanction or approval.

[Now comes (1) through (43) permissible sterilizing solutions, including several with isopropyl alcohol, like:]

(25) An aqueous solution containing elemental iodine (CAS Reg. No. 7553-56-2), potassium iodide (CAS Reg. No. 7681-11-0), and isopropanol (CAS Reg. No. 67-63-0). In addition to use on food processing equipment and utensils, this solution may be used on beverage containers, including milk containers and equipment and on food-contact surfaces in public eating places.

[Then in paragraph (c)(19) the exact concentration of the iodine is specified. Nowhere is the concentration of the isopropanol specified. It can be as strong as desired.]

Fig. 19 US regulations on sterilizing solutions.

Even if there were regulations governing removal of sanitizing solutions, the overwhelming truth is missed: that **nothing can ever be completely removed after it has been added**. Or perhaps the lawmakers didn't miss this fact. Perhaps they believed that small amounts—too small to measure with an ultraviolet spectrophotometer—could surely do no harm.

The good news is that isopropyl alcohol leaves your body, by itself, in five days after you stop getting it.

Isopropyl alcohol is a pollutant in cold cereals. Stop buying all cold cereals. Even the most natural cold cereals are polluted. I haven't tested every cereal on the market, but I have tested so many that you should not take a chance on a single one. See *Recipes* to make your own.

Why is it so important to get rid of isopropyl alcohol if you have already gotten rid of the intestinal fluke, and are on the parasite maintenance program? Because reinfection can occur so quickly! Dairy products and fast-food hamburgers are not heated high enough to kill metacercaria (the shelled stage that can survive extreme heat and cold in ponds). Even when you ask to have your hamburgers cooked very thoroughly, you run

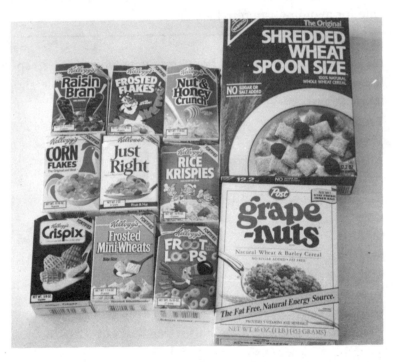

All cold cereals I tested, including health-food varieties, are polluted with solvents such as benzene, carbon tetrachloride and isopropyl alcohol. DON'T EAT THEM.

Fig. 20 Some polluted cold cereals

the risk of having your hamburger removed from the grill with the same spatula that just put the next batch of raw patties on the grill, defeating your efforts. Within 24 hours the fluke stages are in your blood, some of which are "hatching" into adults, and before your next maintenance dose of black walnut tincture they are in your liver and your ortho-phospho-tyrosine is back. But without isopropyl alcohol this doesn't happen. With isopropyl alcohol it is inevitable.

> You should <u>not</u> stay on high doses of parasiticides as a substitute for avoiding isopropyl alcohol.

Read all labels on the body products you buy. Keep a lighted magnifying glass with you for this purpose while shopping.

Isopropyl Alcohol Polluted Products

THROW THESE OUT

<u>even if isopropyl alcohol is not listed on the label!</u>

- **shampoo**, even health brands
- store-bought **fruit juice**, including 100% natural and health store varieties
- store-bought and **bottled water**, including distilled, mineral, health store or self dispensed varieties
- **cold cereals**, including granolas and health food varieties
- **rubbing alcohol**
- **mouthwash**
- **vitamin supplements and herb extracts** unless tested

- all **shaving supplies** including aftershave
- **prescription, and over-the-counter drugs** unless tested
- **white sugar** (use confectioner's sugar or <u>brown</u> sugar, but add vitamin C to detoxify mold)
- **decaffeinated coffee**, postum, herb tea blends (single herb teas are OK)
- **hair spray** and **mousse**
- **carbonated beverages**
- **cosmetics** (see *Recipes*, page 543)

You can make many of these products yourself, free of toxins (see *Recipes*).

Remember that isopropyl alcohol is also called <u>propyl alcohol</u>, <u>propanol</u>, <u>isopropanol</u>, and <u>rubbing alcohol</u>.

Endogenous Isopropyl Alcohol Means Made-In-Your-Body

There is another, even more fiendish source of isopropyl alcohol. Certain bacteria of the *Clostridium* family make it! A portion of our colon bacteria are *Clostridium* varieties. It is considered "normal." Yet, children's bowel contents tested negative[17] for the six *Clostridium* species I searched for. Instead they had *Bifidus* varieties (a "good" bacteria). I think <u>absence</u> of *Clostridium* and <u>presence</u> of *Bifidus* is <u>truly</u> normal, even for adults.

Perhaps only a few varieties of *Clostridium* make isopropyl alcohol. I have found only one reference to this in the classical literature. It states that *Clostridium toacum* makes isopropyl alcohol in its metabolism. Perhaps this species is also present, although I cannot test for it yet. In any case, I usually see <u>all</u> six species of *Clostridium* in the intestinal tract of cancer patients. Only in cancer patients have *Clostridium* species invaded the upper parts of the intestine, too, not only the lower parts, so much more isopropyl alcohol may be made. In fact the esophagus and stomach are frequently colonized as well! The Syncrometer easily detects the isopropyl alcohol being made in the intestines when *Clostridium* is present.

Evidently, the bacteria burrow through the walls of the intestine, find the tumor site, and colonize there, producing isopropyl alcohol. Is it any wonder that the body runs out of detoxifying capability for this antiseptic?

---

[17] Based on 3 children, ages 2, 5 and 6: two specimens tested per child.

Aflatoxin B

Whenever isopropyl alcohol is in the liver, I find **aflatoxin B**, a mold by-product, in the liver as well. Aflatoxin B is known to be extremely carcinogenic. My interpretation of this coincidence is that aflatoxin B is inhibiting isopropyl alcohol detoxification. Of course the reverse may be true: isopropyl alcohol could be inhibiting detoxification of aflatoxin. Either way, if you stop eating moldy foods your aflatoxin B level will be zero.

Some foods with aflatoxin B are beer, nuts, bread more than a few days old, overripe fruit, and many bulk grains. Surprisingly, very moldy foods like cheese show no signs of aflatoxin B. Maybe removal of aflatoxin is the reason there are documented cases of freedom from cancer after changing to the "macrobiotic" diet.

Malignant tumors have both the fluke and isopropyl alcohol present. Before that, the tumor was benign. If you can prevent tumors from forming at all, you would never have to worry about malignant ones.

The Formation of Tumors

A tumor begins as a small overgrowth of tissue. You may notice it simply because it presses against its neighboring organ giving you strange sensations. When it is examined or scanned, the doctor may call it an "adenoma" or "neoplasm," or just plain "mass." Although scientists have worked for 100 years on the causes of such little growths, there is no conclusive explanation yet.

But by analyzing this little growth with the Syncrometer, its composition can be determined qualitatively. When its composition is compared to that of other masses, in other persons, in other organs, common denominators can be found. And if removing these common denominators for patients results in shrinkage of these benign masses, a recipe for curing your "tumor disease" can be formulated.

A brief sketch of how we see tumor disease progress will be given here so you can begin your healing and prevention program.

The Cause of Tumor Disease

These are the common denominators of all the masses or growths I have investigated, even including warts. There are only about a dozen, not hundreds upon thousands as we are told.

- tapeworm stages
- *Ascaris* worms
- *Clostridium* bacteria
- copper (the metal)
- cobalt (the metal)
- vanadium (inorganic)
- malonic acid and derivatives
- fungus species

This is not an unmanageable list. Compared to the thousands of chemicals on the "carcinogen" list compiled by anti-cancer institutions, this is simple.

What Do The Tapeworm Stages Do?

We have already stated that they produce malonic acid or somehow cause it to be made by the host, which is us. Malonic acid stalls the Krebs cycle (the major energy-producing mechanism going on within our cells) an event that leads to tumor formation. But that is not all. Tapeworm stages also host bacteria.

One of the constant companions of tapeworm stages are *Streptomyces*, fungus-like bacteria. There are hundreds of species; they are well known for making streptomycin, an antibiotic. But they should not be making such compounds in our tissues on a steady basis. The side effect of streptomycin is stopping protein formation. This is exactly what happens in the tumor. When *Streptomyces* are present, the Syncrometer can detect no RNA, which is the nucleic acid that leads to protein building. Healthy cells make RNA constantly.

Ozonated oil plus cysteine is the best way to kill tapeworm stages because together they are also effective against *Streptomyces*.

What Does *Ascaris* Do?

The primitive metabolism used by *Ascaris* (and other parasites) is called the **glyoxylate cycle**. *Ascaris'* glyoxylate cycle commandeers our Krebs cycle. (The Krebs cycle is what <u>humans</u> use to burn food into energy.) Killing *Ascaris* stops this, and helps speed up our metabolism in a single day.

Another thing that *Ascaris* does is to destroy all the vitamin C in the organ with the tumor by <u>oxidizing</u> it (removing a hydrogen atom). To be useful, vitamin C must have <u>reducing</u> power (it must be able to pin a hydrogen atom onto other compounds). When *Ascaris* is killed, vitamin C is immediately present again, and in proper reduced form.

Ascaris harbors *Rhizobium leguminosarum*. We have been taught that *Rhizobium* is a rather lovable bacterium, busily changing nitrogen gas into nitrates in the nodules along the roots of legume plants. But in our bodies, the nitrate gets reduced to nitrite, nitrites form nitroso compounds, and these cause mutations. *Rhizobium* is also capable of making DNA, which is necessary for tumor formation. Fortunately, killing *Ascaris* with ozonated oil plus cysteine also kills *Rhizobium*.

Another bacterium harbored by *Ascaris* is *Mycobacterium avium/intracellulare* (two species are mixed on my specimen). Although I have not discovered any of its metabolic pathways, it is easy to notice the big improvements in health when it is killed. Night sweats are immediately gone!

Ascaris has still more tumor-related activities! To understand them you have to know about extensive studies done in the 1930's. At that time the structure of cholesterol was being discovered, and some of its byproducts were suspiciously similar to the coal tar products known to cause "cancerous tumors" in mice. Hundreds of coal tar products were studied over a ten year period, and one of the worst was **20 methyl cholanthrene.**

20 methyl cholanthrene is considered one of the most potent carcinogens ever discovered. One tenth of a milligram (approximately 1/10 of a flyspeck) injected into the skin of a mouse, only once, could produce tumors up to 8 months later, filling the mouse with big round balls that ended its life. Just one dose! To my amazement the Syncrometer detects 20 methyl cholanthrene in tumor cells when *Ascaris* is also present!

How have we escaped our demise by this route for so many years? We have hosted *Ascaris* from our early beginnings as humans, although having household pets is probably a new lifestyle. I don't know the answer, but obviously eliminating *Ascaris* infestation is a most important task.

I believe it can be safely concluded that tapeworm stages and *Ascaris*, together with their associated bacteria, <u>initiate</u> our tumor disease. Later, *Clostridium* bacteria and various toxins and "carcinogens" make their deadly contribution.

What Does Copper Do?

There is no tumor, benign or malignant that does not have inorganic (toxic) copper, that is detected with the Syncrometer. On blood tests, it is easily seen that non-food copper depresses the serum iron level. Ultimately copper is lethal because without sufficient iron (in a properly reduced state, kept that way by vitamin C) our detoxification systems fail, red blood cell formation fails, energy metabolism fails, we fail.

Metallic copper comes into our bodies with water that has run through copper pipes, from metal tooth fillings, and from plastic tooth fillings polluted with copper. Copper has a great affinity for sulfur and uses up our chief sulfur compounds: glutathione, cysteine, taurine, and methionine. And eventually the sulfur that must stay combined with iron in our most vital organs is used up. Fortunately it is easy to eliminate toxic copper from our bodies by removing it from your water pipes and your mouth.

Copper accumulation in cancer patients has been noted for a long time, but it was thought to be due to the cancer itself. My findings show the reverse, that copper accumulation causes tumor growth. And in fact, the accumulation, far from being due to the cancer patient's genetic tendency, can be easily stopped just by changing the water pipes and getting copper-containing tooth fillings removed. Copper levels fall at once, letting iron levels come up in less than a week. Immediately blood building can resume. And as copper levels continue to go down, the invasive fungus growths also decline.

What Does Fungus Do?

Quite a few fungi and their toxic products, called *mycotoxins*, have been studied in connection with cancer. The Syncrometer routinely detects **aflatoxin** and **patulin**, which are mycotoxins, at the tumor site.

Aflatoxin causes liver tumors. All cases of jaundice I have seen in liver cancer patients are due to aflatoxin. The only remedy I know of is to stop eating all grains and nuts, in any form. Other foods, especially fermented foods, could be contaminated with it, too, because the mycotoxin is not alive and is not damaged by cooking.

Patulin also has a history of scientific research and use (as an antibiotic!). I routinely detect it at a tumor site, but its preferred organ is the parathyroid. It plays a detrimental role in the body's defense against tumors.

Tumor Defense in the Body

Every person I have tested who is without tumors, has **tumor necrosis factor** (TNF) in the parathyroids—but nowhere else. Every person with a tumor does <u>not</u> have TNF in the parathyroid glands. But the reason is clear. Patulin is in the parathyroids, somehow preventing TNF from being made. As soon as patulin disappears, and this could happen as soon as one day after killing the fungus and stopping eating it, TNF reappears in the parathyroids, ready to go to work. No sooner is it back in the parathyroids but it shows up at the tumor sites, too, doing its best to shrink the tumors there.

If you should eat or grow *Aspergillus* fungi again (the kind that make patulin), TNF immediately disappears. So it is rather a fragile system. Our habit of eating rotten fruit (not right off the tree) and letting fungus germinate in the intestine (constipation) keeps us inundated with patulin.

The bruised parts of apples may have as much as 1 ppm patulin.[18] Stopping eating bruised fruit and clearing the bowel of fungus with Black Walnut Hull Tincture Extra Strength (two

---

[18] Horubala, A., *Influence of fungal metabolites on the quality of fruit and vegetables and on the quality of resultant products* (Polish). Przemysl-Fermentacyjny-I-Owocowo-Warzywny, 36 (6) 11-13, 1992.

tsp. dose is effective) immediately eliminates patulin in the parathyroids.

Now the tumors <u>can</u> shrink. But the forces favoring growth may still be stronger.

What else is making them grow? Cobalt, vanadium, malonic acid, several bacteria varieties, and assorted carcinogens.

What Does Cobalt do?

Very little is known about cobalt toxicity. It was even given as medication in the past, for anemia. But the treatment was worse than the disease. Inorganic cobalt blocked oxygen utilization so that the body was fooled into believing it was at the top of a tall mountain, where the air is very thin (poor in oxygen). The body's adaptation to altitude is to make more red blood cells. This appeared to cure the anemia by making more red blood cells. But blocking oxygen utilization has the same effect as being anemic, so nothing was gained.

Long ago numerous scientists discovered an important fact. Any lowering of oxygen use by an organ favored tumor formation in that tissue. A steady trickle of cobalt to your tumor could be expected to support tumor growth.

Another toxic effect of inorganic cobalt is in the liver where the two main blood proteins are made: **albumin** and **globulin**. These two must be carefully regulated since they control the osmotic pressure in the blood vessels. They must add up to about 7 gm/dl. The total may get much too high, such as 10 gm/dl in multiple myeloma, or much too low (below 6) when terminal illness has progressed. Cobalt raises the albumin too high and keeps globulin levels too low. These derangements can be seen on a standard blood test.

The toxicity of cobalt to the heart has been known for decades; it was made illegal in nearly all uses then. But gradually it has reappeared in more and more products. By allowing it in dish detergent and laundry detergent we now get a steady dose of it as a residue on our dishes and from our clothing which constantly massages cobalt into our skin.

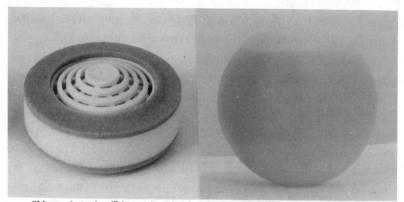

"Non-chemical" laundry devices actually spew surface tension reducers into the water, including cobalt containing chemicals.
Fig. 21 Laundry discs and spheres

A ridiculously obvious and preventable source of cobalt is metal tooth fillings. But by replacing the metal with plastic, we have frequently <u>not</u> removed the cobalt! It is usually present, either as a component or contaminant of the plastic restoration. When both metal and plastics are meticulously removed, blood albumin and globulin levels correct themselves—often in just three days! And a life-threatening situation is turned around to recovery.

What does Vanadium Do?

Vanadium, like cobalt, causes the red blood cell count to go up—much too high. In fact, polycythemia (a rare "blood disease") is primarily vanadium toxicity. How this happens is unknown. But when the red blood cell count is over 4.7, for men or women, the Syncrometer always detects cobalt or vanadium in the bone marrow. Vanadium is asserting its toxicity in other organs, too; in the liver, and in the tumorous organ.

In the liver, vanadium toxicity has the opposite effect of cobalt toxicity. Now the albumin production is too low, while globulin goes too high.[19] Since globulin is less effective than albumin as an osmotic water attractant, water is allowed to leave the circulation and simply seep into the surrounding tissue. It is called **edema** and becomes a fatal condition.

Vanadium is also the cause of the frequent mutations seen in tumors—in the p53 gene. It does this by combining with nucleic acid to make **vanadyl complexes**. A healthy p53 gene is necessary for the gene's tumor suppresser action, which is to produce a substance that prevents tumors from forming.[20] By removing vanadium from your dentalware (both metal and plastic), the vanadyl complexes disappear and p53 gene mutations disappear, too.

Then how could a patient without any tooth fillings develop tumors? We have seen many children with cancers whose dentition was intact. But their tumors were filled with vanadyl complexes! And as the disease became terminal the additional toxic effects of vanadium were easily spotted: much too low albumin and high globulin, and an exceptionally high red blood cell count.

The children's vanadium came from 1) chronic exposure to car exhaust (a source that constantly invaded their home), 2) a household gas leak, or 3) leaking refrigerant (I suspect fossil

---

[19] One might expect that having both toxins would cancel the toxicity. Indeed, the blood proteins are often in normal range for cancer patients, the problem being masked by this dual toxicity. But in other ways they do not cancel their toxicity, and each takes its toll on your health.

[20] Sharon Begley, *The Cancer Killer*, Newsweek, Dec. 23, 1996, pp. 42-47. Hollstein, M., et al, *p53 Mutations in Human Cancers*, Science, vol. 253, July 5, 1991, pp. 49-53.

fuel is often part of the refrigerant). These are important sources of vanadium for adults, too.

Vanadium leaves the body, even from the vital organs, in a week after clean air is supplied and artificial materials are taken out of the mouth. These simple moves can turn around a terminally ill patient.

What Does Malonic Acid Do?

It is toxic, and a lot of research has been done on it (see page 121). Malonic acid was found to inhibit the use of oxygen by animals (respiration) as early as 1900! By 1930, Otto Warburg had found that anything that inhibited respiration could cause tumor formation. But it was never suspected that tapeworm stages release malonic acid, or that plastic teeth seep it, or that we even eat it in certain common foods. The Syncrometer detects it in every tumor (based on approximately 500 tests). New research is needed to clarify the exact role it plays in tumor growth.

What do Bacteria do?

We have seen that some of these common denominators of tumors suppress our oxygen use. Some cause mutations. Some interfere with iron availability. Some lower our detoxifying capability. Some destroy our vitamin C. Some drastically lower our immunity. Some prevent us from making tumor suppressers. But, in spite of all these tumor-promoting forces, a tumor could still <u>not grow</u> unless it had sufficient DNA to grow on. Imagine a garden. It has been tilled, seeded, fertilized, and is completely ready to grow. But each seed needs one more thing: water. For our cells to divide they must have DNA, the gene material with which each gene reproduces itself. Certainly, our cells can make their own DNA from RNA, but resources for this are limited. And it occurs only in the nucleus, at an appropriate time, at a pace that allows for replenishment of the RNA.

In tumors, the Syncrometer detects DNA <u>all the time</u>. This may seem normal, because all of our cells have DNA, but I consider it abnormal because DNA is typically not detectable by the Syncrometer. Perhaps because it is buried in the cell nucleus. Only in tumors (and the ovaries!) does it show up, leading me to believe that when I do detect it, it is out of place and out of control.

How can DNA (the "water") be continually supplied for cell multiplication? The answer is **bacteria**.

Only a few bacteria varieties[21] out of the vast numbers inhabiting this planet are able to make DNA using vitamin B_{12} like humans do. These bacteria are certain species of *Clostridium*, *Rhizobium* and *Lactobacillus*. (There may be more which I have not yet researched, but when these three are banished, DNA formation stops, and abnormal cell division must cease.) These bacteria have found their way into the human body, particularly the intestinal tract and dental crevices. And from there, when low immunity allows, they travel to the young tumor and colonize it.

Clostridium is the hardest to eradicate. Evidently it invades the tumor cells and is not killed. Perhaps immunity is too low. Once inside, I suspect its DNA-making enzymes seep out into the cytoplasm where our copious amounts of RNA are, changing it all to DNA. And with an ever present supply of DNA, the last requirement for unrestrained growth is met.

So some bacteria can cause your "garden" to be "watered" in overabundance.

Another bad thing bacteria can do is transport viruses into your cells. This is because bacteria can themselves be infected

---

[21] Geoffrey Zubay, *Biochemistry*, Addison Wesley Publishing Co., 1984, pp 706-707.

with viruses. So when the bacteria manage to invade your cell by penetrating the membrane (not an easy job), the virus gets a free ride. Periodically viruses get released from those bacteria inside your cell, putting them in position to attack your DNA. When foreign DNA joins yours, it is called *transformation*.

Scientists have studied transformation to determine when and how it causes tumor growth but don't have all the answers. To me, it seems likely that bacteria and their viruses, such as we discuss here, are probably the transforming agents sought by scientists.

Bacteria Implicated In Other Growth Factors

Although the DNA-making bacteria seem most important, other common bacteria contribute to tumor growth. For instance if an organ tests positive to DNA, I assume tumorous growth is occurring. If that organ then tests positive to CA-125 (a cancer marker), I know from experience the Syncrometer will find *Salmonella typhimurium*. Always. The conclusion is that *S. typhimurium* is a causative factor for both CA-125 and the tumor. Here are other correlations I routinely find:

Bacteria	Source	Growth Factors /Markers Detected By Syncrometer
Staphylococcus aureus	Dental	Epidermal growth factor (EGF)
Escherichia coli (E. coli)	Bowel	Cancer associated antigen GI
Salmonella typhimurium	Dairy	Cancer antigens, CA 15-3 and CA-125
Salmonella paraty-phimurium	Dairy	Platelet derived growth factor (PDGF)
Shigella flexneri	Dairy, tapeworm stages	Cancer antigen, CA 15-3, PDGF, Insulin like growth factor (ILGF)
Shigella sonnei	Dairy, tapeworm stages	Alfa Feto protein (AFP)
Shigella dysenteriae	Dairy, tapeworm stages	Cancer antigen, CA 72-4

Vanquish Tumor Causing Bacteria

The *Clostridium* family can be stopped in the digestive tract by taking **betaine hydrochloride** (see *Sources*). 1500 mg a day is an average dose. Of course a dental source will recolonize the digestive tract, so you must stay on this daily dose for protection until the dental source has been removed (see Dental Clean-up, page 73). This will also clear up *Staphylococcus*.

The *Shigellas*, *Salmonellas*, and *E. coli* can be cleared up with the bowel program (page 586). To prevent reinfection, observe safe dairy rules (page 135).

How Benign Tumors Turn Fatal

Tumor growth is a grand conspiracy between parasites, bacteria, fungi, copper, cobalt, vanadium, malonic acid, and assorted carcinogens! Yet the human body is big and strong. There are many mechanisms within our immune systems to fight these intruders. But if the tumor enlarges or new ones arise, we know these mechanisms are failing. We should be coming to our body's assistance rather than shrugging it off as "merely benign."

At some time, the benign little mass may become malignant. This means that I observe ortho-phospho-tyrosine is present. Plus I always observe multiplying *Fasciolopsis* stages as well as isopropyl alcohol now. Did the *Fasciolopsis* stages suddenly discover the tumor the way a hermit crab discovers an unused shell?

My detection of growth factors in tumors and even the presence of a few fluke stages there suggests we should be much more concerned about them. Perhaps the distinction between benign and malignant tumors is deluding. Like the distinction between a loaded and unloaded gun. When ammunition is available, no gun should be ignored.

We should really view tumor formation, or *tumorigenesis*, with the same caution as cancer, even though it is slow at first. It could begin to accelerate, doing more and more harm. Yet the body has coped with tumorigenesis a very long time, from the beginning of humanity, as evidenced by our body's ability to produce tumor necrosis factor (TNF), tumor suppresser genes, and to repair mutations. What has gone wrong in the last century to permit such a flurry of tumors and cancers?

Even though tumor growth is ancient, perhaps <u>malignancy</u> is a recent phenomenon. Perhaps this past century has produced the overload of heavy metals, solvents, and globetrotting parasites required to spark this epidemic.

Yet knowing what starts our tumors gives us the power to stop them, whether benign or malignant.

Preventing Tumors Will Prevent Cancer

Tumors are complex structures, which appear to be associated with fungi, metals, bacteria, tapeworms, *Ascaris* and toxins. Being complex, you would think they would be fragile, and removing just one building block would topple them. But the opposite is true: together they form a highly durable opponent for your immune system. The best way to beat tumors is not allowing them to start.

How To Prevent __All__ Tumors

1. Kill tapeworm stages and *Ascaris* regularly and completely with your parasite killing recipe plus Mop Up.
2. Stop eating foods that contain malonic acid.
3. Get away from coppered water.
4. Stop using cobalt-containing products.
5. Avoid vanadium in fossil fuel contamination of the air <u>in your home</u>!
6. Have only safe dentalware in your mouth since you must suck on this day and night.
7. Stop *Clostridium* invasion with a betaine hydrochloride supplement.
8. Don't eat moldy food.

I have neglected the subject of **carcinogens**, though they are also important. In fact, it may be the carcinogen that chooses the organ to be targeted for a tumor. This role keeps them from being "common denominators". Certainly, urethane pollution of plastic dentalware could be very significant. Urethane was studied intensively for a decade and found to be a very strong tumor inducer, especially in the lungs. Certainly, the legions of chemicals found to "increase the risk of cancer" are playing their roles in obscurity.

I have also neglected the concept of **raising immunity**. This is the practice of giving interferon, giving interleuken, giving thymosin, giving bacterial antigens, and giving many other entities to raise or stimulate the cancer patients' immune powers. The concept is excellent, and would certainly bear results <u>if only</u> the setting were correct. But in a setting of continued parasitism, bacterial invasion, and metal toxicity, it is hopeless, or at best temporary.

Of the eight preventive measures, none is very difficult to carry out.

Review

As a result of our civilized lifestyle we live in petroleum-heated houses, drink water carried in copper pipes, eat food stored to the limit of freshness, wash our clothes in cobalt-containing detergent, are exposed to parasites we disperse all over the globe, place toxins in our teeth to constantly suck, and anoint ourselves with unnatural chemicals. Carcinogens pervade our modern environment.

An overburdened liver gets an overdose of aflatoxin B, reducing its ability to detoxify isopropyl alcohol. *Clostridium* gain a toehold in your bowel, intensifying the isopropyl burden and causing it to accumulate. About this time human chorionic gonadotropin (hCG), one of the first cancer markers discovered, appears. Next *Clostridium* and other bacteria invade one of your weakened organs, and start producing DNA. A small tumor starts to form. It is benign.

The intestinal fluke, *Fasciolopsis*, facilitated by isopropyl alcohol, finds it can leave the intestine for the liver. And, it can reproduce itself from beginning to end inside your body (not needing a snail). Miracidia and other fluke stages swarm in your body. They produce a super growth factor, ortho-phospho-tyrosine, which makes cells multiply. The adult *Fasciolopsis* is in the liver but stages and growth factor are far away in the new tumor. It is now malignant.

If solvents other than isopropyl alcohol are consumed, *Fasciolopsis* follows a different, non-cancerous, path. Just how solvents facilitate the parasite's life cycle needs more research. Do solvents dissolve the shells of parasite eggs in the intestine, letting them all hatch? Do solvents disarm your immune system?

Certainly, the tiny baby stages (miracidia) get into your blood and travel everywhere in your body. They land, become redia, and reproduce into thousands more. They finally turn into cercaria, metacercaria, and finally adults.

- Adults in your liver, if you have isopropyl alcohol in it, causing cancer!
- Adults in your pancreas, if you have wood alcohol in it, causing diabetes!
- Adults in your thymus, if you have benzene in it causing HIV disease!
- Adults in your brain, if you have toluene or xylene in it, causing Alzheimer's disease!
- Adults in your kidneys (Hodgkin's disease), uterus (endometriosis) or prostate (chronic prostatitis) if you have other solvents there!
- Adults in your skin if you have Kaposi's sarcoma.

I had to mention these diseases even though this book is just about cancer because you should know what a scourge this parasite is, and how deadly it is to have both the intestinal fluke and solvents. In every case (100%) of these diseases that I have seen, both have been present.

Part Two: Getting Well Again

You are not transformed magically into a healthy person on the day the malignancy is gone. You must also shrink or dissolve the tumor somehow. Even this will not make you a healthy person. You need to clean up your adverse environment!

So when you have cancer you really have two problems: the cancer itself, and the contributory problems. In Part One we cured the cancer. Now the tumors aren't growing wildly, but they are not gone, either. They won't shrink until we remove the contributory problems. This will be a marvelous adventure.

Getting well will be the most exciting part of your recovery. You will see yourself heal. Healing has a magic about it that is unique. It is the body's secret. No physician can make your body heal. No human being understands healing. But if you remove all obstacles from your body, you can count on it, <u>it will heal</u>! Remind yourself of a wound you once had and how it healed. Splinters of glass or wood had to be removed, dirt had to be scrubbed out. Bacteria had to be killed. Then, by unknown magic, it healed!

Example of Healing

Let us suppose you had lung cancer. Six days ago you started the fluke-killing recipe and threw away everything that had isopropyl alcohol in it, including shampoo and bottled water. Today the fluke and ortho-phospho-tyrosine and cancer are all gone. You are coughing, too fatigued to go shopping, you can't sleep and your mind dwells on the spots that were seen on your X-rays just recently. Can you heal them before your surgery date? Can you avoid chemotherapy? This is how you accomplish both these goals in record time.

1. Stop smoking. Nobody in your house may smoke indoors. Your poor brain may cry out for nicotine. Take ginseng for a calming effect. Chew herbal combinations instead. Eat candy. Enroll in a smoke-out program. Try hypnotism. Pray. Do whatever it takes to succeed. There is no half-way measure. You must stop smoking. Put a sign on the outside door: "Recovering Smokaholic, Please Help By Smoking Outside." Your lungs will begin to heal from the day you stop smoking. It takes 3 weeks of consistent healing for the tissue pathology to improve enough to change the doctors' minds about your need for surgery and chemotherapy.

2. Change your copper water pipes to plastic. If you only have a short section of copper this is easy and inexpensive. If you have all copper pipes with no control over them, move quickly into a new motel, one that has PVC (plastic) plumbing. There is no halfway measure with copper. There must be <u>none</u> in the laundry water, shower water, or dishwater. Filters or distillers cannot remove the amount of copper coming from copper plumbing. Filters were meant to remove the amount in municipal water. Even if you connect three filters in a row, they will all be letting copper through in a week. All cancer cases have copper water pipes, often unbeknownst to them. The faucets themselves and water heater inlets need not be changed. Nor any of the pipes lying outside the water meter. I'm not sure why these don't have more of an effect.

   There is a new process available (see *Sources*) in which an epoxy compound is blown through your copper plumbing.

It coats the pipe, stops corrosion, and best of all eliminates the copper contact. People say it makes the water taste so good they don't buy bottled water anymore! I tested this water and could find no harmful elements.

If you stop your copper exposure, you are removing one of the common denominators I find in all tumors.

I also find copper in every case of leukemia, which means it is probably a factor in non-tumorous cancers also. (The only type of cancer that I have not seen a copper buildup with is Hodgkin's disease.) So I think this shows the importance of avoiding copper: do not have copper plumbing; do not wear copper jewelry; do not use copper cookware, and get the copper dentalware out of your mouth.

---

3. Remove all the chemicals from your house. You may store them in the garage <u>if and only if</u> there is no door between garage and house. If there is a door, you lock it and cover it with a large sheet of plastic so nobody can accidentally use it and let the fumes in from the garage. You remove everything from the basement, kitchen, bathroom. Remove all paint cans, paint or varnish removers, thinners, brush cleaners, even though they are tightly closed. Remove all containers of floor wax or cleaner or polish, and carpet or furniture or window cleaner. Remove nail polish and remover, tile cleaner, rust remover, wall cleaner. Every chemical must go. Keep only distilled white vinegar, borax, and baking soda as cleaning agents. I will tell you how to use them later.

Remove all fragrances from the house. You may store them in the garage in clear plastic bags. Nobody in your house may wear them. Remember, you have a deadline to meet to heal your lungs. To do this, you remove ALL chemicals. Fragrances are chemicals. This includes detergents, potpourri, colognes, candles, room fresheners, wall lamps, soaps, lotions, after-shave, hair spray, anything that you can smell.

4. Board your pets with a friend. They should be started on a parasite program while at your friend's place. Pets carry *Ascaris* (roundworm), a parasite that goes to the lungs and the eggs are picked up by touching the pet's fur. Later on, when your doctor pronounces your lesions healed, you may give some serious thought to whether you should chance getting parasites again from a pet.

5. Get rid of any possible asbestos sources. Put your hair dryer and clothes dryer in quarantine. There is asbestos, too fine to be measured by Public Health Department equipment, and therefore more dangerous, coming from two out of three hair dryers. Don't use one. Don't let the hairdresser use one on you. Don't sit inside a hair dryer or use hair curlers or you'll add tungsten as well as asbestos to your beleaguered lungs.

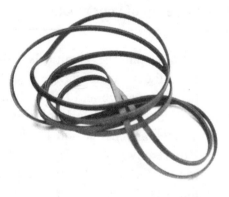

Clothes dryers are our biggest source of asbestos. Check your dryer belt. It should state: "Made in USA"
Fig. 22 Clothes dryer belt

Simply change your hair style. After you're in the clear with your health, buy a Conair

Prostyle Mini 1250™, a 081.A 1600™, or a Vidal Sassoon Misty Tone 1500™; these tested negative to asbestos. **Clothes dryers are our biggest source of asbestos.** It comes from the belt. I suppose our government agencies feel it is safe enough to blow asbestos around inside the machine. However, it comes out through the cracks along the sides and around the exhaust outlet. Install a new belt. How can you pick a replacement belt that does not have asbestos? Choose a "Made in USA" belt. No belt that said "Made in USA" showed asbestos in my tests. All others did! Don't assume that because your clothes dryer is a U.S. brand name that your belt inside is also. Three belts that do not have asbestos are listed in *Sources*. Get a new exhaust hose for your clothes dryer, too, cleaning out all the dust in the machine while installing it; use duct tape around the outlets at both ends. Never exhaust the dryer into your house to save heat, even with a safe belt, because fresh air is best for your lungs. After this, have the whole house from basement to upstairs vacuumed and dusted while you are away for the day.

6. Have the house tested for radon. Buy a 5-day kit from a hardware store and put it in your bedroom. If there is any[22] radon, seal up the cracks in the basement. It is not very difficult to correct a radon problem. Since it takes weeks to get an answer back from the company measuring the radon from your kit, it would be best to go live somewhere else temporarily. Or just tackle the job of fixing cracks. **Your lungs will not heal if there is any radon.** Free pamphlets are available at drugstores to tell you how to seal your home against radon. They make the

---

[22] Government standards allow a certain amount (4 microcuries per liter). This is not safe for a person with lung disease.

job seem more difficult than it really is. Get a quart of black roofing cement and dab it around plumbing pipes and gas pipes where they come through any walls. Dab it on cracks. After a few days, you can go over them with a more attractive caulk. Seal around plumbing pipes upstairs too. Open your crawl space vents and leave them open year round. Don't try to save on your heating bill by keeping them closed. Install a crawl space fan. These measures nearly always work but if a follow-up 5 day test still shows <u>any</u> radon, you will need to <u>move</u>.

7. Remove all possible formaldehyde. If your bedroom is paneled, move out of it and keep the door locked. Move your bed into the cleanest room in the house—no wallpaper, no carpets except the washable kind and no stuffed furniture. Your bedroom should not be above the garage or facing a parking lot. If you have a foam mattress, or pillows, throw them out. Move all new furniture into the locked room out of circulation. Wash all the new clothing hanging in your closets. Don't wear them until they have been washed to remove the sizing, it has formaldehyde.

8. Remove all possible arsenic. Throw out (in outside garbage) any ant killer compound, roach killer, mouse-bait, spray bottle or can, lawn chemicals, house plant spray, every bit of pesticide. Steam clean the carpets yourself (see *Recipes*, page 581); at the same time clean the cloth furniture (stain resistant treatments contain arsenic). If you have it done for you, specify <u>no</u> "stain resistant" treatment and be present to check on the job being done. If there is new wallpaper, close and lock the door to these rooms or have it removed by someone else while you are away for the day. Wallpaper glue contains arsenic and must be carefully washed away. Don't do any painting or remodeling. Don't get new furniture, carpets, or cars.

Much as you may love that new-car smell, it would be chemical suicide.

9. Check your home for exposed fiberglass. If your home is insulated with fiberglass, seal all holes in your ceilings or walls that lead to insulated areas. If your hot water heater has a fiberglass blanket, remove it. Also check for fiberglass insulation around fans and air conditioners.

10. If you have gas heat or a gas water heater or stove, ask your local Health Department to come out to check for leaks. Your gas company does not have sensitive equipment to find small leaks. Also have a furnace repair person check your furnace and flue. Better yet, switch to all electric. Fossil fuels bring with them vanadium. Gasoline and car exhaust similarly bring vanadium. Keep these vapors away from your home.

The biggest obstacle to all these changes is the feeling that you are not worth all this trouble. Of course, you are worth it! And what a fine example you are setting to family members by getting well. You are rewarding them for their efforts to help you. And you are teaching them a valuable lesson about the toxic pollution of our environment. Your recovery will be an inspiration to everybody. You may be saving lives!

Your total cost will probably be under $2,000. These changes will herald a new era in your life. I have seen every one of these tasks done in as little as one week <u>when family and friends pitched in</u>. Healing starts the day they are completed. Count how many times you cough in 5 minutes. It should go down to zero. If it does not go to zero, you have missed something. Go over the whole list. Be more meticulous. Or go on vacation. You may go to a friend or relative's house if they are willing to clean it up for you. This will get you away from asbestos, pets, Freon, copper, chemicals, and fragrance all at once (tell the maid not to spray for bugs, nor use air fresheners) .If you get better while on vacation, stay on vacation. Never come back to your tumor-causing house.

Healing In General

What about other cancer types? Most of the healing tactics for lung cancer apply to other types as well. But for each different organ affected you should focus on its special needs. For skin cancer, you would focus on laundry, soap, lotions and ultraviolet light. Clothing rubs into skin constantly and always has detergent residue in it. Soap and lotions are chemical soups with isopropyl alcohol antiseptic. There are simple replacements for all of these given in the *Recipes* chapter.

Getting well after <u>any</u> cancer depends on cleaning foreign things out of your body so it CAN heal. You have already removed all the parasites from your body and the isopropyl alcohol. That was critical, but don't stop there if you want to get your health back. I have seen people get well whose doctors told them they had only 10% of their lung, or liver, or kidney still functioning!

You can get all your health back from <u>any</u> kind of cancer by removing unnatural chemicals.

1. Remove all unnatural chemicals from your mouth.
2. Remove all unnatural chemicals from your diet.
3. Remove all unnatural chemicals from your body.
4. Remove all unnatural chemicals from your home.

That is all there is to it. Let us look at each step, the mouth, the diet, the body, the home. Make a decision first: that you are worth the trouble. Now that the cancer is gone, your life is not in immediate jeopardy, but do you wish to get well? Do you wish to get rid of your bowel disease with its bloating and gas and discomfort? Do you wish to get rid of fatigue and feel like walking and working again? Do you want your strength back? What about pain? Do you wish to be free of foot pain, hip pain, low back pain, upper back pain, chest pain, knee pain, and other pain? Headaches, too, can be cured by cleaning up.

If you had these health problems before the cancer struck, then you will still have them after the cancer is gone. Getting well again means getting rid of all the problems that brought you to the cancer, such as breast lumps, enlarged prostate, as well as problems resulting from the cancer, such as weight loss.

1. Clean Up Your Dentalware

This section on dentistry was contributed by Frank Jerome, DDS, with comments added by the author. To get an even clearer idea of how to make good dental choices, read his book, Tooth Truth (see *Sources*).

Dr. Jerome: *The philosophy of dental treatment taught in America is that teeth are to be saved by whatever means available, using the strongest, most long lasting materials. Long-term toxic effects are of little concern. The attitude of the majority of dentists is: whatever the ADA (American Dental Association) says is OK, they will do.*

A more reasonable philosophy is that there is no tooth worth saving if it damages your immune system. Use this as your guideline.

The reason dentists do not see toxic results is that they do not look or ask. If a patient has three mercury fillings placed in the mouth and a week later has a kidney problem, will she call the dentist—or the doctor? Will they ever tell the dentist about the kidney problem or tell the doctor about the three fillings? A connection will never be made.

It is common for patients who have had their metal fillings removed to have various symptoms go away but, again, they do not tell the dentist. The patient has to be asked! Once the patient begins to feel well they take it for granted, and don't make the connection, either. If everybody's results were instantaneous, there would be no controversy.

Dr. Clark: Some people are noticing that when they replace metal fillings with plastic they get tumors. It is too early to know if this is a coincidence. My recent tests show that most varieties of dental plastics contain known tumorigens as did amalgams, of course. In fact, I believe that toxic dental materials we suck on day and night are largely responsible for our cancer epidemic and the abnormal T-cell ratio in AIDS. So plastic fillings, at least the varieties in use now, are not the answer. They are very toxic, too.

Dr. J: *Isn't this somewhat of a bombshell?*

Dr. C: Not really, the fact was already known decades ago that even solid materials allow their water soluble components to leach out. That's why fluoride is now added to tooth fillings: it is expected to leach out. When fillings have toxic pollutants or just plain toxic components, like urethane, maleic acid, or an azo dye they will leach out, too. And I find them in the tumors of a cancer sufferer.

Dr. J: *There is no perfect dental material. The best filling is never needing one. The question of toxicity is of degree. If a patient has a terminal disease, they will not be able to tolerate any contaminants. Fortunately, most patients are not in such dire circumstances.*

Finding the right dentist is your first and most important task. The alternative dentists have been leading the movement *to ban mercury from dental supplies. Not only mercury, but <u>all</u> metal needs to be banned.*

If your dentist will not follow the necessary procedures, then you must find one that will. The questions to ask when you phone a new dental office are:

1. *Do you place mercury fillings? (The correct answer is NO. If they do, they won't have enough commitment to do removals properly.)*
2. *Do you do root canals? (The correct answer is NO. If they do, they do not understand good alternative dentistry.)*
3. *Do you remove amalgam tattoos? (The correct answer is YES. Tattoos are pieces of mercury left in the gum tissue, or that settled on the jawbone as it was temporarily exposed during dental work.)*

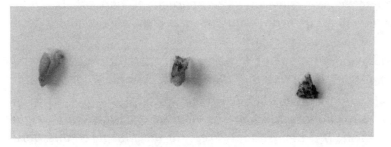

Find the black dot on each bone fragment. That is the tattoo, although the rest of the bone fragment that was removed is also discolored by amalgam.

Fig. 23 Tattoos

4. *Do you treat cavitations? (The correct answer is YES. By cleaning them.) Cavitations are simply holes (cavities) left in the jawbone by an incompletely extracted tooth. A properly cleaned socket which is left after an extraction will heal and fill with bone. Dentists routinely do NOT clean the socket of tissue remnants or*

infected bone. A dry socket (really an infected socket) is a common result. These sockets never fully heal. Thirty years after an extraction, a cavitation will still be there. It is a form of osteomyelitis, which means bone infection.

Dr. C: An X-ray showing a cavitation is on page 90. I often see osteomyelitis (bone infection) in the rest of the body, particularly in bone cancer. It always starts in the jaw bones due to some dental problem. It spreads from the jaw to the rest of the body. Amazingly, when we clean up the jaw, other areas of osteomyelitis clear up, too! *Staphylococcus aureus* is <u>always</u> present in cavitations.

Dr. J: *It will be very frustrating for people to find a dentist who can answer all four questions correctly. Most mercury-free dentists still use many metals in crowns. Many of these metals are carcinogens, such as nickel, chromium, and cobalt. These are the least expensive metals so it is a purely economic decision for the dentist.*

Cavitations are done by very few dentists. Some state dental associations claim that they do not even exist and that it is malpractice for a dentist to treat them. There are few training courses available and even then, dentists are reluctant to try to treat them. If a dentist says "Yes" to the first three questions and "No" to the fourth, they may still be a good choice. The dentist may be able to refer patients to an oral surgeon for treatment for their cavitations.

Dr. C: Something else to be aware of when looking for a new dentist: be considerate of the dentist's feelings when you ask questions. Even the alternative dentist likes to "run the ship" his or her own way. If you can get answers more discreetly, as from a friend or the receptionist, you might get better service. You should also inquire if the dentist uses a magnifying viewer or a camera and monitor device to spot tattoos. The dentist will be delighted to answer this question. It puts the dentist into the class of a select few who aim at perfection in their practice.

Dr. J: *If you choose a dentist who does not understand the importance of these questions, you could end up with new problems. Find the right dentist first even if you must travel hundreds of miles. There are 6,000 to 10,000 dentists who should be able to help. Some can do part of the work and refer you to a specialist for the rest. Five hundred to one thousand of these dentists can do it all.*

Dr. C: What is the treatment for cavitations?

Dr. J: *To prevent a cavitation from forming in the first place, you clean the walls of the socket very carefully at the time of tooth extraction. They must be free of rough edges and bits of tissue; one must use tweezers to carefully remove every tiny bit that might still be stuck. For old cavitations that have become sealed into the jawbone, the simplest way is to make a small access opening. The cavitation is flushed with antiseptic then cleaned using hand and rotating instruments. Then it is flushed again. They heal and fill with bone with few problems for the patient. Larger ones may require a second treatment.*

Dr. C: I recommend squirting in a dilute solution of Lugol's iodine to sterilize the socket instead of commercial antiseptic. Six drops in a quarter cup of tap water gives enough solution to clean up several cavitations or sockets.

Dr. J: *US dentists use standard antiseptics or just salt water. Why not stay with that?*

Dr. C: Nothing is as effective as iodine. We are dealing with very vicious bacteria here, not just Staph, which is friendly by comparison. I often detect six varieties of *Clostridium* bacteria, and assorted *Streptococci*. They have very tough shelled capsules, or spores, inside them. The capsules survive even when the microbe dies. Later the capsules hatch again. But iodine kills the capsules, too. Tooth bacteria infect tumors; that's why I emphasize tooth bacteria so much. Lugol's iodine is easy to make and quite cheap (see *Recipes*). You don't feel any stinging sensation, of course, because your mouth is anesthetized.

Dr. J: *What about antibiotics? Dentists everywhere routinely use antibiotics to help after-procedure healing. It seems quite effective. Many use antibiotics to protect themselves legally, of course.*

Dr. C: *Clostridium* bacteria in the jaw bone do not respond well to antibiotics. They return as soon as the antibiotic is stopped. That is because the wound is rather deep, and there is very little oxygen deep down. This is the classical setting for *Clostridium*. Our "home remedy" antibiotic works better than commercial varieties (see page 101). What often helps as much as antibiotics is just getting every iota of metal <u>and plastic</u> out of the mouth. This in itself restores the mouth immunity so suddenly that infections don't develop. It's quite remarkable.

Dr. J: *The simpler the dental treatment, the better. If the dentist says that he or she can remove your metal fillings but this would leave such a big hole it would be better to CROWN them, say "NO!" A crown is a prescription for disaster. The tooth has to be drilled down to a nubbin to fit the hollow cap (crown) over it.*

Dr. C: The space between that nubbin and the cap is supposed to be completely filled, so no space exists for bacteria. But actually, that doesn't happen. Every crown I have seen removed revealed a gray to black tooth zone. This is where the *Clostridium* was growing right into the tooth. Since *Clostridium* is a "tumor microbe", that is, it can change RNA to DNA, such infected teeth must be quickly extracted for very sick patients. The infection is <u>in</u> the tooth, not <u>on</u> the tooth. You can assume that every crowned or capped tooth has gross infection underneath. The tooth cannot be cleaned up. Crowned teeth and capped teeth must be extracted.

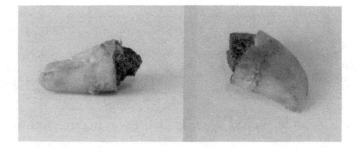

These teeth with their crowns removed reveal a black surface underneath and fine gray lines of further invasion of the tooth. It is invariably *Clostridium* at work.

Fig. 24 Black tooth under crown

Dr. J: *That's a lot of extractions for some people.*

Dr. C: Yes. A mouthful of caps or crowns must be exchanged for dentures or partials. They should not have had crowns put on in the first place. Of course, the hazard was not known at that time.

Dr. J: *Would you suggest different dentistry for healthy and sick people, then?*

Dr. C: I suppose we do this unconsciously, already. When we are sick we stop our bad habits and risk taking. Later, when we are well we return to them. But it isn't logical. It's only a matter of time when we must correct our mistakes. A sick person has only weeks to root out the sources of his or her body's infections, while those who still feel well may have years remaining, depending on body immunity.

Dr. J: *What do you do for yourself? Do you have metal or plastic in your mouth?*

Dr. C: All my large plastic fillings became extractions. I plan to fill the back spaces with partials. At present, there is no filling material safe enough to keep permanently in my mouth, but I am watching the dental marketplace in Germany. They are aware of the toxicity problem from plastics and may be the first to solve it.

Dr. J: *What about the front teeth? Are you carrying plastic in them?*

Dr. C: No, I simply had the plastic taken out by air abrasion. This avoids enlarging the original hole. I am keeping the holes empty and very, very clean. Perhaps a new non-toxic plastic will be developed soon. In fact, I was hoping you would develop it.

Dr. J: *So you took out the plastic I so artistically put in 13 years ago?*

Dr. C: Yes, and I am happy to tell you I had no *Clostridium* infections under them. So it can be done! Maybe your technique was superior. Maybe no open dentine was involved, only enamel! The technique being used everywhere else, though, has to be much better before it is acceptable.

Dr. J: *Then why did you remove them?*

Dr. C: When I originally tested the composite you were going to use for me, I found it free of heavy metals but I didn't test for urethane and bisphenol-A. And I didn't test the base/liner and other little adjunctive materials a dentist uses besides the composite. These become part of the restored tooth and leach their toxins constantly. So my fillings were seeping copper, cobalt and vanadium which I detected in my retina and optic nerve. In addition I detected mercury and silver that was stuck <u>under</u> the plastic fillings–the remains of my previous amalgams. But they came out with the air abrasion.

Dr. J: *Do you think that small amount matters?*

Dr. C: That tiny amount makes the difference between recovery and no recovery for the very sick patient. In healthier people you don't notice the health boost.

Dr. J: *Since you are now extracting mercury-filled teeth instead of refilling them with plastic, do you use any special precautions?*

Dr. C: Extractions should be done carefully, so the amalgam doesn't break up, letting little pieces get away to lodge in crevices in the gums or bone or the hole itself. In Mexico we routinely refer the patient to an <u>oral surgeon</u> for extractions and to a dentist for air abrasion cleaning or temporary cement fillings.

Dr. J: *No dentist in the US would extract a tooth just because it has a large amalgam filling in it.*

Dr. C: The amalgam is very toxic. The available plastic replacements are toxic, too. But to prove this, you would need Syncrometer technology, searching for metals in the bone marrow, spleen, thymus, lymph nodes. That's where it's killing you by blocking iron metabolism. It doesn't chelate out. Your choice is to succumb to illness or extract. Extractions are life-saving. Patients will need to go to foreign countries for their dental work.

Dr. J: *How could you convince a seriously ill patient to do that?*

Dr. C: Words are not convincing so I don't try too hard. But if an MS patient who is disabled sees another MS patient gain ground after tooth extraction it is quite convincing. The results come so quickly that there is no argument. Likewise, for the cancer or AIDS patient. They may be concerned about the "stress" on their bodies from extractions. But when they see similar patients start to eat again, get dressed or go for a walk within days after getting their extractions, it doesn't take persuasion. It's seeing the miraculous recovery of others in the same hopeless situation that's convincing. In fact, I have heard patients say, "Who needs their own teeth in a wooden box?"

Dr. J: *What percentage of patients give such a dramatic response?*

Dr. C: All of them, 100%. Evidently, toxic dentalware was a large part of each person's problem. The patient has run out of detoxifying capability for heavy metals in certain vital organs, and the tiniest bit now tips the scales, even tattoos. The front teeth must be cleaned out carefully, as well, because the plastic still has metal (copper, cobalt, and vanadium). After this, all the teeth are polished clean with the same air abrasion device using baking soda (instead of aluminum oxide). Baking soda will combine with metal oxide in crevices and do a perfect job of cleaning up after amalgam. You do the same for plastic fillings. A dramatic response only comes after the entire job is completed.

Remember to wait until your gums are healed over before doing the air abrasion of front teeth, otherwise particles could lodge in the wound site. It takes four to six days.

Dr. J: *You advise using a rubber dam, don't you?*

Dr. C: Yes, a rubber dam plus a suction device to keep bits of loose amalgam from swimming away to other locations, hiding under gums and settling in extraction sites never to be found again. That's disastrous.

Dr. J: *How do you fill these new holes left after removing metal and plastic fillings?*

Dr. C: You don't.

Dr. J: *Don't they get infected?*

Dr. C: Not in half a year's time. That's plenty of time to get well in. After the patient is well, some risk-taking comes to their mind again and they are determined to fill the holes. After narrowly escaping death, though, would you risk putting anything even slightly suspicious back in your mouth to suck on continuously?

Dr. J: *The answer to that is easy; no, of course. But what about infection? Don't all the open teeth start to ache?*

Dr. C: No, they don't. Patients treasure these last teeth. They keep them squeaky clean by brushing with colloidal silver (five drops on toothbrush), or with white iodine; that saves them from infection. If a tooth does become infected, it becomes an extraction.

Dr. J: *Ultimately, do you fill them?*

Dr. C: Yes, with zinc oxide and eugenol, common ZOE cement.[23]

Dr. J: *That's really going back in time. If you don't mix the zinc oxide and eugenol in the right proportion it will crumble right out.*

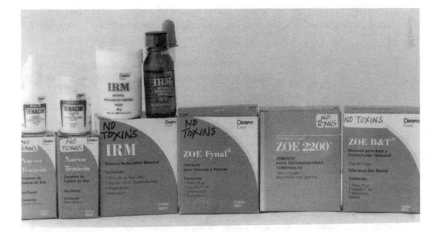

The various ZOE supplies I tested were free of contaminants provided they were sets of powder and liquid, not premixed varieties.
Fig. 25 Good ZOE varieties

Dr. C: We're doing it very well in Mexico. No problem at all. No crumbling. They look bright white, a little too white, but maybe a safe colorant will soon be found. The good thing is that these ZOE fillings clean out easily; with air abrasion you don't even need anesthetic and you don't have to drill the hole

---

[23] ZOE stands for zinc oxide and eugenol. When these two are mixed, the resulting "cement" gets very hard. Eugenol is also antiseptic, so the cavity wall doesn't let infection get started.

bigger every time you exchange it for a new ZOE filling or for safe plastic when that becomes available. It was meant to be temporary, but is holding up very well, as long as enough powder is used in the ZOE mix.

Some people are allergic to ZOE, but this can be tested beforehand, and one of the other cements used instead.

Guidelines For A Healthy Mouth

If you have	then...
Metal fillings Inlays and onlays	Change them to zinc oxide and eugenol. The original powder and liquid come in 2 separate bottles. The ratio of powder to liquid determines the hardness. No premixed or faster setting varieties are safe. Caution, do not use base/liner, adhesive, bonder, primer or other preparatory agents except as discussed later.
Crowns (all types)	Extract tooth entirely.
Bridges	Change to methacrylate partials.
Metal partials	Change to methacrylate partials.
Dentures	Change to methacrylate dentures.
Porcelain denture teeth	Change to methacrylate denture teeth: they must come loose in a bag, not set in a wax bar. The wax adheres and pollutes the whole denture, unless you wash each tooth thoroughly and dry it.
Badly damaged teeth	Become extractions.
Root canals	Become extractions.
Braces and implants	Avoid.
Cavitations	Need to be surgically cleaned and disinfected with diluted Lugol's iodine.
Temporary crowns	Become extractions.
Temporary fillings	Same procedure as for metal fillings.

The guidelines can be summarized as:

1. Remove all metal and plastic from the mouth.
2. Remove all dead or infected teeth and clean cavitations.

Dr. C: Removing all metal and plastic means removing all root canals, fillings and crowns. Take out all bridge work or partials made of metal or plastic and change them into methacrylate. But you may feel quite attached to the gold, so ask the dentist to give you everything she or he removes. Look at the underside. You will be shocked at the corrosion.

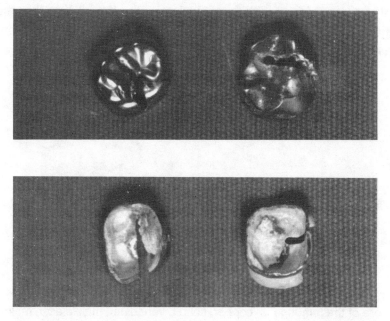

The top surfaces of tooth fillings are kept glossy by brushing (you swallow some of what is removed). Underneath is tarnish and foulness. Ask to see your crowns when they are removed.
Fig. 26 Tops and bottoms of some metal crowns.

The stench of the infection under some teeth may be overwhelming as they are pulled. *Clostridium* gases are particularly offensive. Bad breath in the morning is due to such hidden tooth infections, not a deficiency of mouthwash!

All metal must come out, no matter how glossy it looks on the surface. Metal does not belong in your body. It is toxic to your metabolism and your immunity. Do this as soon as you have found a dentist able to do it. Find a dentist with experience and knowledge about this subject. It is more than replacing acknowledged culprits like mercury-amalgam fillings. This is toxin-free dentistry. Only non-toxic plastic should be put back in your mouth. At present, only methyl methacrylate has been found to be safe, along with the cements, zinc oxide and zinc phosphate. More varieties could be on the "safe" list, like the silicates and carboxylates, if these compounds are ordered from a chemical supply company, rather than a dental supply.

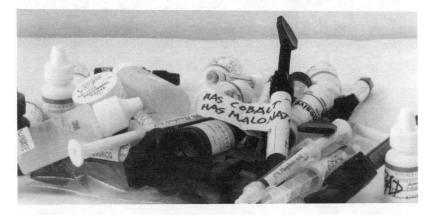

These are a few of the dental supplies I tested. They contain one or more of the tumorigens: copper, cobalt, vanadium, maleic acid, malonic acid, urethane, or scarlet red azo dye.

Fig. 27 Dental materials

Dental plastic, to be safe, must not contain malonic and maleic acids, nor urethane or bisphenol-A, nor a carcinogenic "azo" dye, nor polluting heavy metals. Not only the restorative material, but the liner/adhesive, bonder, primer, etc. must be free of these toxins. An analysis for these toxins should be a requirement for all dental materials.

Dr. J: *If your dentist tells you that mercury and other metals will not cause any problems, you will not be able to change his or her mind. <u>Seek treatment elsewhere</u>!*

Your dentist should do a complete X-ray examination of your mouth to begin with. Ask for the panoramic *X-ray before starting dental work. The* panoramic *X-ray shows the whole mouth including the jaws and the sinuses. This lets the dentist see impacted teeth, root fragments, bits of mercury buried in the bone and deep infections. Cavitations are visible in a panoramic X-ray that may not be seen in the usual tooth by tooth "full mouth series."*

Dr. C: Here is a sample of a panoramic X-ray.

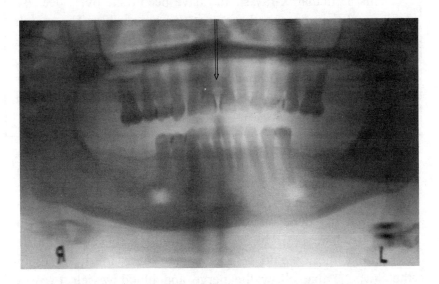

Fig. 28 A print of a medium-good quality panoramic X-ray

A print of an X-ray reverses the light and dark areas. Since you will be comparing this print with your own X-ray, you must convert light areas on the print shown here to dark areas on your X-ray.

To read your panoramic X-ray, tape it up on a window. First find the angles of your jawbone, noting left and right side and top and bottom. Use a hand magnifying glass to study it.

You Be The Judge

It doesn't take an advanced degree in dentistry to judge whether it is a good or bad X-ray. Are all the root tips visible? If not, you wasted your money; you got the panoramic so you could see the root tips and beyond! Since the X-ray can be viewed right at the time it is made, you can request a retake (it costs very little extra).

This particular X-ray should have been done over, because looking at the upper teeth no root tips are visible. The mouth was not correctly positioned for the X-ray. Also, the teeth at the ends are a solid black, so nothing can be deduced about them. The intensity setting on the X-ray machine was not correct for them. A duplicate X-ray at a different setting would have been wise.

Next, look at the lower teeth: The root tips are on the print, but not very clear. The X-ray machine produced two dark vertical lines at the centers, obscuring the roots further (a good reason to get it redone on the spot). Under each end-tooth is a roundish white spot. On the X-ray film, which you would be examining, these would be dark spots. These are the holes in the jawbone that allow the nerve and blood vessels to pass through. Note that a tooth was pulled three months ago on the lower left side. The bone has already filled in almost to the top, so that a nearly flat line is seen to mark the ridge of the jaw bone from one side to the other.

Locate the center. You have four small flat teeth in front on the lower side. The center is between them so two are on the left side and two on the right. The center on the upper side is easier to find; see the arrow.

The fifth tooth from the center at upper left has a black cloud emerging from the root tip like a swarm of gnats above it. This is an infection, the bacteria are parading up towards the brain. Brain tumors are made of such events. Trying to save such a tooth would be a bad mistake, even though it "looks good and was giving no trouble." Plastic (black edges) can be seen on the inner edge of the top center teeth; this was done for cosmetic purposes. A few more bits of plastic are seen here and there. No cavitations are seen in the bottom half where the visibility is good.

A large tattoo did not show up on this X-ray although the dentist spotted it easily while working on the mouth.

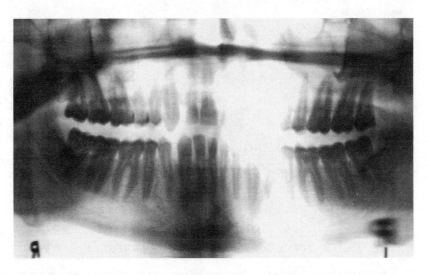

No fillings, no crowns, no cavitations, but perhaps a dead tooth led to the abscess at the white spot above the R. Drainage revealed mere mush, implying infection, as far as the probe could reach.
Fig. 29 Good quality panoramic

The second panoramic shows all the root tips. There are no cavitations seen. Notice the round white spot (black on the X-ray film) just above the R. This was an abscess, far removed from the teeth, but probably stemming from a dead or infected tooth. An X-ray cannot identify dead teeth. They should have been tested for vitality. A dead tooth always harbors *Clostridium*. Such a "silent" infection will reach vital organs such as thymus, bone marrow, and spleen, besides the tumor! All dead teeth should be extracted.

The last panoramic, although poor quality, shows a large cavitation at the lower right. One or two teeth extracted there long ago left a large hole with infection (dark area) along the sides. Thorough cleaning would have allowed it to fill in with

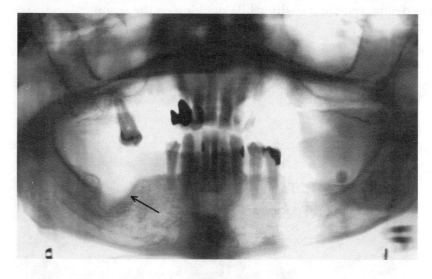

Fig. 30 Panoramic showing large cavitation at lower right.

bone again and stop the chronic illness (including cancer) this patient suffered from. At the upper right, a solitary tooth is sitting in a bed of infection. The dark black areas are metal. Syncrometer tests of this patient showed that the tooth bacteria, *Staphylococcus* and *Clostridium,* were both present at the breast, producing growth factors and turning RNA into DNA to spur the tumor there.

Dr. J: *White areas on the print (black on the negative) are either overlapping teeth or plastic fillings. The dentist is the best judge of this. Ask the dentist to interpret them for you.*

Dr. C: We are accustomed to thinking that plastic is metal-free. This is wrong. Modern plastic contains metal both as components and as contaminants, even including mercury. A possible explanation is that manufacturers are using recycled chemicals. It is particularly important not to get copper,[24] cobalt, or vanadium seeping from the plastic since these cause bone marrow, liver, spleen, and thymus toxicity. They diffuse out into the saliva and from there to the tumor or other unlucky organ. Most of the time metals are purposely added to the plastic to make it harder and give it sheen or color.

Dr. J: *The chief reason is a frivolous one; so the fillings are visible on X-rays! Dentists are not given information on metals added intentionally. The information that comes with dental supplies does not list them either. Many are listed on the Material Safety Data Sheets (MSDS). Dentists are required to keep these in their office. The ADA, also, has a library full of such information.[25]*

Dr. C: There are many lanthanide (rare earth) metals used in dental plastic. Their effects on the body from constantly

---

[24] Copper and other metals were found to be pollutants of plasticware as early as 1975. See *Trace Element Contamination 1. Copper From Plastic Microlitre Pipet Tips*, Benjamin, M. and Jenne, E., Atomic Abs. Newsletter, Vol. 15, No 2, Mar-Apr 1976 or *Trace Metal Contamination Of Disposable Pipet Tips*, Sommerfeld, M et al, Atomic Abs. Newsletter, Vol. 14, No 1, Jan-Feb 1975.

[25] Call the American Dental Association at (800) 621-8099 (Illinois (800) 572-8309, Alaska or Hawaii (800) 621-3291). Members can ask for the Bureau of Library Services, non-members ask for Public Information.

sucking on them have <u>not</u> been studied. Only metal-free plastic is safe. And of course it should not have urethane, bisphenol-A, or a carcinogenic dye, either.

Dr. J: *At present there is only one acceptable <u>denture plastic</u>; it can be procured at any dental lab and is used to make both dentures and partials.*

- *Plastic for dentures: methyl methacrylate. Available in clear and pink. <u>Do not use pink.</u>*
- *Plastic for partial dentures: methyl methacrylate. Available in clear and pink. <u>Do not use pink.</u>*

Dr. C: The pink color is from mercury, cadmium, or scarlet red dye which is added to the plastic. This dye is also called **Sudan IV**, and is a potent carcinogen. It was used by surgeons in World War I. Rubbing it into the wound made it "heal" faster. Much later, it was noticed that tumors grew from the wound and the practice was stopped.[26]

Plastic teeth that are made from methacrylate do not have metal, maleic, bisphenol, scarlet red dye, or urethane pollution. I tested many with the Syncrometer.

Dr. J: *I think the reason methacrylate products are not polluted is that the supplies for making them consist of only 2 bottles, one with powdered methyl methacrylate and one with the liquid "monomer". The monomer is a two-molecule bit of methacrylate which forms the solution. Powdered methacrylate is added to the liquid according to the recipe and the whole thing polymerizes into a solid.*

---

[26] Greenstein, Jesse P., *Biochemistry of Cancer*, 2nd edition, Academic Press, NY, 1954, p. 88. IARC Monograph 8, 1975, pp. 217-224.

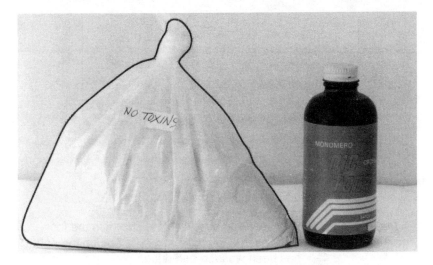

The bag contains methyl methacrylate powder, very cheap when purchased in bulk. The bottle contains the liquid monomer.
Fig. 31 How simple to make dental acrylic!

Dr. C: Teeth themselves come in many styles and sizes that the dentist or lab technician picks from a catalog. Make sure the dentist orders <u>loose</u> teeth in a bag for you, <u>not</u> teeth set in a wax bar (called a "card"). The wax from the bars I tested characteristically had nine tumorigens: copper, cobalt, vanadium, malonic acid, methyl malonate, maleic acid, maleic anhydride, D-malic acid and urethane in addition to bisphenol-A, an estrogenizer! Or ask for your teeth in advance so you can clean them up yourself (pay for them in advance, too, in case you lose one down the sink). After prying them out of the wax bar, wash with plain tap water; then dry very thoroughly until perfectly polished.

Methacrylate teeth, called "acrylic", bond very well with the methacrylate denture plate or partial, still it will be tempting for your dentist to apply "just a dab" of special adhesive. The adhesive has tumorigens and, once again, your efforts to have safe dentalware will be foiled. That little <u>dab</u> or touch-up is extremely important. <u>Make sure</u> no adhesive or anything else is used to stick the teeth in their places.

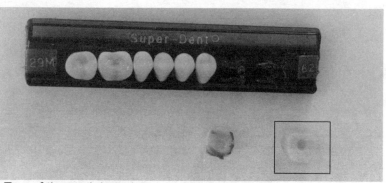

Two of the teeth have been removed and are shown in the foreground. The left one shows the adhering wax. The one on the right has been washed and dried.

Fig. 32 Wax card plus two removed teeth

If your dentist <u>did not</u> use anything but methyl methacrylate powder and monomer and <u>did not</u> use teeth straight from the wax card and <u>did not</u> use adhesive to stick them in their places, you will have safe dentalware.

But you cannot expect a dental lab to do all this. And dentists are accustomed to sending all dentures and partials to dental labs for manufacture. You are left with four options:

1. Your dentist gets into the business of making non toxic dentures or arranges for a dental lab to do so.
2. You take it up as a hobby yourself–take a course in dental technology.
3. You organize a co-op to do this work for the alternative dental trade.
4. You send your dental impression, "bite block", or old dentures to a specialized lab for denture making (see *Sources*). The bite block assures proper alignment, occlusion, etc.

The materials themselves are very cheap. If you change your mind about appearance of teeth or need a better fit, you could have them changed or even have a second "Sunday" set made.

Dr. J: *Many people (and dentists too) believe that porcelain is a good substitute for plastic. Porcelain is aluminum oxide with other metals added to get different colors (shades). The metal <u>does</u> come out of the porcelain! It has many technical drawbacks as well. Porcelain is not recommended.*

Dr. C: The new glass ionomers are even more polluted than plastic. Yet, the underlying concept is a good one; simple glass is not toxic. Remember, though, that toxicity isn't the only problem with dentalware. Even if a perfect, non-toxic filling material is developed, we would still need a perfect, non-toxic bonding technique that solves the infection problem.

Dr. J: *"Microleakage" is the dental term used to describe the penetration by bacteria into the microscopically small space*

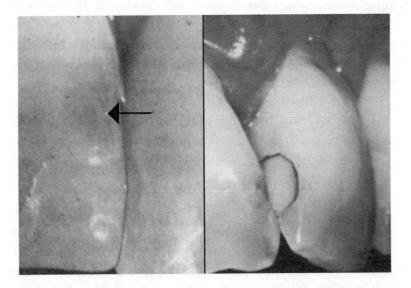

The left tooth has a plastic repair up to the faint wavy line. Above this is gray discoloration due to bacterial invasion. The plastic filling in the tooth on the right has a black outline of bacteria.

Fig. 33 Teeth with visible bacteria

left under fillings, due to poor adhesion. This crevice shouldn't be there.

Dr. C: In Germany, the dentists feel they have the microleakage problem solved for adhesion to enamel.

Dr. J: *That's the easy part. I had that solved when I filled your teeth—it's getting adhesion to the dentine that's the problem! The new bonding techniques are meant for the dentine as well as enamel.*

Dr. C: But it's just not successful. The tiniest microscopic flaw in the bond between the natural tooth surface and the dental material gives *Clostridium* bacteria a chance to start. And they are present in **every patient with large fillings**. The adhesive technology must be improved to be safe.

Dr. J: *It's an old truth: If the public demands plastic restorations that <u>don't</u> leach toxins and that adhere to the tooth <u>without</u> microleakage, the industry will develop it. The secret is in the public being knowledgeable about the issues. People could organize their own safety groups and exchange information. People need to be protected by others like themselves, not corporate executives.*

Dr. C: I'd like to thank Dr. Jerome for his contribution to this section, and his pioneering work in metal-free dentistry. I hope more dentists acquire his techniques.

Horrors Of Metal Dentistry

Why are highly toxic metals put in materials for our mouths? Because not everyone agrees on what is toxic at what level. Just decades ago lead was commonly found in paint, and until recently in gasoline. Lead was not <u>less</u> toxic then, we were just less informed! The government sets standards of toxicity, but those "standards" change as more research is done (and more people speak out). You can do better than the government by dropping your standard for toxic metals in your mouth to zero! Simply remove all metal.

The debate still rages over mercury amalgam fillings. No one disputes the extreme toxicity of mercury compounds and mercury vapor. The ADA feels that mercury amalgam fillings are safe because they do not vaporize or form toxic compounds to a significant degree. Opponents cite scientific studies that implicate mercury amalgams as disease causing. Many dentists advocate mercury amalgam fillings simply because they are accepted by the ADA, which they believe protects them from malpractice litigation. Why risk your health and life on their opinions? Remember everything corrodes and everything seeps, so dental materials must too.

Amalgams also contain copper, cobalt, and vanadium. This combination at a steady slow trickle from our teeth, poisons the liver, bone marrow, thyroid, thymus, spleen and parathyroids. These organs have regulatory functions: they must regulate how much albumin or globulin is made, how high or low the calcium level goes, and so forth. These regulatory organs have active centers containing iron and sulfur. Evidently the heavy metals compete with these to knock out the regulatory center. When these organs fail we die. We die from anemia, heart failure, edema, uremia or sepsis, although technically it is called cancer or AIDS.

Often mercury amalgam tooth fillings also test positive to thallium and germanium with the Syncrometer. Inorganic germanium is extremely toxic, while thallium causes leg pain, leg weakness, and paraplegia. If you are in a wheelchair without a very reliable diagnosis, have all the metal containing teeth removed from your mouth. Don't try to restore them. Search carefully for tattoos. Even the tinniest speck makes the difference between getting out of the wheelchair or staying in it. Small fillings could be cleaned out by air abrasion. Don't refill them until your condition improves. Ask the dentist to give you the grindings. If you are curious, try to have them analyzed for thallium using the most sensitive methods available, possibly at a research institute or university.

I was astonished to find thallium in mercury amalgams! It couldn't be put there intentionally, look how toxic it is:

TEJ500   **HR: 3**
THALLIUM COMPOUNDS
Thallium and its compounds are on the Community Right To Know List.

THR: Extremely toxic. The lethal dose for a man by ingestion is 0.5-1.0 gram. Effects are cumulative and with continuous exposure toxicity occurs at much lower levels. Major effects are on the nervous system, skin and cardiovascular tract. The peripheral nervous system can be severely affected with dying-back of the longest sensory and motor fibers. Reproductive organs and the fetus are highly susceptible. Acute poisoning has followed the ingestion of toxic quantities of a thallium-bearing depilatory and accidental or suicidal ingestion of rat poison. Acute poisoning results in swelling of the feet and legs, arthralgia, vomiting, insomnia, hyperesthesia and paresthesia [numbness] of the hands and feet, mental confusion, polyneuritis with severe pains in the legs and loins, partial paralysis of the legs with reaction of degeneration, angina-like pains, nephritis, wasting and weakness, and lymphocytosis and eosinophilia. About the 18th day, complete loss of the hair on the body and head may occur. Fatal poisoning has been known to occur. Recovery requires months and may be incomplete. Industrial poisoning is reported to have caused discoloration of the hair (which later falls out), joint pain, loss of appetite, fatigue, severe pain in the calves of the legs, albuminuria, eosinophilia, lymphocytosis and optic neuritis followed by atrophy. Cases of industrial poisoning are rare, however. Thallium is an experimental teratogen [used to induce birth defects for study]. When heated to decomposition they [sic] emit highly toxic fumes of Tl [thallium]. See also THALLIUM and specific compounds.[27]

Fig. 34 Thallium excerpt

Even if you do not have cancer, it would make sense to have all your metal fillings out if you have several of the listed symptoms.

Thallium pollution frightens me even more than mercury, because it is completely unsuspected. Its last major use, rat poison, was banned in the 1970s. One current use for thallium is in Arctic/Antarctic thermostats. When added to mercury the mercury will stay liquid at lower temperatures. Are mercury suppliers then providing the dental industry with tainted amalgam?

Who tests for the purity of dental mercury? What is tested for? As recently as 1972, mercury was considered <u>pure</u> if you simply <u>looked</u> at it.

> The purity of dental mercury in the American Dental Association specification is defined by its surface appearance, its residue after pouring and its nonvolatile residues. The tests for surface appearance and pouring residue can determine the presence of 0.001 percent or more of base metal impurities. The addition of 0.001 percent of copper, zinc, tin, lead, bismuth, cadmium, arsenic or antimony caused an immediate change in the appearance of the surface of mercury. The mercury lost its mirror-like appearance and a film or "skin" formed on the surface. The contaminated mercury wetted the glass container and the container could not be completely emptied. The effect was very pronounced and could be readily detected in each case.

---

[27] *Dangerous Properties of Industrial Materials* 7th ed. by N. Irving Sax and Richard J. Lewis Sr., Van NOSTRAND, Reinhold N.Y. 1989.

> However, the addition of 0.001 percent of silver or gold did not cause a change in the appearance of the mercury.[28]

Fig. 35 "Pure" mercury excerpt

The question is: how would you detect other, more toxic metals, like thallium or germanium, at <u>lower</u> concentrations? If they are present, why have they not been found? Either no one has looked for them or they are hard to find. (Thallium and mercury are next to each other in the periodic table of elements, meaning their mass is almost identical, which may contribute to the difficulty.)

The cancer causing action of metals has been studied for a long time, although it doesn't get attention by our regulatory agencies. A scientific book on this subject was published in 1980.[29] One table from this book is shown on page 144. We can see that chromium and nickel compounds are the <u>most</u> carcinogenic metals. Nickel is used in gold crowns, braces and children's crowns!

Note that the form of the metal is very important. Some metals have an essential/toxic duality. For instance, chromium is an essential element of *glucose tolerance factor*, but most of its other compounds are extremely toxic. In general, xenobiotic compounds (foreign) are to be avoided! Metal doesn't belong in our foods or in our bodies.

---

[28] *American Dental Association Guide to Dental Materials and Devices*, sixth edition, copyright 1972, p. 31.

[29] *Carcinogenicity and Metal Ions*. It is volume 10 of a series called *Metal Ions in Biological Systems*, edited by Helmut Sigel. A university chemistry library should have this book. It has a fascinating chapter on the leukemias by two scientists from the Academy of Sciences of the USSR, E. L. Andronikashvili and L. Mosulishvili.

Dental Aftercare, Prevent Infection

One of the chief purposes of doing the dental cleanup is to kill all *Clostridium* bacteria that have invaded the deeper regions of the jaw bone. They come originally from the crevices under plastic tooth fillings. Antibiotics are not successful in such a task because they only inhibit the bacteria until your immune system has time to rally and mount a big response. In a cancer patient, this immune response never happens. And as soon as the antibiotic is stopped, new, more serious bacteria surface to bewilder and defy attack.

A very vigorous program is needed to clear up infection after the infected teeth are pulled because deep wounds are the preferred locations of *Clostridium*.

Just removing the tooth does not automatically clear up the small abscess at the tip of the root, even with antibiotics. Not when *Clostridium* is the inhabitant. Cleaning the socket thoroughly can prevent *Staphylococcus* invasion but does not prevent *Clostridium* invasion which is deeper down.

This Dental Aftercare program is successful in killing *Clostridium*, *Staphylococcus*, and *Streptococcus* bacteria all together. (*Streptococci* go to your joints to cause arthritis.)

You will need:
- A water pick.
- Lugol's iodine solution (see *Recipes*) six drops in ½ glass water four times per day.
- Colloidal silver (see *Sources*), take as directed by provider.
- Inositol, a supplement, 500 mg, take two four times a day.
- Betaine hydrochloride, a supplement, about 300 mg (see *Sources*), take two three times a day.

101

- Baker's yeast cakes (keep refrigerated) ½ cake once a day with breakfast.
- Raw garlic, one clove a day, or germanium (carboxyethyl germanium sesquioxide only, see *Sources*) one a day.
- Hot water.

Acquire these before your dental appointment. Practice using the water pick and making the colloidal silver. The most important of all these is the hot water!

The immune power of your arterial blood is much greater than in your veins. How can you bring arterial blood into the jaw area to heal it faster after dental work? Simply by hot-packing it from the start!

The first day of dental work is critical. If you miss this, a massive spread of infection can occur because the mouth is always a "den of bacteria," and the abscessed teeth are themselves the source. As soon as you get home from the dentist you need to bathe your mouth with hot water. The heat brings in arterial blood. Swish gently. Keep the cotton plug in place for you to bite down on and reduce bleeding, even while swishing. Don't <u>suction</u> the water around your mouth, you could dislodge the clot that needs to form in the socket. Gently move the hot water about your mouth. At the same time apply a hot pack to the outside of your face where the dental work was done. Wring a wash cloth out of the hottest water you can endure. Or fill a plastic baggie halfway with hot water, zipping it shut securely. Do this for 30 minutes four times a day, for a few days. Then three times a day for a week—even when there is no pain. Don't suck liquids through a straw for 24 hours; the sucking force is especially risky, it could dislodge the healing clot. Don't allow your tongue to suck the wound site, either; and <u>don't put fingers in your mouth</u>.

As the anesthetic wears off there will be very little pain if the bacteria in the tooth sites have been killed. But you could introduce the bacteria yourself, by <u>eating</u>, and by putting fingers into your mouth. Consider your mouth a surgery site. Anywhere else on your body, the surgery site would be scrubbed first, then painted with iodine or other strong antiseptic, and later sprayed again and bandaged to keep everything out—certainly food particles and fingers!

But the mouth cannot be bandaged and you must eat! So eat a big meal just before your dental appointment. Afterwards, for the rest of the day, drink only clear liquids, such as tea with honey or confectioner's sugar. You may need a pain-killer on the first night; choose a non-aspirin variety to minimize bleeding.

Take the supplements described above.

Bleeding should be considerably reduced by bedtime. The cotton plug put in your mouth by the dentist may be thrown away. However, if bleeding is still substantial, make a new plug for yourself by rinsing the fresh gauze the dentist gave you, then rolling it into a wad shaped like your finger. If the dentist did not give you any gauze, use paper towel. Place the wad on top of the bleeding gum and bite down hard.

The next day you need to be well fed, yet without eating solids or liquids with particles in them. The particles lodge too easily in your wound. Your choices are:

1. Chicken broth, strained, skimmed of fat.
2. Milk, boiled, cooled with vitamin C added.
3. Eggnog, made with boiled milk.
4. Plain ice cream made with boiled cream (see *Recipes*).
5. Pudding made with cornstarch or flour.
6. Fruit and vegetable juice, strained.

Immediately after "eating" (drinking), water pick your mouth with very hot salt water. Do not be afraid to start some bleeding; this could be expected and is desirable if an infection has already started. Water picking never dislodges the healing clot, only strong suction or infection dislodges it.

Continue taking the supplements described above.

If pain increases instead of decreases on the second day, you have an infection. Water pick continuously for an hour! If the pain subsides, the infection has cleared. Water pick until the pain is completely gone. It could take four hours!

On the third day you may drink blended food (particulate); do not try to chew solids. Water pick after each meal. Floss the front teeth and brush them with white iodine or colloidal silver (hydrogen peroxide is not strong enough).

Continue taking the supplements described above.

If the pain level is increasing and water picking has not succeeded, you must <u>hurry</u> back to the dentist to search for food particles. He or she will open the wound and clean it out again.

Continue to hot pack, hot swish, water pick, floss, brush, and take the supplements for one week. If you detect an odor from your mouth, at any time, it is *Clostridium* making a comeback, even without pain. Try water picking for a half day, if that doesn't help, hurry back to the dentist. Assuming no problems, however, you may reduce the supplements by half and stay on them for three more weeks.

If your dentist carefully cleans the sockets and rinses them by squirting Lugol's solution into them, and if you are doing the Dental Aftercare program conscientiously, you will not need an antibiotic or extra pain killer. This conclusion is based on over 500 cases of dental work, all free of antibiotics and infection. In every case of failure (infection), trapped food particles were the cause.

It is common for dentists to recommend cold packing to reduce swelling after dental work. I recommend hot packing because I consider swelling less important than infection or pain, especially if you are not on an antibiotic.

Antibiotics are too unreliable for cancer patients, with one exception, heart disease. Here, *Staphylococcus* plays a major role, and antibiotics should always be added. Typically, however, you can look forward to your jaw healing stronger than ever, a boost of health, and no antibiotics or side effects!

Dental Aftercare, Heal The Jaw

To heal your jaw bone after dental work you need extra **calcium**, **magnesium** and **vitamin D**. Because most supplements are highly processed, and therefore contain trace amounts of solvents and heavy metals, it is wiser to use the food nature intended for growing bones. Namely baby food. Mother Nature provides milk for this purpose. Goats' milk or cows' milk has the extra calcium (one gram per quart) you now need. But milk can not be consumed as it arrives from the grocery store. Many harmful bacteria ride along from the dairy barn, through the milk tanks and into your milk container. *Salmonellas* and *Shigellas* are two very harmful bacteria <u>always</u> found in every milk sample I test. *Clostridium* and *Rhizobium* are other common types. Besides bacteria, one can find eggs of parasites, such as tapeworms and flukes in milk. And since cheese, yogurt, ice cream and butter are made from milk, they too are contaminated, in spite of pasteurization. Of course, you could test your dairy products with a Syncrometer to try to find a good one.

But there is a simple way to correct this sanitation problem. Boil the milk with a pinch of salt. Ten seconds is minimum. This would not be long enough for some exceptionally hardy bacteria, but it is enough to kill the tapeworm cysts and bacteria varieties I commonly detect. The salt raises the boiling temperature just enough to kill *Rhizobium leguminosarum*, too, which is extra hardy.

Milk also has traces of malonic acid, a strong metabolic inhibitor, and boiling does not detoxify it. It must be detoxified with a small amount of vitamin C powder, 1/8 tsp. per pint. This could curdle some milk, so an equal amount of baking soda may be added first. These treatments actually improve the flavor.

Persons with anemia should buy raw milk in order to obtain the factor, *lactoferrin*. Raw goat milk is best because it has some of the same factors as shark cartilage in addition to lactoferrin. It must still be boiled. (More on lactoferrin and treating milk under Clean Up Your Diet, page 116.)

Besides milk, canned salmon or other fish also have extra calcium you need to heal dental work. It is in the bones. There are numerous tiny bones, too small to see or taste throughout fish.

So, to upgrade your dental health, begin by increasing your calcium intake with milk and fish. You need one to two grams of calcium (elemental) per day. One quart of milk has one gram. For canned fish, read the label. Make up any deficit with a safe calcium supplement (see *Sources*).

Get the extra **magnesium** you need from leafy green vegetables plus a supplement (magnesium oxide, 300 mg daily). Eat a green vegetable every day, during and after dental work. You may need to blend it in a blender until your dentures or partials are ready.

There are three hazards with eating greens: pesticides, *Ascaris* eggs and sprays. If you are not sure whether pesticides have been used, then only buy Swiss chard, cabbage, collards (large leafed greens) that can be easily washed. Eat them every day or make coleslaw or raw salad.

To kill *Ascaris* eggs and any other live parasite stuck to the greens, you must briefly soak the greens in iodine-water. One drop of Lugol's iodine in one quart of water is strong enough to kill on contact. If you leave this out you will have wasted the Mop Up parasite program. (It would be better not to eat greens!) All the lettuce, cabbage, and strawberries I tested had live *Ascaris* eggs, even after washing. Evidently, the fertilizer used on these crops is raw manure! <u>A one minute soak in Lugol's kills everything</u>.

If you see spray nozzles in the produce section, you must detoxify any benzene that may be present with ozone. Rinse your greens and put them in a plastic bag. Insert the air hose from your ozonator. After 20 minutes the benzene is changed to phenol. To get rid of the phenol, soak the greens for five minutes in a bowl of water with a pinch of baking soda added.

The extra **vitamin D** you need can be made by your own kidneys! The very dental work you are doing helps the kidneys make it. The kidney cleanse (page 591) also helps. Commercial supplies are too polluted to risk. The recipe on page 602 is safe.

Dental Aftercare Summary

You are hot-packing, hot-swishing, and water picking many times a day. You are flossing and brushing your remaining teeth with white iodine or colloidal silver.

You are taking Lugol's, colloidal silver, inositol, betaine HCl, baker's yeast, and garlic or germanium.

You now have the extra calcium, magnesium and vitamin D you need to heal your jaw bone.

You will return to take out stitches <u>on time</u>, as your oral surgeon advises. If bleeding and pain do not stop by the third day, you will return to your doctor <u>before</u> your stitch-removal appointment day.

The M-Family

As if avoiding metal were not enough, we must also avoid toxic plastic. The toxins I am referring to I call the "M-Family" and consist of **malonic acid** (also called **malonate**), **methyl malonic acid, maleic acid, maleic anhydride**, and **D-malic acid**. Malonic acid is widely used in organic chemical manufacturing[30] and most dental plastics test positive to it, too, making it a common pollutant. Maleic acid is a component of some bonding agents[31] (meant for bonding the plastic to the tooth). You could be jumping from the frying pan into the fire if you trade your amalgams for plastic that contains malonic acid or any one of the M-family.

Malonic acid also occurs in certain foods, see page 120.

Malonic and maleic acids, seeping from composites, glass ionomer or porcelain teeth, soon reach the tumor where metabolism is then slowed down, and *glutathione* is used up in order to detoxify them. Glutathione is critical, because without it bacteria and viruses grow unchecked in your cells, making you sick. (The M-Family has many other bad effects, too. See page 116.)

Wherever I observed any of the M-Family to be present, glutathione was absent. And where all of the M-Family was absent, glutathione was present (provided heavy metals were absent, too). Evidently, glutathione sacrifices itself to detoxify the M-Family.

To spare glutathione, your body has other detoxification mechanisms. Using vitamins and minerals, your body detoxifies malonic acid by converting it to methyl malonate. Then methyl

---

[30] Common malonic acid reactions are described in many college texts including *Introduction to Organic Chemistry* by Fieser and Fieser or *Chemistry of Organic Compounds* by Carl Noller.

[31] *Skinner's Science Of Dental Materials 9th ed.*, Ralph W. Phillips, M.S., D.Sc., W.B. Saunders Company, 1991, p 240.

malonate to maleic acid. Then maleic to maleic anhydride. And maleic anhydride to D-malic acid. That is why I call them a "family," and there are more family members I haven't researched yet.

Only dental materials known to be free of the entire M-Family as well as copper, cobalt, vanadium, urethane,[32] and scarlet red dye, are safe in your mouth. Having something in your mouth has the same effect as sucking on it constantly. Things like that should be as safe as food.

How would you know which dental materials are free of these? Don't expect your dentist to understand this problem. You can test electronically for them, like I do (page 453, and Lesson 2 in particular), or use only the materials that I have found to be reliably safe, listed in the previous table.

One Step At A Time

As stated above, if you have a mouth full of metal or plastic and are ill with cancer, get it all removed. Extract teeth with large fillings. Don't put back <u>anything</u>. You will have holes and gaps in your teeth. But those holes could save your life!

It's hard to believe, but removing a dab of plastic or tiny speck of amalgam can mean the difference between getting well again or sinking.

---

[32] Urethane was researched decades ago and found to be a particularly potent carcinogen. Hundreds of research reports on urethane reside in the biology libraries of our universities. If you wish to research this, you could begin with: *The Carcinogenic Action and Metabolism of Urethane and N-Hydroxyurethane*, Sidney S. Mirvish, Advan. Cancer Res., 11, 1-42 (1968)

After removing everything, get a new panoramic X-ray. Search the X-ray for tattoos and plastic <u>again</u> using a hand magnifier. Tattoos appear as tiny specks of light. Some specks are merely artifacts from dust on the cartridge. Plastic is hard to identify. Your dentist can tell the difference. These are very important findings.

After searching the new X-rays, also have your mouth searched by a dentist who uses a magnifier. I have seen that a meticulous <u>visual</u> search for leftover bits of metal or plastic can reveal some that were <u>missed</u> on X-ray and change a deteriorating trend to recovery. Just one bit!

Always keep your final X-rays. Your earlier ones are obsolete, of course. If your dentist refuses to give them to you, offer to pay to have a copy made. You might want to take your copy to another dentist to study. Even <u>several</u> dentists could miss something important on your X-rays. This is not the dentists' fault. X-rays are an inadequate tool in many ways.

Choose a dentist who uses **air abrasion technology** for the final cleanup of leftover traces of amalgam and plastic. Don't refill the holes. Only after you are well and have regained strength and weight should you begin to plan your restorations.

If you are extremely ill,

and have little time left, but have only a few natural untouched teeth, extract <u>all</u> your teeth. Don't bother with X-rays, removing fillings, or finding safe materials. Get general anesthesia to minimize the trauma. Don't try to "save" those few good teeth because you risk your life missing just one unsuspected filling. Dentures are much safer than fillings, and a complete set fits better than partials. (Get fitted for dentures before the extractions.)

Follow the Dental Aftercare program diligently. You will notice an immediate improvement in appetite and blood building ability. The stress of the surgery is negligible compared to the benefit of removing the toxicity.

Unfilled cavities in remaining teeth require you to keep your mouth perfectly sanitary. Sterilize them before going to bed by putting one drop of straight Lugol's or white iodine on each "open" tooth and then brushing it around. If you are worried about staining, use white iodine although it is only half as strong as Lugol's. Open teeth treated this way are surprisingly resistant to infection. Rubbing baking soda on Lugol's-stained teeth removes stain. Alternatively, you may brush with colloidal silver (five drops on toothbrush).

Don't chew at an extraction site; drink as much of your food as possible (blend it). Rinse your mouth after eating <u>anything</u>. Before going to bed inspect your mouth for bits of food that got lodged. Flush them out with a water pick.

If you feel yourself getting better, don't rush to put back some kind of filling. Wait until you have maximized your improvements, at least six weeks. Get used to how this feels, so you can judge if your new fillings will harm you. Keep notes so you can be objective. Get a new complete blood test so your doctor can assess your overall health improvement.

When going to the dentist to get teeth filled, beware of the plastic "strips." These are just strips of plastic the dentist places between your teeth to keep the goop and chemicals off neighboring teeth. They also give a smooth finish to your filling. But, commercial strips I tested were polluted with cobalt, copper, vanadium and the M-family! Perhaps they were dipped into a chemical solution to make them spot-free. These toxins <u>do</u> wash off. You could use the dentist's supply of strips if you took

111

them to the washroom, washed them under the cold faucet and dried them. Don't neglect this detail.

Because there are no safe plastic restorations at present, your cavities are best refilled with a temporary material, zinc oxide and eugenol (ZOE) cement. It is safe to use pure calcium hydroxide $Ca(OH)_2$ solu-

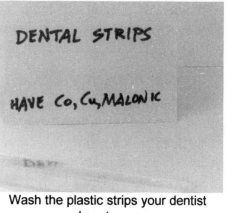

Wash the plastic strips your dentist plans to use.

Fig. 36 Dental strips

tion in the raw cavity first. It is painted over the nerve and the open ends of the dentine; it seals the cavity.

Don't be surprised or annoyed if a zinc oxide filling drops out. It wasn't meant to hold up to great pressure. Just have another one put in. At least the hole doesn't have to be made larger and no anesthetic is needed. Your dentist will soon master the new (in reality, old) skill.

If your dentist wishes to use additional substances like phosphoric acid or calcium phosphate, they should be ordered only from chemical supply companies (see *Sources*), dental sources are too polluted. But so far, I have not found pollutants in zinc oxide, eugenol, zinc phosphate or methyl methacrylate ordered from dental supply companies. If there is no way to test the supplies, stick with chemical supply companies.

If you have a Syncrometer, there is a way to test your present plastic teeth to see if they really do contain copper, cobalt, vanadium, the M-family, urethane, bisphenol-A, or scarlet red dye. You simply get emery boards used for filing nails. Then brush your teeth with plain water first. File one of your teeth, straight across the top and on the side. File hard. Then break the tip of the emery board where the filing marks are and place it in a reclosable plastic bag. Add a tsp. of filtered tap water. Test for these toxins electronically using pure standards (like Lesson Seven in *How To Test Yourself*). Do these tests in triplicate; that is, make three emery board samples of each tooth to be sure you are correct in identifying "bad" teeth. Don't be surprised to find all of them bad. Dentists regularly put a dab of plastic here and a dab there, just to "fix them up" as an extra favor to you while other work is being done. The toxins from all bad plastic are accumulating in your thyroid, liver, spleen, tumor, and bone marrow. You cannot tolerate these little "beautifications." Fortunately, air abrasion with baking soda removes it all in seconds.

Naturally, you would not deliberately <u>eat</u> malonate-containing food when you are going to a great deal of trouble to clean it out of your teeth. Which foods are good are shown on page 117.

Dental Rewards

After your mouth is free of metal and toxic plastic, notice whether your sinus condition, ear-ringing, enlarged neck glands, headache, enlarged spleen, bloated condition, knee pain, foot pain, hip pain, dizziness, aching bones and joints improve.

Keep a small notebook to write down these improvements. It will show you which symptoms came originally from your teeth. Symptoms can come back! So go back to your dentist, to search for a hidden infection under one or more of your teeth, or <u>where your teeth once were</u>! That infection can be the cause of tinnitus, TMJ (Temporal Mandibular Joint), arthritis, neck pain, loss of balance, and heart attacks! Most importantly, these tooth bacteria easily find their way to your tumor. Pull infected or dead teeth. Do not try to save them.

Dentures can be beautiful. Of course, methacrylate plastic isn't natural, but it is the best compromise that can be made to restore your mouth. At least it isn't positively charged like metals; it can't set up an electric current nor a magnetic field in your mouth, nor cause tumors to grow.

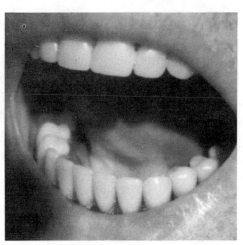

Which are plastic teeth? Ans. pg. 116
Fig. 37 Beautiful plastic mouth.

Do not be swayed by arguments that "noble" metals like gold and platinum and silver are OK, that they are "inert" and do not tarnish or seep. Nothing could be more untrue. **Everything tarnishes and everything seeps.** You may be keeping them glossy by the constant polishing action of your toothpaste. But if you look at the underside of metal crowns, the view is frightful. Your mouth is quite corrosive! You wouldn't expect a handful of metal, even noble metal, that was dropped in a well 50 years ago, to be intact. As it corrodes your body absorbs it!

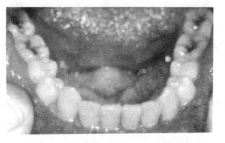

Fig. 38 Ugly metal in mouth.

In breast cancer, especially, you find that metals from dentalware have dissolved and accumulated in the breast. They will leave the breast if you clear them out of your mouth (and diet, body, home). **The cysts will not shrink until the metal is gone.**

Getting well is the magic you can expect from removing unnatural chemicals. To do this for your mouth, get started immediately, since your dentist may need more than one day to complete it. Get started the day you read this book! Don't wait until the parasite program is completed.

You now have accomplished 5 things:

1. You have killed the intestinal fluke, and all of its stages, and cured the cancer.
2. You have killed all your other parasites, done the Mop Up program, and have yourself on a maintenance program to keep killing them. Your pet has been loaned to a friend.
3. You have gotten rid of all isopropyl alcohol sources.
4. You are attacking the causes of tumors.
5. You have started getting well by cleaning up your dental-ware and eliminating bacteria, especially *Clostridium*. You have also partially eliminated copper, cobalt, vanadium, malonic acid, urethane, and scarlet red dye. You are measuring your progress against a list of all your symptoms.

One final tip: many dentists are now offering intravenous (IV) treatments. <u>Do not accept them</u> unless you can test the IV injectable and the IV bag for isopropyl alcohol and bacteria. <u>Over half</u> of the injectables and about a tenth of the IV bags I have tested (over 1,000) are polluted! The injectables are bottles of vitamins or ampoules of various health factors. These are injected into the IV bag, which contains either salt (saline) or blood sugar (dextrose). Then it is injected into you. The effect of any pollutant is much greater when it is injected than if taken by mouth. You are <u>mainlining</u>!

The injectables and IV bags are manufactured using the same antiseptics used for foods. Bottles and tubing are sterilized with isopropyl alcohol and not necessarily rinsed! Pumps that fill bottles and bags are greased with food lube containing benzene. I often find wood alcohol and heavy metals, too. Some injectables have live bacteria in them, most often the albumin and vitamin C. Persons who "get a reaction" to their IV are reacting to *Salmonella* or *E.coli*, not some mysterious "allergens." Of course, the bottles state "Do not use if contents are cloudy"—but should one ever expect bacteria?

2. Clean Up Your Diet

This is the easiest part of your get-well program because YOU are completely in charge.

The fundamental rule is:

EAT CHEMICAL-FREE AND MALONATE-FREE FOOD.

Why Is Malonic Acid Bad?

Malonic acid is not natural for humans; nothing in the scientific literature indicates that it is a metabolite. It <u>is</u> natural for plants. Certain plants, about 24 families of them, make malonic acid as a step in making their oils! Higher plants pack their seeds with a little oil; some, like the avocado plant, make a lot of oil. But <u>animals</u> only make *malonyl Coenzyme* A (a relative

---

*Answer: all of them.

of malonic acid). There is never any <u>free</u> malonic acid in healthy animals.

There is a very important reason for never having free malonic acid in our bodies anywhere. Malonic acid is an extremely potent metabolic inhibitor. In whatever organ it is found, your metabolism is slowed down. In fact it almost grinds to a halt. Then this organ can't use as much oxygen, nor make as much energy (body energy is called **ATP**) as it should. Consequently we make fewer amino acids and can't make as much protein as we should. This leads to lowered immunity by reducing glutathione. The organ is extremely handicapped. There is even a direct effect of malonate on immunity.[33]

Although the malonate forming food plants have other fine properties and are otherwise nutritious, the presence of malonate puts them off limits to anyone trying to improve their health. Fortunately, plants <u>without</u> malonates are in the majority!

Malonate-Free Foods

Here is the malonate-free food list; stick to it; do not eat foods that are not listed. The fastest way to recover the health of the tumorous organ, or any other organ, is to stop poisoning it with malonic acid. You may notice the difference in a few days.

There is an extra benefit for persons who switch to a malonate-free diet. You may notice a higher body temperature after a few weeks, which brings with it a rosier complexion. Overweight persons may experience a slow, steady weight loss!

---

[33] *The Effect of Malonate on Salmonella typhimurium Infection in Mice*, Berry, L. Joe and Mitchell, Roland B., Science, Vol. 118, p 140 (1953)

Eat Only These

Remember, that a food may be malonate-free and still not be good for you for other reasons. Remember, too, that this is a <u>plant</u> list, since animals do not make it. But milk is an exception; it has traces. So dairy foods are listed as safe, but only with special treatment.

acorn squash (with peel)
allspice
almonds (including brown skin)
aloe vera
amaranth
apples (red delicious, golden delicious, green)
apricot kernels
artichokes
avocados
bananas
banana squash (without peel)
bean sprouts
beans, adzuki
beans, pinto
bee pollen
beet tops
beets, red
bell peppers (red, green)
black pepper
black-eyed peas
blueberries
bok choy
brazil nuts
brewers' yeast
Brussels sprouts
buckwheat
butter (add salt, boil, add vitamin C)
butternut squash (without peel)
cabbage (purple, white)
cactus (nopalitos)
cantaloupe (and seeds)

capers
cardamom
carob powder
cauliflower
cayenne pepper
chayote squash (with peel)
cheese (add salt, boil, add vit. C)
cherries (Bing)
chili peppers (California, jalapeno, pasilla, serrano, yellow)
chili peppers - red (dried)
cilantro
cinnamon
currants
coconut (without the milk)
collards
corn (yellow & white)
cornmeal
cranberries
cream (add salt, boil, add vitamin C)
cucumbers
cumin
dairy products (add salt, boil, add vitamin C)
dandelion (greens)
dill (fresh)
dulse (sea vegetable)
eggplant
eggs (wash, do not store in original carton)
extract of wintergreen
eyebright herb (dried)

fenugreek
figs (dried)
flax seed
flour (unbleached white)
garbanzo beans
garlic cloves
ginger capsules
ginger root (inside only)
goldenseal
grains and legumes from India (see Sources), chana dal, split urad chilka, split moong chilka, whole urad, moth, whole moong USA green with skins, masoor, chori, kabu fee chana, whole val, moong zib, whole moong dal, toor dal, yellow peas, split val, oily toor (the dals are legume-like)
grapefruits
grapes (green, red & purple)
green bean thread
green beans
green olives (in jar)
grits
hazel nuts
hominy (white canned)
jicama
kale
Kamut (grain)
kiwi
kumquats
leeks
lemon grass tea
lemons
lentils
lettuce (iceberg, green leaf and red leaf)
loquats
maple flavoring
maple syrup
masala (spice)
millet
mint leaves
miso (sweet)
mullein flowers

mushrooms (common white)
nectarines
nutmeg
oats
olive leaves (for tea, see Sources)
onions (white, yellow, green)
paprika
parsley
Pau d'Arco
peaches
peanut butter
peanuts (without red skin)
pears (Bartlett, Bosc)
peas (green)
peas (split green)
peas, black-eyed
peas, green (in shell)
peas, snow
peppermint
pimentos
pineapple
plums (red and blue)
pomegranate
potatoes (russet, red, sweet)
psyllium seed husks
pumpkin
pumpkin seeds
quassia
quinoa
radishes (red)
raspberries
rhubarb
rice (white, cooked in pressure cooker)
salsa picante hot sauce
sesame seed
shave grass
soy lecithin
soybean (whole)
spearmint (dried)
spinach
strawberries
sunflower seeds
sweet basil
Swiss chard

tahini	watermelon (ripe inside portion only,
tapioca (pearl)	including seed)
thyme	wheat berries, flour
tomatillo	yellow split peas
turnip greens	zucchini squash (yellow, pale green,
Uva Ursi capsules	mottled, with peel)
walnuts	zucchini squash blossoms

The presence of malonic acid in plants was reported as early as 1925.[34] Yet, it has never been suspected that we are eating it daily in significant amounts! Here are some popular foods that contain it.

Foods That Contain Malonic Acid

Be aware that in <u>packaged</u> foods, the processing could contribute the malonic acid.

alfalfa sprouts	green zucchini (dark)
apricots	Kombo (seaweed)
araica (dried)	limes
beans (black)	mangos (large, small yellow)
beans (great northern)	Nori sea weed, packaged
beans (lima)	onions (purple)
beans (mung)	oranges, all kinds
beans (navy)	papaya (Mexican)
beans (red kidney)	parsnips
black olives (canned)	passion fruit
broccoli	persimmons (Fuji, regular)
butternut squash peel	radish (daikon)
carrots	red skin of peanuts
chaparral (dried)	Tamari soy sauce
chocolate	tomatoes
ginger root skin	turnips, rutabaga
grape jam, commercial	wheat grass

---

[34] Turner, W.A., and Hartman, A.M., J. Amer. Chem. Soc., 47, 2044 (1925)

Note: these lists were made using the Syncrometer. I have not found any similar lists in the scientific literature. A short list published in 1952 only tested leaves.[35] But the parts you eat are often roots. So when I discovered malonic acid in <u>carrots</u> (root portion) I was so unhappy I searched to find a confirming study. It was reported as early as 1964.[36] Malonic acid in fruit juices, including orange juice, was also reported in various scientific articles.

What happens to malonic acid that you eat? It must either be used by the body (metabolized), detoxified, excreted, or left alone to create havoc!

Toxic Effects Of Malonic Acid

The need to detoxify any free malonic acid quickly is obvious when you read the effects it has.

A lengthy and excellent review of malonate research has been published in <u>Enzyme And Metabolic Inhibitors</u>.[37] Here is a partial list of topics reviewed.

◊   Malonate inhibits uptake of glycine and alanine.
◊   Malonate may chelate iron so it can't be incorporated into hemoglobin.
◊   Malonate inhibits healing.
◊   Motility of sperm is reduced by malonate.

---

[35] Bently, L.E., *Occurrence of Malonic Acid in Plants*, Nature 170: 847-848 (1952)

[36] Harmon M. Kellogg, E. Brochmann-Hanssen and A. Baerheim Svendsen, *Gas Chromatography of Esters of Plant Acids and Their Identification in Plant Materials*, J. of Pharmaceutical Sciences 53: 420-423 (1964).

[37] *Enzyme And Metabolic Inhibitors, Vol. II*, by J. Leyden Webb, Academic Press, NY, 1966, pp. 1-244. This book can be found in most university libraries.

◊ Bacterial phagocytosis by human neutrophils is depressed by malonate.

◊ Malonate chelates calcium.

◊ Malonate drops the resting potential of muscle.

◊ Malonate causes air hunger (dyspnea).

◊ Methyl malonate is toxic to the kidney.

◊ Acetoacetyl Co A can transfer its Co A to malonic acid to make malonyl Co A. This could lead to acetoacetate buildup, namely ketonuria and possibly a block in fat utilization of even numbered carbon atoms, leaving odd numbered carbons to predominate.

◊ Malonic acid reacts with aldehydes.

◊ Thallium is chelated by malonic acid into a stable compound. (This could explain accumulation effect in a tumor.)

◊ A color test for malonates is tetra hydroquinoline-N-propinal to form blue-violet compounds. It is sensitive to 0.01 mg malonate.

◊ Malonate complexes with zinc and magnesium, thereby depleting them.

◊ A fall in malate concentration due to malonate causes depletion of NADP.

◊ Malonate induces ketonemia.

◊ Malonate reduces oxygen uptake. Coenzyme Q10 is required to make ATP.

◊ Malonate raises cholesterol.

◊ D-malic acid complexes with malic dehydrogenase and NADH, but is enzymatically inactive.

◊ Maleic acid is competitive inhibitor of succinic dehydrogenase.

◊ Synergism between rotenone and malonate occurs in mitochondria.

◊ Malonate causes oxidation of NADH and cytochromes.

◊ Rats can convert malonate to acetate in the presence of malonyl Co A.

◊ Malonate reduces survival of infected animals.

◊ Malonate fed to dogs is recovered as methyl malonate in urine.

◊ Malonate can pick up an amino group from glutamine, thereby destroying it.

◊ Hemolysis of red blood cells may be caused by malonyldialhyde (MDA), a derivative of malonic acid.

◊ Malonate catalyses renal glutaminase; with less glutamine, uric acid levels fall.

◊ Malic acid (apple juice) may be an antidote to malonic acid. (But commercial sources contain patulin which depletes cellular glutathione.)

◊ Malonic acid is present in urine.

◊ Malonate depresses the reduction of GSSG to glutathione.

◊ Malonate inhibits protoporphyrin formation 32%.

◊ Malonate inhibits insulin stimulation of muscle respiration.

◊ Malonate inhibits acetylcholine synthesis.

◊ *Mycobacterium phlei* respiration is stimulated by malonate. (All schizophrenia cases I see test positive to this bacterium in the brain!)

◊ Malonate is put into soy sauce in Japan.

◊ Malonate stimulates *Entamoeba histolytica* growth.

◊ Malonate inhibits phosphate entry into cells.

◊ Potassium transport into cells is inhibited by malonate.

◊ Malonate causes systemic acidosis.

◊ Calcium and iron transport by rat duodenum is severely reduced by malonate.

◊ Malonate inhibits pyruvate oxidation.

◊ Malonate causes increased utilization of glucose due to the Pasteur effect of a blocked Krebs cycle.

◊ Lactic acid formation is increased with malonate inhibition of respiration.

◊ Glycolysis is stimulated by malonate.

◊ Malonate has different effects on different tissues.

◊ Much less glucose goes to form amino acids and proteins in the presence of malonate.

◊ Malonate induces the appearance of the pentose phosphate shunt. (This is the pathway to nucleic acid formation.)

◊ Malonate diverts fatty acid metabolism to acetoacetate.

◊ Malonate increases the formation of fatty acids up to 10-fold.

◊ Maleic acid is a potent inhibitor of urinary acidification.

◊ Malonate inhibits oxidation of fatty acids.

◊ Malonate fed to dogs produces acetoacetate, acetone and alcohol.
◊ Malonate can reduce the concentration of magnesium and calcium to 25% or 50%.
◊ The methyl derivative of malonate depresses renal function.
◊ Malonic acid can form malonyl coenzyme A, which is very stable, thereby depleting the system of coenzyme A. (Coenzyme A has a nucleic acid base, adenine, plus pantothenic acid and sulfur in its makeup. You will have an increased need for these nutrients.)
◊ Malonate inhibits urea formation by reducing the supply of oxalacetate.
◊ Malonate inhibits cell cleavage (the formation of a wall between 2 dividing cells; multinucleate cells are the hallmark of cancer).
◊ Benzaldehyde reacts with malonic acid.

It's no wonder that the body tries frantically to detoxify malonic acid that reaches the tumorous organ, or any other part of the body.

Detoxifying Malonate

One way the body detoxifies unwelcome substances is called *methylation*. But it is costly to the body's resources, requiring large amounts of vitamin B_{12}, folic acid, methionine, betaine, glycine, taurine, cysteine, lecithin, and vitamin C. Keeping up the supply means depleting the rest of the body.

Not only the organ under siege, but the rest of the body is becoming very malnourished.

The actual amounts of vitamins needed to replenish your body will be given in the section on supplements. What is needed most is to stop stealing these nutrient factors from your body just to detoxify malonic acid.

With your new malonate-free food list in hand, you are ready to shop for breakfast supplies.

Breakfast

Cook your cereal from scratch. Don't eat cold cereal; it has numerous solvents and added chemicals. Even the hot cereals can be polluted with mercury and thallium from the cardboard box. Evidently it was contaminated or sterilized with mercury compounds, and mercury products bring with them thallium pollution. Select a cereal that you have tested or see pictured. Cook it with milk to add nutritive value. Add salt while cooking in order to reach a higher temperature that will kill *Rhizobium leguminosarum*. Later add vitamin C; not so much that it spoils the flavor.

Make granola from a recipe, there are three in this book (page 551). Use honey or confectioner's sugar. Add raisins that aren't sulfited and cook them with the cereal to kill mold. Don't use nuts; they carry aflatoxins. Use whipping cream or half and half if you need to gain weight. These are very easy to boil and de-malonate with vitamin C. Isn't this a delicious way to start your day! Use ground cinnamon to flavor, or frozen fruit and honey.

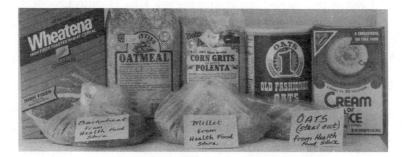

Fig. 39 Unpolluted breakfast cereals

> The biggest obstacle to eating natural food is time. Find a friend who has the time to cook for you, if you are not up to it.

Or start your day with fried potatoes and an egg and glass of milk. Don't worry about cholesterol while you are recovering.

Eat the simplest dairy products you can find, not flavored milk, not whipped butter, not cream cheese, not kefir. Choose milk and butter without coloring added. **Always sterilize the milk, first** (page 135) and later, after cooling, add vitamin C. Try to find raw certified milk at a health food store. It has a special blood building factor in it, called *lactoferrin*. Cooking does not destroy it but–and I can't explain this–pasteurized varieties do not contain it. If you could find goat milk, you would also get some of the same rare and valuable factors that are found in shark cartilage. But these factors are damaged by heating, so count the ten seconds for boiling carefully. Milk should be 2% or more butterfat because the calcium in milk cannot be absorbed without at least this much fat. Eat homemade yogurt and add honey or homemade preserves yourself. You need 3 cups of a milk product each day. If you don't tolerate milk, and get diarrhea from it, try a milk digestant tablet to go with it, or cook your milk into your foods. Start with only ¼ cup at a time. Do not choose chocolate milk.

Cheese can be used in baked dishes with vitamin C added.

Butter can be treated like milk (boiled ten seconds, then add vitamin C).

Yogurt is not easily boiled, but it can safely be made from boiled milk.

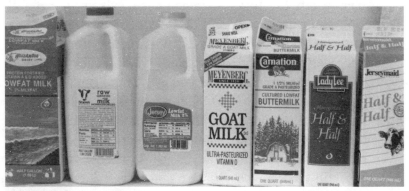

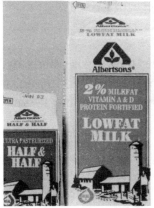

Most dairy products found in supermarkets or natural food stores were polluted with copper, cobalt, vanadium, urethane, tartrazine,[38] and scarlet red dye. Those pictured were free of them. Of course, they must still be boiled and vitamin C-ed. Unless the chemicals used in processing milk are carefully evaluated for purity, such widespread pollution cannot be stopped. Test your local varieties with a Syncrometer.

Fig. 40 Good dairy products

No food is perfect.

You don't have to be perfect in your food selection to get well.

---

[38] Also known as FD and C Yellow #5 or Acid Yellow 23, a food dye.

It can be difficult to know which chemicals are unnatural. This book can't go into a long discussion of different definitions of "natural" and "unnatural." What counts for a cancer patient is whether the immune system will be called upon to remove something from the food you eat. Your immune system is precious. You have (or had) 5000 white blood cells in every little dot of blood.[39] They have the job of keeping you clear of parasites, bacteria, viruses, fungi, and unnatural chemicals. Even if the unnatural chemicals you eat do not do great harm, they must still be <u>removed</u>. White blood cells that are busy removing aluminum, nickel, mercury, copper, flavors, fragrance, or even soap are not free to fight bacteria, viruses, parasites, and fungi.

Give your immune system a chance to heal your body by removing the burden on it: the burden of countless, frivolous cleaning-up jobs. Clean yourself up so your immune system does not have to.

Lunch

Cook your food from scratch. Don't start with cans or packages or frozen items to make some recipe. In fact, don't bother with <u>any</u> fancy recipes. Just cook two or three vegetables for lunch and eat them with butter[40] and salt (use pure salt, see *Sources*). Bread and milk rounds it out, plus fruit. Soup is a nice change. Cook it with all the vegetables you can find that don't have malonate. Don't start with a packet or cube. Use a bit of onion and genuine herbs to give it zest.

---

[39] 5000 white blood cells per cubic millimeter.

[40] Butter is our only source of butyric acid in the intestine. There is some evidence that butyric acid favors beneficial bacteria in the intestine! Butyric acid has been advanced as a cancer therapy; perhaps it intervenes in isopropyl alcohol's biochemical reactions!

If all this is too much work, select the easiest to prepare items from the menu given (see page 561) and have that with bread and yogurt or milk.

Never try to lower your cholesterol while regaining your health from cancer.

This is a rule based on common sense. Synthetic eggs, margarine and cholesterol-reduced products are extremely "chemical" foods.

Bake your own bread! I found aflatoxins in commercial bread after just four days in my refrigerator, but none in homemade bread stored in a paper bag even after two weeks! Aflatoxin is extremely toxic; it is made by mold. **Zearalenone** is another very toxic substance found on grains and produced by mold. In fact, zearalenone is the toxin that keeps the liver from clearing benzene from your body! Bread goes moldy easily. Don't <u>ever</u> eat moldy food, whether it is fruit, breads or leftovers in the refrigerator. Throw them out. <u>Buy a bread maker</u>. It can do everything, including baking the bread. Use unbleached (unbrominated) flour; I never found aflatoxin or zearalenone in packaged flour. And add ½ tsp. vitamin C powder per loaf to help retard mold further. (It also helps the bread rise!)

Do not toast your bread! This makes 4,5 benzopyrene which inhibits benzene detoxification. Pan fry in butter to toast.

One big advantage of making your own bread, ice cream, and beverages is that you avoid the commercial machinery that stirs, pumps, kneads, holds, and scoops it all. All machinery requires regular lubrication, and "food-safe" lubricants are well defined by US regulations. <u>They are petroleum products!</u> This is a sample regulation.

21 CFR 178.3570 (4-1-94 Edition) Lubricants with incidental food contact.

Lubricants with incidental food contact may be safely used on machinery used for producing, manufacturing, packing, processing, preparing, treating, packaging, transport, or holding food, subject to the provisions of this section:

(a) The lubricants are prepared from one or more of the following substances:

(1) Substances generally recognized as safe for use in food.

(2) Substances used in accordance with the provisions of a prior sanction or approval.

(3) Substances identified in this paragraph (a)(3).

Substance	Limitations
Here you find 39 chemicals like BHA, BHT, Polyethylene, 2-(8-Heptadecenyl)-4,5-dihydro-1H-imidazole-1-ethanol, and also including:	
Mineral oil	Addition to food not to exceed 10 parts per million.
Petrolatum	Complying with §178.3700. Addition to food not to exceed 10 parts per million.

(b) The lubricants are used on food-processing equipment as a protective antirust film, as a release agent on gaskets or seals of tank closures, and as a lubricant for machine parts and equipment in locations in which there is exposure of the lubricated part to food. The amount used is the minimum required to accomplish the desired technical effect on the equipment, and the addition to food of any constituent identified in this section does not exceed the limitations prescribed.

(c) Any substance employed in the production of the lubricants described in this section that is the subject of a regulation in parts 174, 175, 176, 177, 178, and §179.45 of this chapter conforms with any specification in such regulation.

Fig. 41 "Safe" lubricants that could be in your processed foods, but not on the label of the product

Notice the mineral oil and petrolatum which are petroleum oil products. How was it decided that they "may be safely used"? Safe for the machinery, but not for you. Petroleum

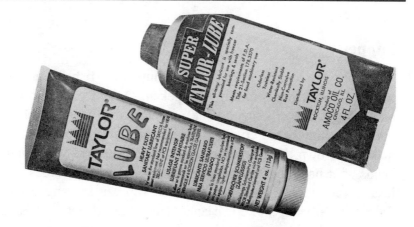

"Food lube" for heavy-duty machinery like ice cream and dough mixers and "food oil" for light-duty equipment like cheese and meat slicers are petroleum products that introduce benzene into our foods.

Fig. 42 Examples of commercial "food lube."

products should not be in our food, not even in minutest amounts. This is because there would always be tiny traces of benzene and other petrochemicals left in them. These are not negligible even though test instruments can't find them. Even our best test instruments are very crude compared to our body's ability to detect. Benzene is very difficult to detect, costing thousands of dollars for a single test. Manufacturers would resist such added expense. Yet, the cancer epidemic is upon us. We must demand new, more sensitive testing for toxins in our foods. Wouldn't it be wonderful if our lawmakers required only chemicals that didn't show up in our immune systems to be used in manufacturing foods. Lubricants would then be things like olive oil, beeswax and cornstarch. And under "Limitations" would be "none."

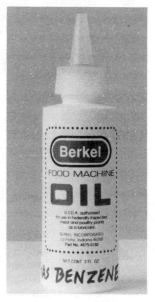

Fig. 43 Example of "food oil"

131

Supper

Cook your supper from scratch. Emphasize fish for animal food, not beef, pork, turkey or chicken. Do not grill, broil or barbecue (it makes benzopyrene); instead, fry, bake, poach or boil. Don't buy bread crumbs, use your own. Don't buy batter, make your own. Use genuine eggs, not substitutes. Wash your hands after handling raw eggs or meat. Cook real potatoes, not instant varieties. Always peel them so you can see any potato fungus underneath and cut it away (red skinned potatoes have less fungus). Make your own salad, not prepackaged or from a salad bar. Make salad dressing out of olive oil, lemon juice, white distilled vinegar (not apple cider vinegar which has afla-toxins) honey, salt, and herbs to flavor.

If your digestion isn't strong enough for raw vegetables or fruit, make juice. Get a sturdy juicer and make your juice from any vegetable that is malonate free. First dip for one minute in Lugol's iodine water. Avoid greens that have been sprayed in the grocery store to keep them fresh looking. Shop at small, lo-

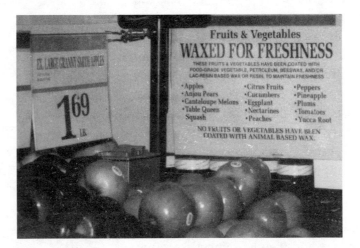

If the apples seem shinier than usual in your grocery store, inquire if they have been sprayed.

Fig. 44 Glossy produce

cal grocery shops that do not spray their produce. The spray contains petroleum products. Add herb seasoning. Make lemonade in the blender leaving it whole, but peeling it first with a sharp knife to remove the sprayed surface; then strain. Scrub the lemon carefully first, just with water. Lemon peel and seeds have **limonene**, useful for weight gain. But don't overdo it. Use only one lemon a day. Exact instructions are given in *Recipes*.

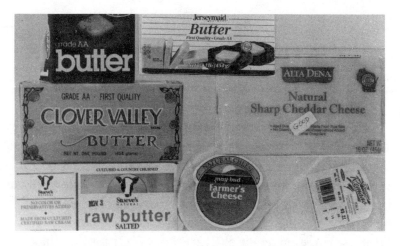

Find dairy products that do not list color as an ingredient—not even annatto seed. Evidently a company that uses both artificial and natural colors cannot keep them totally apart.

Fig. 45 Good butter and cheese

Make mashed potatoes from scratch—not box potatoes, nor chips nor French fries. Box potatoes have added chemicals. Chips and fries were made in chemical grease called "hydrogenated vegetable (or other) oil." There is a large amount of nickel in hydrogenated fats.[41] Fry your potatoes in butter, lard or olive oil. Find butter that is not wrapped in foil

---

[41] 114 mcg/100 g. Taken from *Food Values* 14ed by Pennington and Church 1985.

and is not salted.[42] Salt your own butter, using pure salt. Add salt to the butter while you're boiling it; this raises the temperature of boiling so the hardy bacteria, *Rhizobium leguminosarum*, are killed. Butter should not have color added. Even the annatto seed (a natural colorant) varieties tested positive on the Syncrometer to tartrazine (a yellow food dye), and scarlet red dye (a red food azo dye)! Do not eat dairy products that list color as an ingredient.

> # Eat no meat that hasn't been cooked as thoroughly as if it were pork.

Other animals are as parasitized as we, full of flukes and worms and *schistosomes* in every imaginable stage, and since the blood carries many of these, would we not be eating these live parasites if we eat these animals in the raw state? We have been taught to cook thoroughly any pork, fish or seafood. Now we must cook thoroughly any beef, chicken or turkey. It must be at cooking temperature (212°F or 100°C) for 20 minutes after salt has been added. Freezing is not adequate. Canned meats are safe from living parasites, but are not recommended due to added chemicals.

Of course, you are protecting yourself with a parasite killing maintenance program. But killing a parasite AFTER it is IN your tissues will not keep you healthy; you must avoid parasites.

---

[42] Salt has aluminum in it to keep it from caking. Test your salt for aluminum silicate. Or buy pure sodium chloride that laboratories use (see *Sources*).

If you have been very ill, the best advice is to be a "seafood vegetarian" eating fish, eggs and dairy products to supply you with protein.

Beverages

Drink 6 kinds of beverages:
- milk
- water
- herb teas
- malonate-free fruit juices
- malonate-free vegetable juices
- homemade (see *Recipes*)

This means getting off caffeine. And if you are already fatigued, this means you might be even more fatigued for a short time. You might have headaches from withdrawal, too. But they will only last 10 days. Mark your calendar and count off the days. Headache medicine, like all medicine, is likely to have benzene pollution from the colorant used; avoid it. For energy, to replace caffeine, take one arginine (500 mg) upon rising in the morning and before lunch. Soon you won't need it.

Cutting down on coffee, decaf, soda pop and powdered drinks won't do. You must be completely off. They contain very toxic solvents due to the processing.

Although grain (drinking) alcohol is the recommended antiseptic for household use, that doesn't mean you may safely drink it. It is inadvisable to drink any form of alcohol at least until you are fully recovered (two years). This is why black walnut hull tincture, which is 20-50% grain alcohol, is taken in a lukewarm beverage (to evaporate some of the alcohol) and followed by a dose of niacinamide.

1. **Milk**: 2%, in plastic container (paper containers tested positive to dioxane, which is a well studied carcinogen). Drink three 8 oz. glasses a day. Homemade yogurt is fine. Goat milk is better. Start with ¼ cup and increase

gradually, if you are not used to it. If you do not drink milk because it gives you more mucous, switch to a different kind. If you have other reactions, like diarrhea, try milk digestant tablets (available at health food stores). Milk is too valuable to avoid: there are many unwanted chemicals in most brands of milk, but it is solvent-free and very nutritious. The only exception should be for serious symptoms, like colitis, bloating, flu, or chronic diarrhea. Do not use powdered milk; it is heavily polluted with solvents. All milk should be sterilized, then cooled and vitamin C-ed.

Pasteurization is not sterilization.

Milk goes sour after the expiration date on the carton even when refrigerated and unopened. Although souring isn't caused by *Salmonella* or *Shigella* (other bacteria are responsible), my point is that it is obvious that milk isn't sterile.

Boil milk for 10 seconds with a pinch of salt to kill Salmonellas and Shigellas. It will also kill the tumor causing bacteria species, *Clostridium* and *Rhizobium*.[43] Then refrigerate. But what about the malonic acid in milk? You must do one more thing. Add vitamin C (1/8 tsp. per pint). If your taste buds detect this or you are afraid the milk might curdle, add baking soda first (again 1/8 tsp. per pint). If you are making yogurt, buttermilk or cottage cheese, you do not need baking soda. Treat butter and whipping cream the same way. Do not undercook or you will reinfect with parasites! Many people prefer the

---

[43] It only kills the *Clostridium* and *Rhizobium* varieties if salt is added when boiling because salt raises the boiling point.

taste of such "treated" milk. And many people can tolerate dairy products for the first time after making this change.

Of course, milk is not a plant food. How does malonic acid get into milk? I have preliminary evidence that tapeworm stages make malonic acid and killing these by boiling does nothing about the malonate already present. Perhaps the vegetable matter of the feed brings it into the milk, too. More research is needed here.

If you simply cannot tolerate dairy products, try making cottage cheese (see *Recipes*). Separate the curds and whey. Whey is a traditional, delicious beverage with all the calcium of milk in it.

There is no substitute for milk; calcium tablets are not satisfactory. Vegetable matter, although high in calcium, does not give you <u>available</u> calcium either. Eating fish can give you a lot of calcium, but it is in the tiny bones hidden in the fish. Don't try to remove them. Canned salmon has a lot of calcium. On a day that you eat fish, you would not need milk. Goats' milk is better for you than cows' milk because it has beneficial factors in it that are similar to shark cartilage and speeds up your ability to make amino acids. It needs to be boiled and vitamin C-ed, too. Dairy products are <u>too important</u> to your recovery to abandon. But cheese varieties are too difficult to sterilize; avoid unbaked cheese completely.

2. **Water**: 2 pints. Drink one pint upon rising in the morning, the other pint in the afternoon sometime. The cold water faucet may be bringing you cadmium, copper or lead, but it is safer than purchased water, which usually has solvents in it. Let it run before using it. Filters are rather useless because water pollution comes in surges. A single surge of PCB contaminates your filter. All the water you use after this surge is now polluted, so you will be getting it chronically, whereas the unfiltered

water cleans up again after the surge passes. Until you can test your own water for solvents, PCBs and metals, no expensive filter is worth the investment.[44]

An inexpensive carbon filter that is replaced <u>every month</u> may improve your tap water, though. Plastic pitchers fitted with a carbon filter pack are available. Never buy filters with silver or other chemicals, even if they are "just added to the carbon." If you have copper or galvanized pipes, switch to PVC to be safe from cadmium, copper and lead. (See the section on Cleaning up the Environment.)

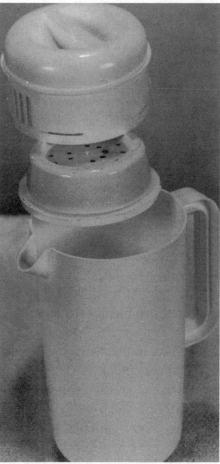

Fig. 46 Water pitcher with filter.

3. **Herb tea**: fresh or bulk packaged if available. If only tea bags are available, cut them open and dump out the tea. Throw away the bag, it is full of antiseptic. Buy a

---

[44] Even reverse osmosis water is polluted with thulium and ytterbium which must be coming from the filtration membrane.

non-metal (bamboo is common) tea strainer. Sweeten with confectioner's sugar or honey. Honey obtained from the bulk tank in a health food store never had solvent pollution when I tested it. Be careful <u>not</u> to buy foil packs of tea or <u>tea blends</u>. Tea blends are mixtures of herb teas; these have solvents in them from the extracts used to improve flavor!

4. **Fruit juice**: fresh squeezed only. Some stores make it while you wait. If they freeze some of it, you could purchase the frozen containers. Bottled fruit juices have traces of numerous solvents, as do the frozen concentrates, as do the refrigerated ones, <u>don't buy them</u>. You have to <u>see it being made</u>, but watch carefully: I recently went to a juice bar where they made everything fresh, before your very eyes. And I saw them take the fruit right from the refrigerator and spray it with a special wash "to get rid of any pesticides", then put a special detergent on it to clean off the wash! So instead of getting traces of pesticide, I got traces of isopropyl alcohol![45] More recently I stepped into a San Diego juice bar for a "smoothie." The banana that was going into it was half black, and I expected the black part to be cut off, but <u>the whole thing</u> was thrown in the blender! You can not <u>trust</u> commercially prepared food, even if it is a health food store or juice bar. Best of all, buy a juicer, peel the fruit and make your own juice (enough for a week—freeze it in half-pint used plastic bottles). Try pineapple, pear, peach, nectarine, cantaloupe, and grapefruit. For stronger flavor add a bit of fresh lemon to each variety to give it more zip.

---

[45] Yes, I took a sample of the wash to test.

5. **Vegetable juice**: Buy a juice-maker. Start with head lettuce and other broad-leafed greens. Fine-leafed greens cannot be washed free of spray and regularly test positive for benzene! If you cannot test for benzene, and are not sure if the greens have been sprayed, <u>ozonate</u> them.

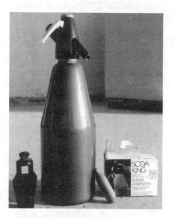

Jazz up your favorite homemade juice with seltzer water. It is not harmful to you.

Fig. 47 Seltzer maker

Wash greens and place in a plastic bag. Ozonate for 20 minutes. Rinse again in water with a pinch of baking soda and a drop of Lugol's iodine to kill *Ascaris* eggs. Drink ½ glass of vegetable juice a day. After you are accustomed to this, add other vegetables to double the amount. Use cabbage, cucumber, beet, pale zucchini, squash, anything malonate-free. <u>But never anything with soft spots!</u> And peel everything that has a peel. Add herbs and fruit for extra zest.

6. **Homemade beverage**. If you will miss your coffee or decaf, try just plain hot water with whipping cream or lemon. Sweeten with honey. See *Recipes* for many more suggestions.

Horrors In Commercial Beverages

Commercial beverages are especially toxic due to traces of solvents left over from the manufacturing process. There are solvents found in decaffeinated beverages, herb tea <u>blends</u>, carbonated drinks, beverages with artificial sweetener, <u>flavored</u> coffee, diet and health mixes, and fruit juices, even when the label states "not from concentrate" or "fresh from the orchard," or "100% pure."

Some of the solvents I have found are just too toxic to be believed! Yet you can build the test apparatus yourself (How To Test Yourself, page 453), buy foods at your grocery store, and tabulate your own results. I hope you do, and I hope you find that the food in your area is cleaner than mine! Remember that the Syncrometer™ described later can only determine the presence or absence of something, not the concentration. There may only be a few parts per billion, but a cancer patient trying to get well cannot afford any solvent intake. For that matter, none of us should tolerate any of these pollutants:

- **Acetone** – in carbonated drinks
- **Benzene** – in store-bought drinking water, store-bought "fresh squeezed" fruit juice
- **Carbon tetrachloride** – in store-bought drinking water
- **Decane** – in health foods and beverages
- **Hexanes** – in decafs
- **Hexane dione** – in flavored foods
- **Isophorone** – in flavored foods
- **Methyl butyl ketone** and **Methyl ethyl ketone** – in flavored foods
- **Methylene chloride** – in fruit juice
- **Pentane**– in decafs
- **Propyl alcohol** – bottled water, commercial fruit juices, commercial beverages.
- **Toluene** and **xylene** – in carbonated drinks
- **Trichloroethane**(TCE), **TCEthylene**– in flavored foods
- **Wood alcohol** (methanol) – in carbonated drinks, diet drinks, herb tea blends, store-bought water, infant formula.

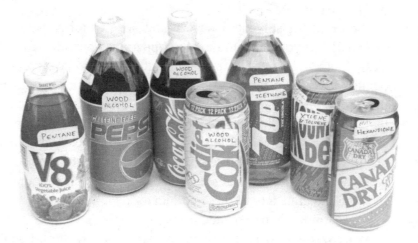

Fig. 48 Unsafe beverages

If you allowed a tiny drop of kerosene or carpet cleaning fluid to get into your pet's food every day, wouldn't you expect your pet to get sick? Why wouldn't <u>you</u> expect to be sick with these solvents in your daily food? These solvents are just tiny amounts, but tiny amounts are nevertheless <u>billions</u> of molecules! Your body must detoxify <u>each</u> molecule.

Flavors and colors for food must be extracted somehow from the leaves or bark or beans from which they come and I suspect benzene contaminated solvents are used for this. Until safe methods are invented, such food should be considered unsafe for human consumption (or pets or livestock!).

Food Preparation

Cook your food in glass, enamel, ceramic or microwavable pots and pans. Throw away all metal ware, foil wrap, and metal-capped salt shakers since you will never use them again.

If you don't plan to fry much (only once a week), you might keep the Teflon™ or Silverstone™ coated fry-pan, otherwise get an enamel coated metal pan. Stir and serve food with wood or plastic, not metal utensils. If you have recurring urinary tract infections, you should reduce your metal contact even further; eat with plastic cutlery. Sturdy decorative plastic ware can be found in hardware and camping stores. Don't drink out of styrofoam cups (styrene is toxic). Don't eat toast (many toasters spit tungsten all over your bread besides making benzopyrenes). Choose baked goods sold in paper or microwavable pans, not aluminum. Don't run your drinking water through the freezer, fountain, or refrigerator. Don't heat your water in a coffee maker or metal tea kettle; use a saucepan. Don't use a plastic thermos jug—the plastic liner has lanthanides, which break up your RNA and DNA molecules. The inside must be glass.

Why are we still using stainless steel cookware when it contains 18% chromium and 8% nickel? Because it is rustproof and shiny and we can't see any deterioration. **But all metal seeps!** Throw those metal pots away.

Many bacteria and yeast(!) varieties have a requirement for nickel so that their enzyme **urease** will work for them. Urease attacks urea, present in all our body juices, and makes ammonia from it. Ammonia is a utilizable nitrogen source (food) for bacteria and yeasts. If our bodies weren't polluted with nickel, many of our yeast invaders couldn't grow! Why do we take in nickel and supply our bacteria and yeast? Nickel is in the soil, where bacteria and fungi belong, too. But if we insist on keeping plenty of nickel in our tissues, we have only ourselves to blame for our invasion.

It is hard to believe that metals we handle every day in our coinage, food and beverage containers, body products, and home and garden products could be hazardous. Yet this has been well studied. The real question is: why don't we heed our own research that we funded so dearly?

An Index Of Carcinogenicity Among Metal Carcinogens
By C. Peter Flessel et al. From *Carcinogenicity and Metal Ions*, volume 10 of a series called *Metal Ions in Biological Systems*, edited by Helmut Sigel.

Metal	Human studies		Animal Studies		Short-term bioassays			
	Positive results	Points	Positive results	Points	Positive results	Negative results	Net points	Total points (a)
Arsenic	>3	12	0	0	4	0	3	15
Beryllium	~1	6	3	6	4	1	3	15
Cadmium	1	6	3	6	5	0	3	15
Cobalt	0	0	2	5	3	1	2	7
Chromate	>3	12	>3	6	5	0	3	21
Iron (Fe)	~1	6	~1 (b)	3	4	2	2	11
Nickel	>3	12	>3	6	4	1	3	21
Lead (Pb)	~1	6	~2	5	4	1	3	14
Titanium	0	0	~1	3	0	0	0	3
Zinc	0	0	2	5	3	1	2	7

(a) See pp. 41-43 [not shown] for scoring rules.
(b) A number of studies have confirmed that only iron-carbohydrate complexes, among a variety of iron compounds tested, are carcinogenic in animals.

Fig. 49 Metal carcinogenicity

Again, I want to emphasize that the amount and the form of the metal is very important. For instance, zinc <u>metal</u> is carcinogenic (cancer producing). However an appropriate dose of zinc sulfate is anti-carcinogenic.[46] **Get your essential minerals from foods, not cookware.**

Never, never drink or cook with the water from your hot water faucet. If you have an electric hot water heater the heating element releases metal. Even if you have a gas hot water heater, the heated water leaches metals from your pipes. If your kitchen tap is the single lever type, make sure it is fully on cold. Teach children this rule.

---

[46] *Inhibition of Carcinogenesis by Dietary Zinc*, Nature, Vol. 231, No. 5303, pp. 447-448, June 18, 1971.

Food Guidelines

It is impossible to remember everything about every food, but in general do not buy foods that are highly processed. Here are a few foods; see if you can guess whether they should be in your diet or not.

breads	Yes, but not fancy varieties that have flavor listed in the ingredients, nor "day-old", or "cholesterol-reduced" bread.
cheese	Yes in baked dishes only. It must have no mold (throw it out if you see any). Trim away the outside ¼ inch, in case petroleum products or azo dyes were used on the exterior. Rotate brands. Add vitamin C.
chicken	Only if cooked for 20 minutes at boiling point, as in soup, or canned (never prepare raw chicken yourself).
wine with dinner	No.
peanut butter	Yes if you grind it yourself, adding vitamin C (¼ tsp. per pint) as you grind, to remove aflatoxins.
cottage cheese	Yes if sterilized by baking or cooking. Add vitamin C.
desserts	Yes, but again, only if not flavored with extracts (maple and vanilla are OK).
rice	Yes, white rice if cooked in pressure cooker to kill bacteria. Add vitamin C.
pasta	Yes, with homemade sauce (tomato free) and vitamin C.
jello	No, it has artificial flavor and color.
egg dishes	Yes, but not "imitation", cholesterol-free or cholesterol-reduced varieties.
popcorn	No, it has zearalenone, a mold toxin. (If you have an ozonator, you can put the air hose in the bag of kernels for five minutes and detoxify the zearalenone!)
fish, seafood	Yes!

soy foods (tofu)	No. It's the extensive processing that taints it.
soup	Yes, if seasoned only with herbs (no bouillon cube) and malonate free.
cheesecake	Yes, if homemade and baked thoroughly. Add vitamin C to recipe.
rice cakes	No. Processing pollutes them.

Fig. 50 Some good foods

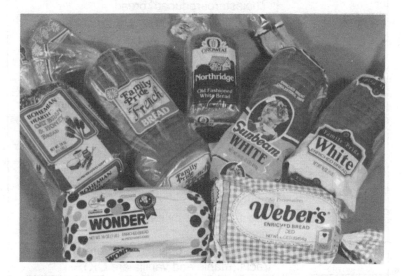

Fig. 51 These breads had solvents

Other guidelines are: choose brands with the shortest list of ingredients. Alternate brands every time you shop.

If friends are cooking for you, give them a copy of these pages about the diet. The support of your family and friends is very valuable to you, but don't eat with <u>their</u> dishes (dish detergent is on them). You can always eat off paper plates, use plastic cutlery and a plastic cup you wash yourself under the tap. Keep a set of everything handy to take out with you. Carry your own pure salt and vitamin C. Your friends are not made ill by these pollutants—YOU ARE. They can excrete them efficiently—YOU CAN'T. They go to your tumor.

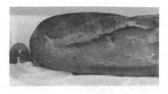

Fig. 52 No solvents found in bakery bread so far

Because you cannot supervise restaurant chefs, many normally safe foods should not be ordered. Here is a list of things that are generally safe to order:

pancakes, French toast, waffles	But ask your waiter to bring the syrup to boiling. This kills mold spores. Add vitamin C to any natural syrup.
eggs	Not scrambled—the added milk or cheese does not get sterilized, and not soft boiled—the white should be solid.
hash browns	If lightly fried, not deep fried.
soup	Only if nothing else is available. (It probably came in a can and was cooked in an aluminum pot. Do not order soups made from items on the malonic list, like tomato soup or cream of celery.)
vegetarian sandwiches	But no soy products, cheese, or tomatoes.
baked or boiled potatoes	With olive oil, bring your own salt, don't eat the skin if it was wrapped in foil or has black spots.
cooked vegetables	Cauliflower, Brussels sprouts, beets, corn, squash, and so forth.
vegetable salads	You must kill *Ascaris* eggs. Add one drop Lugol's to your water glass. Pour over salad to immerse for one minute. Drain.
vegetarian dishes	Especially Chinese food, but no soy ingredients.
bread and biscuits	But not "cholesterol-free" varieties.

fish and seafood	Anything but deep fried (the oil may have benzene) is fine: baked, steamed, fish cakes with tartar sauce.
fruit cup	With honey, no whipped cream.
fruit pies, cobblers	But not with ice cream (it has not been sterilized and flavoring has benzene).
lemon meringue pie	Indulge yourself.

Fig. 53 Good restaurant foods

The only beverages you should order in a restaurant are water and boiled milk (not just steaming). Add the vitamin C yourself (just a pinch). Herb teas are all right if they are single herbs, if you dump the bag, and make sure the hot water comes from a non-metal pot.

If you order food "to go", ask the chef to line the aluminum or styrofoam containers or cups with plastic wrap. Clear plastic containers are OK, but do not store leftovers in them.

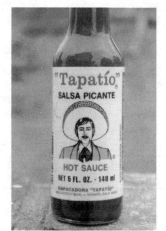

This sauce is not made with tomatoes and repeatedly tested free of the M-family, benzene, isopropyl alcohol, and wood alcohol, a tribute to the manufacturer.

Fig. 54 Good sauce

148

Check Your Progress

You now have accomplished 7 things:

1. You have killed the intestinal fluke and cured your cancer.
2. You have Mopped Up all your other parasites. You are zapping regularly and are on the parasite program.
3. You have removed all products with isopropyl alcohol in them from your house and are eating no foods with isopropyl alcohol pollution.
4. You have taken out all the metal and plastic from your mouth and are waiting (patiently?) for safe partials or dentures. Teeth with large fillings or crowns have been extracted. You are hot packing.
5. You have switched from eating food concoctions to eating simple foods, free from solvents and malonic acid. You are starting to strike symptoms off your list.
6. You no longer have any tumor-forming common denominators.
7. You have found a new home for your pet.

As you see your symptoms disappear, one after another, you will feel the magic of healing. Most cancer patients have 50 or more symptoms to start out! They could fill two sheets of paper, one symptom to each line. It can be quite shocking to see a list of all your symptoms.

Sometimes a new symptom appears as fast as an old one disappears. The coincidence makes it tempting to believe that one symptom turns into a different one. But it is not so. If a new symptom appears, it is because another pathogen has become activated due to a new toxin. Try to identify the new item. Stop using any new food, supplement, or body product, even if it is a health variety, and see if it goes away.

3. Clean Up Your Body

We are living in a very fortunate time. We are not expected to all look alike! The 60's brought us this wonderful freedom. Freedom to dress in a variety of styles, use make-up or no make-up, jewelry or no jewelry, any kind of hair style, any kind of shoes.

You will need to go off <u>every</u> cosmetic and body product that you are <u>now</u> using. Not a single one can be continued. They are full of titanium, zirconium, benzalkonium, bismuth, antimony, barium[47], strontium[48], aluminum, tin, chromium, not to mention pollutants such as benzene, PCBs, and azo dyes.

Do not use any commercial salves, ointments, lotions, colognes, perfumes, massage oils, deodorant, mouthwash, toothpaste, even when touted as "herbal" and health-food-type. See *Recipes* for homemade substitutes.

People are trying desperately to use less toxic products. They seek health for themselves. So they reach for products that just list herbs and other natural ingredients. Unfortunately, the buyers are being duped. The Food and Drug Administration (FDA) requires all body products to have sufficient antiseptic in them for your "protection." Some of these antiseptics are <u>themselves</u> substances <u>you must avoid</u>! But you won't see them on the label because manufacturers prefer to use quantities below the levels they must disclose. And by using a variety of antiseptics in these small amounts they can still meet sterility requirements. The only ingredient you might see is "grapefruit seed" or similar healthy-sounding natural antiseptic. This is sad for the consumer of health food varieties. Here are some problems I have seen:

---

[47] Barium is described in the *Merck Index* as "Caution: All water or acid soluble barium compounds are POISONOUS." 10th ed. p. 139 1983.

[48] This element goes to bones.

- Rocks sold as "Aluminum-Free Natural Deodorant". You rub the rock under your arms. It works because the rock is made of magnesium-<u>aluminum</u> silicate.
- Men's hair color with lead in it.
- Lipstick with barium, aluminum, titanium, scarlet red dye.
- Eye pencil and shadow with chromium and cobalt.
- Toothpaste with benzene, tin, and strontium.
- Hair spray with isopropyl alcohol and PCBs.
- Shampoo with isopropyl alcohol!
- Cigarettes with lead, mercury, nickel, benzene[49] and Tobacco Mosaic Virus.
- Chewing tobacco with ytterbium.

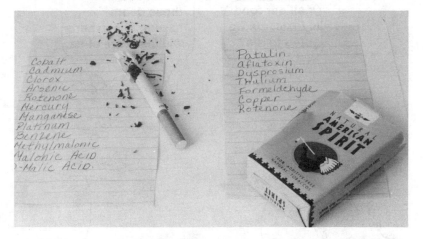

The list of pollutants in these "natural" cigarettes was obtained with a Syncrometer. Use a magnifying glass to read them.

Fig. 55 Health food store cigarettes

---

[49] The higher level of benzene in the blood of smokers was measured in 1989. The title of this report is: *Benzene in the Blood and Breath of Normal People and Occupationally Exposed Workers* by F. Brugnone, L. Perbellini, G.B. Faccini, F. Pasini, B. Danzi, G. Maranelli, L. Romeo, M. Gobbi, A. Zedde: Amer. J. Industrial Medicine, 16:385-399 (1989)

- Marijuana with benzene.

Some of the unnatural chemicals listed were detected with the Syncrometer™ and are probably present because of residues from the manufacturing process, but others you will actually see listed on the label!

How can isopropyl alcohol in shampoo get into your body in significant amounts? The skin is more absorbent than we realize, and time and time again I see clients who have gone off every body product <u>except</u> their favorite shampoo. They have isopropyl alcohol until they make that final sacrifice. It is better

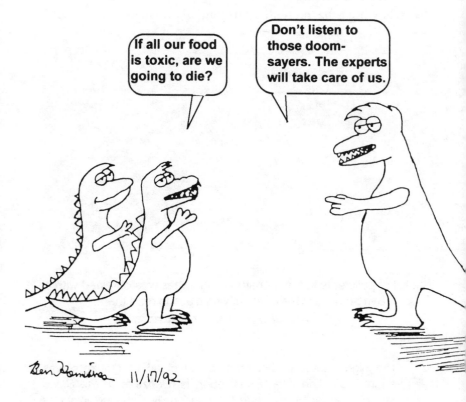

Fig. 56 Our future, unless we act

to switch shampoos than to not need any due to radiation and chemotherapy!

See *Recipes* for easy-to-make, natural substitutes. But you might consider just stopping them all. Especially if you're going on vacation.

Use nothing that you wouldn't use on a new-born baby. This is a permissive age. You will be the only one feeling "naked." Others won't even notice. Don't forget advertising is aimed at you, even if other people's eyes are not!

Don't even use soap unless it is homemade soap (see *Recipes*) or borax[50] straight from the box. Borax was the traditional pioneer's soap. It is antibacterial and can be made into a concentrate. It is also a water softener and is the main ingredient in non-chlorine bleaches. Borax has excellent solvent power for grease. But even borax is not natural to your body and it is therefore wise to use as little as necessary. See *Recipes* for antibacterial natural borax soap.

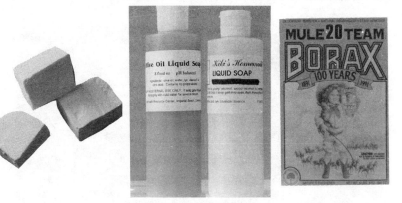

homemade soap   2 homemade liquid soaps   pure borax

Fig. 57 Three safe soaps

[50] 20 Mule Team Borax™ works well for soap and is free of metals and other pollutants. Borax inhibits the bacterial enzyme *urease*. Urease is used by bacteria and yeasts that live in us to utilize our urea as a source of nitrogen for themselves.

Don't use toothpaste, not even health-food varieties. To clean teeth, use salt—but dissolve it in water first, otherwise it is too abrasive. Or brush with hydrogen peroxide <u>food grade</u>, not the regular variety (see *Sources*). To floss before brushing, use unwaxed, unflavored floss that has been soaked in plain cold water for half an hour, then wash. If you don't do this, you could be getting a meal of all 9 tumorigens plus solvents! Throw away your old toothbrush—solvents don't wash out (see Brushing Teeth, page 571).

Don't use mouthwash. Use saltwater (pure salt) or food grade hydrogen peroxide (just a few drops in water).

Don't use hair spray.

Don't use massage oils of any kind. Even olive oil occasionally has benzene pollution, probably due to adulteration with other oils. The varieties shown on page 550 never tested positive for benzene.

Don't use bath oil. Take showers, not baths, if you are strong enough to stand. Showers are cleaner.

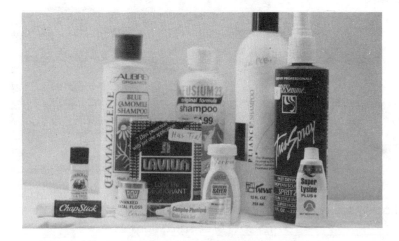

Our household, health, and body products, and drugs were found to be polluted with solvents, heavy metals, PCBs and lanthanides using the Syncrometer.

Fig. 58 Some polluted body care products

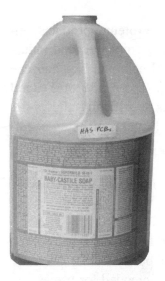

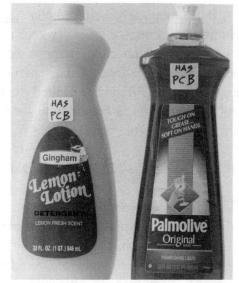

Fig. 59 You can't even trust health-store brands.

The Syncrometer detected PCBs in all the popular detergents, making dishes and clothing our primary source of PCBs.

Fig. 60 Detergents with PCBs.

Don't use perfumes or colognes.

Don't use lotions or personal lubricants except homemade.

Banish Benzene

Benzene deserves special attention not only because it is <u>the AIDS-related solvent</u>, but because it is presumed to be absent from our consumer environment. Yet I have found traces in everything from bottled water to toothpaste! It is so toxic its concentration is even regulated and tested in gasoline and dry cleaning fluid to reduce exposure to it in the air. Can you imagine <u>eating it or putting it on our bodies</u>, even in minute quantities?

It is commonly believed that <u>all</u> petroleum products, including benzene, are carefully kept away from the food industry. And under no circumstances would solvents like benzene be allowed near food. This is wrong. The Code of Federal Regulations (CFR) in the United States <u>specifically allows</u> petroleum products to be added to food. Mineral oil is an example; it is made from petroleum.

21 CFR 172.878 (4-1-94 Edition) White mineral oil.

White mineral oil may be safely used in food in accordance with the following conditions:

[Paragraphs (a) and (b) describe purity levels]

(c) White mineral oil is used or intended for use as follows:

Use	Limitation (inclusive of all petroleum hydrocarbons that may be used in combination with white mineral oil)
1. As a release agent, binder, and lubricant in or on capsules and tablets containing concentrates of flavoring, spices, condiments, and nutrients intended for addition to food, excluding confectionery.	Not to exceed 0.6% of the capsule or tablet.
2. As a release agent, binder, and lubricant in or on capsules and tablets containing food for special dietary use.	Not to exceed 0.6% of the capsule or tablet.
3. As a float on fermentation fluids in the manufacture of vinegar and wine to prevent or retard access of air, evaporation, and wild yeast contamination during fermentation.	In an amount not to exceed good manufacturing practice.
4. As a defoamer in food	In accordance with §173.340 of this chapter.
5. In bakery products, as a release agent and lubricant	Not to exceed 0.15% of bakery products.
6. In dehydrated fruits and vegetables, as a release agent	Not to exceed 0.02% of dehydrated fruits and vegetables.
7. In egg white solids, as a release agent	Not to exceed 0.1% of egg white solids.

8. On raw fruits and vegetables, as a protective coating	In an amount not to exceed good manufacturing practice.
9. In frozen meat, as a component of hot-melt coating	Not to exceed 0.095% of meat.
10. As a protective float on brine used in the curing of pickles	In an amount not to exceed good manufacturing practice.
11. In molding starch used in the manu-facture of confectionery	Not to exceed 0.3% in the molding starch.
12. As a release agent, binder, and lubri-cant in the manufacture of yeast	Not to exceed 0.15% of yeast.
13. As an antidusting agent in sorbic acid for food use	not to exceed 0.25% in the sorbic acid.
14. As release agent and as sealing and polishing agent in the manufacture of confectionery	Not to exceed 0.2% of confec-tionery.
15. As a dust control agent for wheat, corn, soybean, barley, rice, rye, oats, and sorghum.	Applied at level of no more than 0.02% by weight of grain.

Fig. 61 Lawful uses of white mineral oil in food.

All of the following petroleum products are also "safely used in food" subject to similar conditions of purity and use: petrolatum (21 CFR 172.880), synthetic isoparaffinic petroleum hydrocarbons (21 CFR 172.882), odorless light petroleum hydrocarbons (21 CFR 172.884), petroleum wax (21 CFR 172.886), petroleum naphtha (21 CFR 172.250).

There is even one food that benzene can be used with directly:

21 CFR 172.560 (4-1-94 Edition) Modified hop extract.

The food additive modified hop extract may be safely used in beer in accordance with the following prescribed conditions:

(a) The food additive is used or intended for use as a flavoring agent in the brewing of beer.

(b) The food additive is manufactured by one of the following processes:

(1) [describes a hexane extract]

(2) The additive is manufactured from hops by a sequence of extractions and fractionations, using benzene, light petroleum spirits, and methyl alcohol as solvents, followed by isomerization by potassium carbonate treatment. Residues of solvents in the modified hop extract shall not exceed 1.0 part per million of benzene, 1.0 part per million of light petroleum spirits, and 250 parts per million of methyl alcohol. The light petroleum spirits and benzene solvents shall comply with the specification in §172.250 except that the boiling point range for light petroleum spirits is 150°F-300°F.

[(3) through (8) go on to describe other allowable manufacturing processes using methylene chloride, hexane, methyl alcohol, sodium hydroxide, butyl alcohol, ethyl acetate, potassium carbonate, ethylene dichloride, isopropyl alcohol, trichloroethylene, palladium, hydrochloric acid, sulfuric acid, peracetic acid, sodium borohydride and other chemicals.]

Fig. 62 Lawful ways of making hop extract for use in beer.

Ironically, the law mandates the purity of the benzene used (§172.250). It's hard to imagine what worse chemicals the government agency is concerned about! And if you think one part per million doesn't sound like a lot, keep in mind that the government maximum allowed level in drinking water is five parts per <u>billion</u>, 200 times less concentrated. Of course it's assumed that by the time the hop extract is added to the rest of the beer ingredients, the concentration will be much less. But what really counts is the total amount consumed, over days, months and years.

Allowing the use of petroleum products (whose raw form contains benzene), in food has undoubtedly led to the worldwide lowering of immunity that is so apparent. The immune lowering effect of benzene has been studied for many years by scientists. We just didn't know that we were eating it!

I find benzene is present in foods and products that have been colored, flavored, stabilized, conditioned, defoamed, coated, or preserved. Although our regulatory agencies have been vigilant in checking gasoline, dry cleaning fluid, and outdoor air for benzene, the most toxic route, food, has escaped detection. The present extent of benzene pollution is unthinkable and overwhelming.

These are the foods and products which I have found to be polluted with benzene. STOP USING THEM IMMEDIATELY. DO NOT FINISH UP ANY ONE OF THEM. THROW THEM OUT NOW! Throw them into the garbage and take the garbage out of your house.

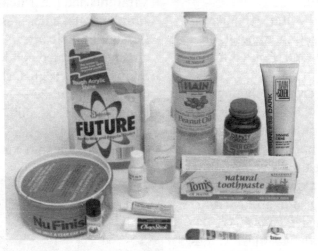

BEWARE! Our household products, body products and even foods have benzene pollution in them.
Fig. 63 Some benzene-polluted products

Benzene Polluted Products

THROW THESE OUT

<u>Your health is worth more than the fortune you spent on them!</u>

- **Flavored food,** yogurt, jello, candies, throat lozenges, store-bought cookies, cakes
- **Cooking oil** and shortening (use <u>only</u> olive oil, butter and lard)
- **Bottled water**, <u>whether distilled, spring, mineral, or name brand</u>. Bottled fruit juice.
- **Cold cereal**, including granola and health brands
- **Toothpaste**, including health brands
- **Ice cream**, frozen yogurt
- **Rice cakes,** even plain ones
- **Baking soda and cornstarch** (see *Sources*)
- **Pills and capsules**. At least a third of all I test are polluted. This includes herbal extracts and prescription drugs. Test yours and switch brands until you find a safe one.

- **Vaseline products** (noxzema, Vick's, Lip therapy), chap stick, hand cleaners.
- **Chewing gum**
- **Vitamins** and other **health supplements**, unless tested.
- **Personal lubricant**, including lubricated condoms
- **Soaps, hand creams**, skin creams, moisturizers
- Flavored pet food, both for cats and dogs
- Bird food made into cakes

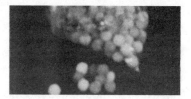

Fig. 64 Mexican made candy with no benzene.

It is impossible for me to have tested every batch of every food and product, but so many test positive you simply can not risk <u>any</u> of the foods and products on the list.

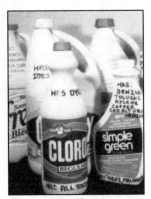

Tear out the benzene list, put it on your refrigerator, and make a copy to stick on your medicine cabinet.

Learn to use the Syncrometer to do your own testing. While you are learning, observe the rules perfectly. There is no half way measure with benzene.

Fig. 65 Pollutants are in unlikely places

Stop using benzene-polluted products as soon as you read this. **This includes health brands!** Don't wait until you have low immunity. If you can't believe this extensive pollution with benzene and wish to have this verified by our government agencies first, set the items aside. <u>Use other products while you are waiting!</u>

You could also check your benzene consumption by doing a <u>urinary phenol test</u> (request one from your clinical doctor, see *Sources*). Choose the test that is meant to identify <u>chronic</u> benzene exposure, not acute. The normal range will be included with your test results. If yours is high, let this galvanize you into action.

Make your own replacements from our recipes!

The body rids itself of benzene in three to five days after stopping the use of polluted products.

Why do only some people accumulate benzene although we all use benzene polluted products? The answer, of course, lies in how much benzene we get. But is that all? Since aflatoxin causes isopropyl alcohol build up could another mycotoxin cause benzene buildup? A search of 13 mycotoxins showed that one was 100% correlated with benzene buildup.

Zearalenone, a corn mold toxin, is responsible. It is in corn chips, popcorn and brown rice. Persons with benzene buildup have been eating these foods. Stop eating them. Eat white rice. The toxicity of zearalenone is much more important than the nutritional difference.

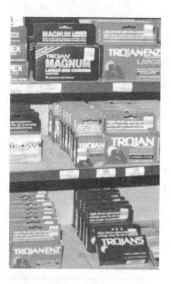

Fig. 66 Lubricated condoms have benzene.

Because benzene accumulates in the thymus and bone marrow, our two most important immune building organs, we would expect a drop in immunity. All persons with AIDS have a benzene buildup. As benzene pollution worsens, many more people must experience immunity loss.

Vitamin B_2 specifically helps the body detoxify benzene to phenol. If your immunity is low, that is, your white blood cell count is below 5000 per mm^3, take 300 mg with each meal. If you already have AIDS take 600 mg with each meal. And don't visit tanning booths. Ultraviolet light destroys the B_2 already in your body.

Stop Using Supplements

Stop using your vitamin supplements. This is the saddest, most tragic part of your instructions. They, too, are heavily polluted with the same solvents used in food processing: benzene, isopropyl alcohol, wood alcohol, xylene, toluene, methylene chloride, methyl ethyl ketone, methyl butyl ketone, and others. I also see **heavy metals** and **malonic acid** in 90% or more of the popular vitamin and mineral capsules and tablets I test. These substances will do more harm in the long run than the supplement can make up for in benefits.

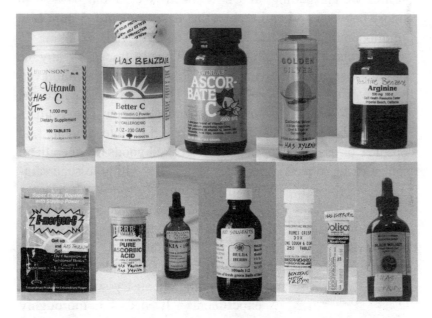

Fig. 67 Assorted supplements

Supplements are a gamble. The most recent tests using the Syncrometer unfortunately showed that many popular varieties of vitamin C now are polluted with **thulium** (a harmful lanthanide). Similarly, all homeopathic medicines had traces of benzene, isopropyl alcohol and wood alcohol. Even some newly organized companies selling Black Walnut Tincture had isopropyl pollution. And a Self Health product was found polluted in 1995 and immediately removed from the shelves. All supplement manufacturers should do Syncrometer testing of their final product.

Until all vitamins and minerals and other food supplements have been analyzed for pollutants, <u>after they are encapsulated or tableted</u>, they are not safe. We need <u>processing</u> disclosure on our products. No manufactured product is absolutely pure. We can't expect that. But at least we should be able to tell what impurities we are getting, and how much. We should be able to choose between a vitamin tablet that has less than 0.5 ppm lead pollution and one that has less than 0.05 ppm lead.

The source of a pollutant can be easily traced by anyone who has mastered the Syncrometer. Manufacturers should avail themselves of this new technology. The future belongs to the ethical business that discloses the chemicals they use to sanitize, lubricate, defoam, release tablets from the tablet punch, seal capsules, or use as release agents for baked goods (to keep them from sticking to pans), etc. They should be willing to send samples for testing.

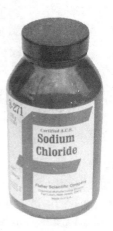

It <u>is</u> possible to do detailed analysis of foods or products at a reasonable price. Look at the bottle of common table salt, sodium chloride, that is used by beginning chemistry students to do experiments. It had be thoroughly analyzed for them because minute impurities affect their results. (Those minute impurities, like lead, affect <u>you</u>, too.) Look at all the information given in the label on the bottle in the picture. Even after all these tests, the cost of

Fig. 68 Pure salt

laboratory salt is only $2.80 per pound.[51]

It is most important not to be fooled by ingredient claims, like "made from organically grown vegetables". That's reassuring, but the analysis *I* trust would be done on the final, cleaned, cooked and packaged product on the shelf. The package itself is a major <u>unlisted</u> ingredient when it leaches pollutants into the food.

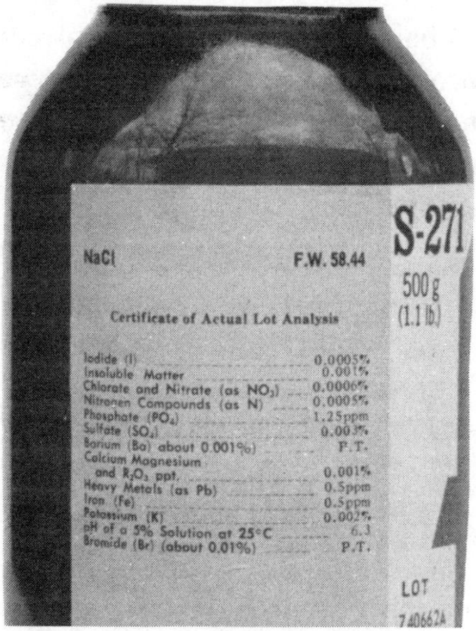

Toxic solvents like decane, hexane, carbon tetrachloride and benzene will get more flavor or fat or cholesterol out of things than nontoxic grain (ethyl) alco-

Common table salt for student use is thoroughly analyzed for pollution. The label gives you the final "Actual Lot Analysis" of the product. It is not expensive.

Fig. 69 Laboratory salt label

hol. Of course, the extraction process calls for washing out the toxic solvent later. But it can't all be washed out, and a detailed analysis <u>on the final product</u> would give the public the information they need to make informed choices.

---

[51] You will pay about $8.00 per pound (Spectrum Chemical Co.) for USP (United States Pharmaceutical) grade. But the same analyses are done on the cheaper grades, and my point is that the analysis is cost effective enough that it should be done on our <u>daily</u> foods.

Use NO supplements

unless they are tested for solvents. Those listed in *Sources* at the end of this book have been repeatedly tested up to publishing time. What we really need are manufacturers who are committed to using ethyl alcohol or old-fashioned steam to extract and sterilize.

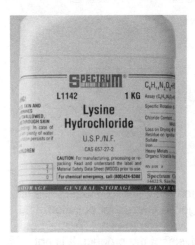

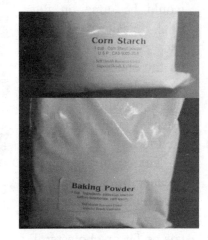

Pure supplements can be obtained from chemical supply companies but must be purchased in bulk–a good project for food co-ops.

Bulk supplies may be repackaged like these samples of baking powder and corn starch.

Fig. 70 Safe products in bulk

Safe Supplements

There are, no doubt, lots of safe supplements to be had. The problem is knowing which are polluted. The nature of pollution is such that one bottle might be safe, while another of the same brand is not. In view of this, as I found a polluted bottle, I stopped using any more of that brand. Only safe ones are listed in *Sources*.

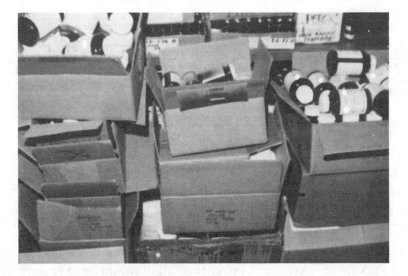

Fig. 71 Boxes of vitamins I discarded

The De-malonating Supplements

The following supplements have been divided into two sets. These in the table are related to malonate consumption. The remainder, below the table, have other purposes.

Supplement	Dosage
Biotin, 1 mg	Take one a day
Calcium, 500 mg	Take one a day at beginning of meal. Replaces calcium lost by chelation with malonic acid.
Coenzyme Q10, 400 mg	Take in morning upon rising.
Cysteine, 500 mg	Take one three times a day
Folic Acid, 0.9 mg	Take one a day, but see text.
Glutamic acid, 500 mg	Take two three times a day
Glutamine, 500 mg	One a day.
Glutathione, 500 mg	You only need one a day if not ill. If you are very ill, take 2 three times a day before meals. Glutathione is particularly important to restore immunity.

167

Glycine, 500 mg	Take 1 three times a day
Lecithin	½ Tbs. daily. Supplies methyl groups, also choline.
Methionine, 500 mg	Take one a day
Pantothenic acid (as calcium pantothenate, 500 mg.	Take three a day, makes coenzyme A
Taurine, 500 mg	Take 1 three times a day. Detoxifies cholesterol, formaldehyde.
Vitamin B_6, 250 mg	Take 1 a day. It is inactivated by malonic acid.
Vitamin B_{12}, 1 mg	Take 1 three times a day if ill, once a day if not ill.
Vitamin C, 1000 mg (1/4 tsp. powder)	Take 6 a day until all malonic acid has been removed from your diet and the dental plastic is out of your mouth. Then reduce to three a day. Take only one a day with food if diarrhea is present.

The dosage of folic acid supplements is regulated by the FDA to be no more than 1 mg. This is because higher doses could mask a B_{12} deficiency. Of course, when using both together, this could not happen. There is considerable research evidence that _much_ higher doses of both B_{12} and folic acid would benefit us all, perhaps even prevent multiple sclerosis and Parkinson's disease. A better regulation would be to require that they always be sold together. Much higher doses than a few mg are needed to detoxify malonic acid. Typically, it takes 25 mg of folic acid to detoxify the malonic acid seeping from plastic tooth fillings. Even higher doses are needed if it is seeping into the brain. This happens in Parkinson's disease and brain tumors.

As soon as dental plastic is gone and the diet is free of malonic acid, the requirement for B_{12}, folic acid, and vitamin C drops dramatically. Perhaps even all the way down to the recommended daily allowance (RDA). After you are well, you could cut all dosages of all supplements in half or less.

The remaining supplements in the list are for other purposes.

General Health Supplements

Vitamin C in powdered form, is a must in your lifestyle. It helps the liver, and possibly other organs, detoxify things. I have not seen it help to detoxify benzene, though. It does help retard mold. Keep some next to your refrigerator so it is handy when you put away groceries. Add 1/8 tsp. to maple syrup, vinegar, cooked cereal, pasta, leftovers. Have at least ¼ tsp. (1 gram) with each meal. This much can be stirred into milk without changing the flavor. If you take it straight, it can give you diarrhea.

Vitamin B$_1$, 500 mg per meal, is essential for the cancer patient to help restore health to the tumorous organ. It also improves appetite and liver function.

Vitamin B$_2$, 300 mg per meal. All B vitamins help oxidize food, something for which cancer sufferers have reduced capability, causing fatigue. B$_2$ also detoxifies benzene to phenol.

Magnesium oxide, 300 mg, is another must. It can detoxify phenol to magnesium phenyl phosphate, allowing it to leave through the kidneys. Take one a day, but not during a bout of diarrhea. It is a major mineral; all of our cells need lots of it. Only leafy vegetables provide it. The green drinks on page 545 can supply some and do not pose a pollution risk nor aggravate diarrhea.

Choline, too, is easily obtained from food, so there is no need to risk taking a tablet or capsule. It is plentiful in eggs, lentils, lecithin granules and milk. It supplies methyl groups.

Ornithine and Arginine, both 500 mg, are very important detoxifiers of ammonia via the *urea synthesis cycle*. But they do much more. We have seen them specifically help to eliminate *Clostridium* bacteria.

Hydrogen peroxide, food grade. It is advantageous to kill bacteria and viruses to some extent every day. Hydrogen peroxide lets you do this. It should never come in contact with metal, including its container or metal tooth fillings. If you get a few drops on your skin it may turn white and sting, but does no harm, so simply wash it off.

Herbs. These are excellent supplements, in <u>bulk</u>. There are many books that describe their medicinal properties. If the herbs are in <u>capsules</u> you must test for petroleum pollution (benzene and other solvents). Don't purchase extracts or concentrates because they are invariably polluted (unless you can test them, of course). The powdered form is also frequently polluted. Buy "c/s", which means cut and sifted.

Lugol's Iodine Solution (see *Recipes*, page 601) is made of potassium iodide and plain, pure iodine. It is made this way because plain iodine does not dissolve well in water; it dissolves much better in potassium iodide. Potassium iodide dissolves well in water and stays clear; for this reason it is also called "white iodine." By mixing the two, we can get stronger concentrations of iodine than either can provide by itself. Commercially available Lugol's was polluted with isopropyl alcohol and other solvents when I tested them with the Syncrometer. Make it yourself from scratch. Be careful not to use bottled water or you will pollute it yourself!

DO NOT TAKE LUGOL'S IODINE IF YOU ARE ALLERGIC TO IODINE. IT COULD BE FATAL.

How do you know if you are allergic to iodine? You can become allergic from having a large amount of iodine poured into you during a special clinical thyroid or kidney procedure. Your doctor or nurse will already have told you if you became allergic. If in doubt, call your doctor.

Iodine has a distinctive trait: it hangs up on anything and everything. In fact, it attaches itself so quickly we consider everything it touches as "stained." This is just the property we want to make it safe for use. The amount you use is immediately hung up, or attached, to your <u>mucous</u> and can not be quickly absorbed into the blood or other organs. It stays in the stomach. And for this reason it is so useful for killing vicious bacteria like *Salmonella*.

Salmonella and *Shigella* are two stomach and digestive tract bacteria. They can give you terrible bloating and gas which is often misdiagnosed as *lactose intolerance.* Younger persons often have a fever when *Salmonella* attacks. "Summer flu" or "24-hour flu" is really *Salmonella* getting you. It comes into you with deli food, chicken, dairy food, not to mention picnic food that has stood around for a while. Hands carry these two bacteria, so always wash hands before eating and after shaking someone's hand. People can have <u>chronic</u> *Salmonella* and *Shigella* infections. Every new strain they eat or drink evidently forms hybrids with the old strain they already had in their stomachs. This results in much more vicious strains which actually make you feel sick. *Shigella*, especially, makes you feel angry, irritable, and short-tempered as a mule. *Shigella* goes to your nervous system. All cases of multiple sclerosis I have seen had rampant *Shigella*!

Six drops of Lugol's solution can end it all for *Salmonella*. If you have gas and bloating, pour yourself ½ glass of water. Add 6 drops of Lugol's (not more, not less), stir with wood or plastic, and drink all at once. The action is noticeable in an hour. Take this dose 4 times a day, after meals and at bedtime, for 3 days in a row, then daily at bedtime. This eradicates even a stubborn case of *Salmonella*. For prevention use one drop in a glass of water at mealtime.

Notice how calming 6 drops of Lugol's can be, soothing a manic stage and bringing a peaceful state where anxiety ruled before.

Lugol's is <u>perfectly safe</u> (if not allergic) to take day after day, when needed, because of its peculiar attaching property. It arrives in the stomach, reattaches to everything in proximity. Doomed are *Salmonella* and other local bacteria; doomed also are eggs (cysts) of parasites that might be in the stomach.

Naturally, one would not leave such medicine within the reach of children. Also, one would not use anything medicinal, including Lugol's, unless there were a need, like digestive distress. Store it in a perfectly secure place. In the past, 2/3 of a teaspoon (60 drops) of Lugol's was the standard dose of iodine given to persons with thyroid disease. Six drops is small by comparison, but you need no more.

Shigella is not killed by Lugol's after it leaves the stomach to reside in the bowel.

Amazingly, the two teaspoon dose of Black Walnut Hull Tincture Extra Strength used in the Parasite Killing Program is also effective against many bacteria, including *Salmonella, Shigella*, and *Clostridium*.

If the tincture doesn't bring total relief in 24 hours, search for a source of reinfection. Then eliminate it. Don't just keep taking the tincture. These bacteria come to us in dairy foods, or perhaps you are self infecting by putting your fingers in your mouth.

A traditional, more gradual method of conquering digestive bacteria is with two herbs (which are also common spices!): *turmeric* and *fennel*. Follow the Bowel Program (page 586).

Another traditional treatment for digestive problems is yogurt and acidophilus beverages. But modern commercial varieties are actually contaminated with *Salmonella* and *Shigella* strains. Test them yourself. It is just too hazardous to risk using them.

Other supplements. The concept of supplementing the diet is excellent, but the pollution problem makes it prohibitive. In

How To Test Yourself you learn how you can test any product, including supplements, to make sure they are safe.

4. Clean Up Your Home

There is only one job left. Clean up your environment. This is an easy task because it mostly involves throwing things out, so it was left to the last. But don't delay for a minute to get this done. Hopefully your family and friends will jump to your assistance.

- The refrigerator gets changed.
- The basement gets cleaned.
- The garage gets cleaned.
- Every room in the house gets cleaned.

Special Clean-up For Freon

Your refrigerator is the most sinister toxin in your home!

In the past, various refrigerants were used. Ammonia was especially efficient. And the tiniest leak alerted you by its odor. The mechanics were engineered to be foolproof.

But switching to **Freon** as a refrigerant, which is nearly odorless, brought a new threat: unsuspected leakage. Cancer patients <u>all</u> have especially high levels <u>right in their tumorous organs</u>!

Wheel your refrigerator outside the same day you read this. You may leave it on an extension cord and use it until you find a new <u>non-Freon</u> variety.

What is so damaging about Freon in your body? After all, it is non-biodegradable. If it has no biological interactions, how could it hurt us? By being non-degradable, however, the liver has no chemical reactions with which to detoxify it so it can leave the body! It builds up, therefore. Healthy people accumulate it in their skin. Sick people accumulate it in their sick organ.

I call this phenomenon *morbitropism*. "Tropism" means there is an attraction. "Morbi" means sick. Toxic things are attracted to sick organs. Although everybody in the health professions know this, it is never discussed in scientific circles. Perhaps morbitropism has a magnetic or electronic explanation, and will soon be a legitimate subject for study.

Freon's contribution to carcinogenicity has been studied.[52] I find the damaging effect of Freon is that it can act like a trap for other fat soluble items like PCBs, metals, and dyes. Particularly, copper is seen at Freon sites. Water that has run through copper pipes carries copper. Your body absorbs the copper which gets trapped by the Freon already there. Obviously, you must remove Freon from your body. But how?

Only one useful reaction with Freon comes to mind. Freon is thought to be responsible for the ozone "hole" at the South Pole. Would Freon react with ozone supplied to your body and thereby become biodegradable? Indeed, it does! But only if you drink it as ozonated water. Other ozone routes, as intravenous or rectal, have not been observed to be as effective.

If you have cancer

buy a small ozonator (see *Sources*) as suggested earlier. Drop the hose into a glass of cold tap water. Two or three minutes is enough to be effective. Drink three glasses a day for the first week, then two glasses a day for six more weeks.

---

[52] Mahurin, R.G., Bernstein, R.L., *Fluorocarbon-enhanced mutagenesis of polyaromatic hydrocarbons*, Environ.-Res. vol. 45, no. 1, 1988, pp. 101-107.

If you are following your progress with the Syncrometer, you will see that Freon now appears in the liver for the first time. Before this, it was marooned in several organs. You may also detect a feeling like indigestion. You must come to the assistance of your liver. Even ozonated Freon is extremely burdensome to the liver.

A combination of herbs (Liver Herbs in *Recipes*, page 594) rescues the liver from its plight, and prevents the indigestion. Drink one to two cups over the course of the day. After drinking liver herbs you will see that the Freon now appears in the kidneys. Yet it is marooned there unless you assist them. Take the kidney cleanse (page 591) to assist the kidneys so they can finally excrete the Freon into the urine.

It's an elaborate detoxifying program of ozonated water, liver herbs, and kidney herbs taken together for six to eight weeks. This gets most of the Freon out. Afterward, continue the program at one third dosage for half a year.

Forane is one of the new refrigerants. Although toxic, at least I observe it in the liver directly, suggesting that your body is capable of handling it. Remember your new refrigerator will still be using a toxic coolant, and it would be best to keep it outside or at least <u>vented</u> to the outside.

Another source of Freon is the air conditioner in your home or car. You must test a dust sample taken from a flat surface in your car or home (after changing your refrigerator) to find out if it is leaking. Fortunately, the success rate on fixing air conditioners is quite good, in contrast to fixing refrigerators.

If you are very sick, find a home without air conditioners and move the refrigerator outside.

Special Clean-up for Fiberglass

Fiberglass insulation has microscopically small bits of glass that are free to blow into the air. When house drafts pull it into the air you will inhale them. They cut their way through your lungs and organs like millions of tiny knives, spreading through your body, since there is no way out for them. You smell nothing and feel nothing. This makes it a very sinister poison. Your body, though, recognizes these sharp, pointed bits and tries to stop their spread by sequestering them in cysts.

Most solid malignant tumors contain fiberglass or asbestos, another glass-like particle. In nearly all cases a hole can be found in the ceiling or walls, leading to fiberglass insulated parts of the house. When these holes are sealed in an air-tight manner the house air no longer is positive for fiberglass. Covering with paneling is not sufficient. Check your dwelling for uncovered fiberglass. Repair immediately. Search for small screw holes intended for pictures, or electric outlet plates that are missing.

Also remove fiberglass jackets from your water heater and fiberglass filters from your furnace and air conditioner. Replace with foam or carbon. Best of all, hire a crew to remove it all from your home, and replace insulation with blown-in shredded paper or other innocuous substance.

Never build a new house using fiberglass for any purpose.

Clean Basement

To clean your basement, remove all paint, varnish, thinners, brush cleaners, and related supplies. Remove all cleaners such as carpet cleaner, leather cleaner, rust remover. Remove all chemicals that are in cans, bottles or buckets.

You may keep your laundry supplies: borax, white distilled vinegar, chlorine bleach and homemade soap. You may keep canned goods, tools, items that are not chemicals. You may move your chemicals into your garage. Also move any car tires and automotive supplies like waxes, oil, transmission fluid, and the spare gas can (even if it is empty) into your garage or discard them.

Seal cracks in the basement and around pipes where they come through the wall with black plastic roofing cement. In a few days it will be hard enough to caulk with a prettier color. Spread a sheet of plastic over the sewer or sump pump.

Clean Garage

Do you have a garage that is a separate building from your home? This is the best arrangement. You can move all the basement chemicals into this garage. Things that will freeze, such as latex paint, you may as well discard. But if your garage is attached, you have a problem. <u>Never, never use your door between the garage and house</u>. Walk around the outside. Don't allow this door to be used. Tack a sheet of plastic over it to slow down the rate of fume entrance into the house. Your house acts like a chimney for the garage. Your house is taller and warmer than the garage so garage-air is pulled in and up as the warm air in the house rises. See the drawing.

In medieval days, the barn for the animals was attached to the house. We think such an arrangement with its penetrating odors is unsavory. But what of the gasoline and motor fumes we are getting now due to parked vehicles? These are toxic besides! This is even more benighted.

If your garage is under your house, you cannot keep the pollution from en-

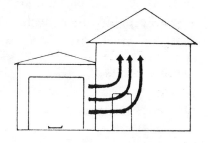

Fig. 72 Garage fumes

tering your home. In this case, leave the cars and lawnmower <u>outside</u>. Remove cans of gasoline, solvents, etc. Put up a separate shed for these items.

Clean House

To clean the house, start with the bedroom. Remove everything that has any smell to it whatever: candles, potpourri, soaps, mending glue, cleaners, repair chemicals, felt markers, colognes, perfumes, and especially plug-in air "fresheners". Store them in the garage, not the basement. Since all vapor rises, they would come back up if you put them in a downstairs garage or basement.

Next clean the kitchen. Take all cans and bottles of chemicals out from under the sink or in a closet. Remove them to the garage. Keep only the borax, white distilled vinegar and bottles of concentrated borax and 50% vinegar you have made. You may also use homemade soap. Use these for all purposes. For exact amounts to use for dishwasher, dishes, windows, dusting, see *Recipes*. Remove all cans, bottles, roach and ant killer, mothballs, and chemicals that kill insects or mice. These should not be used anywhere in your house. They should be thrown out. Remember to check the crawl space, attic and closets for hidden poisons also. To wax the floor, get the wax from the garage and put it back there. A cancer patient should not be in the house while house cleaning or floor waxing is being done.

To keep out mice, walk all around your house, stuffing holes and cracks with steel wool. Use old-fashioned mouse traps.

For cockroaches and other insects (except ants) sprinkle handfuls of boric acid[53] (not borax) under your shelf paper, behind sink, stove, refrigerator, under carpets, etc.

Use vinegar on your kitchen wipe-up cloth to leave a residue that keeps out ants. Pour vinegar all around your house outside, using one gallon for every five feet, to deter ants. Do this several times a year. Keep foliage trimmed next to the house. You may also use an electronic pest deterrent (see *Sources*).

Remove all cans and bottles of "stuff" from the bathroom, to the garage. The chlorine bleach is stored in the garage. Someone else can bring it in to clean the toilet (only). Leave only the borax-soap, homemade soap, and grain alcohol antiseptic. Toilet paper and tissues should be <u>unfragranced, uncolored</u>. All colognes, after shave, anything you can smell must be removed. Family members should buy unfragranced products which <u>must not</u> contain isopropyl alcohol. They should smoke outdoors, blow-dry their hair outdoors or in the garage, use nail polish and polish remover outdoors or in the garage.

Do not sleep in a bedroom that is paneled or has wallpaper. They give off arsenic fumes and formaldehyde. Either remove them or move your bed to a different room. Leave the house while this is being done. If other rooms have paneling or wallpaper, close their doors and spend no time in them.

Take taurine and cysteine to help your body recover from formaldehyde damage (same dosages as given on page 167).

Do not keep new foam furniture in the house. If it is less than one year old, move it into the garage until you are well. It gives off formaldehyde. <u>Wash new clothing</u> for the same reason. And do not sleep on foam pillows or a foam mattress.

---

[53] Boric acid is available by the pound from farm supply stores or see *Sources*. Because it looks like sugar, keep it in the garage, <u>labeled</u>, to prevent accidental poisoning.

Turn off radiators and cover them with big plastic garbage bags, or paint them, or remove them. They give off asbestos from the old paint.

Do not use the hot water from an electric hot water heater for cooking or drinking. It has tungsten. Do not drink water that sits in glazed crock ware (the glaze seeps toxic elements like cadmium) like some water dispensers have. Do not buy water from your health food store or any other dispensing place. All holding tanks, all stills, all pumps, must be periodically cleaned, sterilized and greased. Petroleum derived products are used for this. These pollute the water. You can identify them with a Syncrometer. It would be interesting to find out who is servicing your health food store's supply and with what.

Change all the galvanized or copper water pipes to PVC plastic. **All cancer patients have a buildup of copper.** If you are already anemic, this is your top priority. Copper prevents iron from being used by the body to make hemoglobin. Copper uses up your glutathione. Copper causes mutations. It would be wise to switch to plastic plumbing before anybody in your home develops illnesses. Although PVC is a toxic substance, amazingly, the water is free of PVC in three weeks!

If you have a water softener, by-pass it immediately and re-place the metal pipe on the user side of the softener tank. Softener salts are polluted with strontium and chromate; they are also full of aluminum. The salts corrode the pipes so the pipes begin to seep cadmium into the water. After changing your pipes to plastic, there will be so little iron and hardness left, you may not need a softener. If the water comes from a well, con-sider changing the well-pipe to PVC to get rid of iron. While the well is open, have the pump checked for PCBs. Call the Health Department to arrange the testing. If you must have softening after all this, check into the new magnetic varieties of water softener (although they only work well when used with plastic plumbing).

Another option is to coat the inside of your copper pipes with epoxy (see *Sources*). The coating hardens in a day; it did not appear in the white blood cells later when I tested with the Syncrometer.

Metal from your water pipes can not be filtered out or distilled out. Filters were only meant to remove the amount of metal in city water. Corrosion overburdens it. A new filter may work well for only the first 5 days! Filters even <u>add</u> to the water pollution unless they are made of only carbon. Reverse osmosis water usually contains <u>ytterbium</u> and <u>thulium</u>!

The cleanest heat is electric. Go total electric if possible. If you must stay with gas, have a furnace repair person check your furnace and look for gas leaks before the heating season starts. Don't call the gas company even though it is free. The gas company misses 4 out of 5 leaks! The Health Department does not miss any; call them!

Don't stop because you are already feeling better. Illness can return with a vengeance. Get every clean-up job completed so you can feel secure for your next doctor's checkup and for your future.

It is possible to get most of this house cleaning done in one day. Do all you possibly can. The more difficult jobs may take a week. This is a week of lost time if you are scheduled for a biopsy.

Suppose you have nobody who is willing to clean up the house, basement, garage for you, or take on your pets for a month while you find them a new home. Don't delay for a minute if you should be invited to stay with a friend or relative who is willing to clean up their place for you and take you to the dentist. Remember it is your <u>own</u> home that is the most toxic place for <u>you</u>. If there are no invitations, go on vacation or put yourself into a non-paneled, smoke-free motel room (bring your own soap, sheets, and pillowcases, and ask that they not "clean" your room or spray it). If you have a camper, remember to clean it up first. Foam and paneling must be out of it. Gas lines should be checked or closed off. Simply being outdoors is your safest place. A sunny beach, with shady places, where you can rest all day is ideal. Remember not to use any sunscreen or suntan lotions; make your own (see *Recipes*) or simply wear a hat.

Unnatural Chemicals

...and where I found them.

ARSENIC

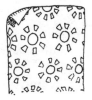

in ant & roach hives,
grains of pesticide

in carpet & furniture "treated"
for stain resistance

in wallpaper

BARIUM

MOLYBDENUM

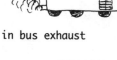

in lipstick

in bus exhaust

in "molys"

COBALT

in laundry
detergent

in dishwasher
detergent

in skin bracer

in mouthwash

ANTIMONY

CADMIUM and COPPER

TITANIUM

in eye liner

in water running
through old metal pipes

in face powder &
other powders, and
in metal dental ware

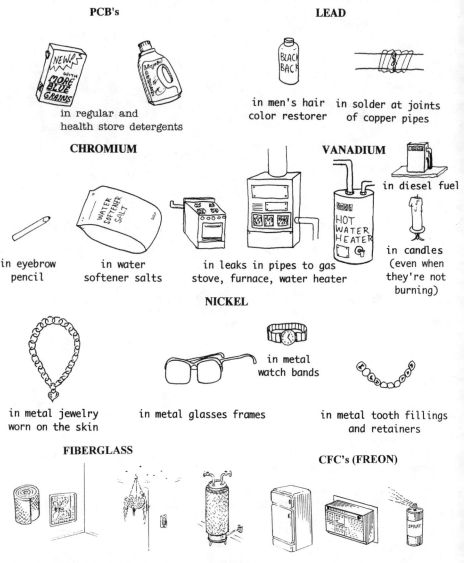

PCB's

in regular and health store detergents

LEAD

in men's hair color restorer

in solder at joints of copper pipes

CHROMIUM

in eyebrow pencil

in water softener salts

in leaks in pipes to gas stove, furnace, water heater

VANADIUM

in diesel fuel

in candles (even when they're not burning)

NICKEL

in metal watch bands

in metal jewelry worn on the skin

in metal glasses frames

in metal tooth fillings and retainers

FIBERGLASS

from insulation behind holes in ceiling or uncovered outlets, water heater jackets, stuffed around fans and air conditioners, insulation

CFC's (FREON)

in refrigerators

in air conditioners

in spray cans

MERCURY and THALLIUM

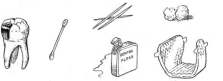

in tooth fillings, sanitary napkins, cotton balls
dental floss, toothpicks, cotton swabs

THULIUM

in most brands of
vitamin C I tested

DYSPROSIUM and LUTETIUM

in paint, varnish,
shellac

HOLMIUM

in hand cleaners

HAFNIUM

in nail polish
& hair spray

RHENIUM

in spray starch

BISMUTH

in cologne and
stomache aids

CESIUM

 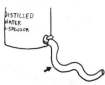

in clear-as-glass
plastic

after running through
long plastic hose

TIN and STRONTIUM

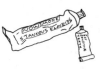

in toothpaste

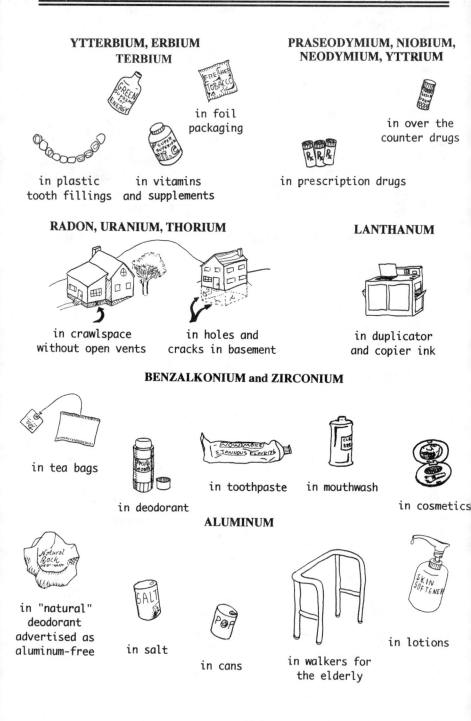

YTTERBIUM, ERBIUM TERBIUM

in foil packaging

in plastic tooth fillings

in vitamins and supplements

PRASEODYMIUM, NIOBIUM, NEODYMIUM, YTTRIUM

in over the counter drugs

in prescription drugs

RADON, URANIUM, THORIUM

in crawlspace without open vents

in holes and cracks in basement

LANTHANUM

in duplicator and copier ink

BENZALKONIUM and ZIRCONIUM

in tea bags

in deodorant

in toothpaste

in mouthwash

in cosmetics

ALUMINUM

in "natural" deodorant advertised as aluminum-free

in salt

in cans

in walkers for the elderly

in lotions

186

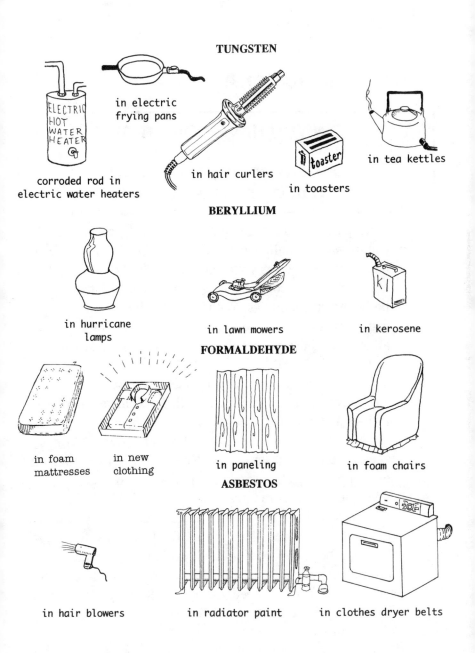

TUNGSTEN

in electric
frying pans

in hair curlers

in toasters

in tea kettles

corroded rod in
electric water heaters

BERYLLIUM

in hurricane
lamps

in lawn mowers

in kerosene

FORMALDEHYDE

in foam
mattresses

in new
clothing

in paneling

in foam chairs

ASBESTOS

in hair blowers

in radiator paint

in clothes dryer belts

187

Visit Your Doctor Again

> ## NOW YOU HAVE DONE IT ALL!
>
> ## Look forward to your next visit
> ## with your cancer doctor!

- Your parasites are gone. Without *Fasciolopsis* stages you cannot have a malignancy. Without *Clostridium*, *Ascaris*, and tapeworm stages your tumors can shrink.
- You have cleaned out the isopropyl alcohol from your body and surroundings. Without this solvent you can't get cancer again. Notice from the case histories how isopropyl alcohol disappears from the body simply by removing the sources.
- You have changed your copper plumbing.
- You have extracted the teeth with large metal or plastic fillings and have replaced them with methacrylate partials. Small fillings have been removed by air abrasion. You are keeping them squeaky clean. You are no longer sucking on copper, cobalt, vanadium, malonic and maleic acid, urethane or scarlet red dye.
- You have switched to foods that are malonate-free and not moldy or processed. This means foods that are fresh and have not been chopped, ground, extracted and mixed with other chopped, ground, extracted foods to create concoctions. You have stopped using supplements unless you know they have been tested for isopropyl alcohol pollution. You are using only safe supplements.
- You have stopped putting chemicals on your skin, in your mouth, on your hair, in your armpits, on your eyelids, on

your teeth, on your scalp, on your nails, in your nose, or lungs.

- You have cleaned the house of all the chemicals that your body considers toxic.
- You have gotten rid of your Freon-containing refrigerator.
- You are zapping every day.

Congratulations, this is a big accomplishment!

I hope you did all this in the first week after you bought this book and started on the parasite killing program. You stand an excellent chance of turning your surgeon's verdict around!

If you have had three weeks of this healthful lifestyle, you should ask your doctor for a fresh evaluation of your situation. The three weeks is counted from the time you finished all the clean-ups. Most patients are too intimidated by their doctors to speak up for themselves. Always take a family member or friend with you to give you courage. If lumps are going down or pain is reduced, tell your doctor about this, so he or she has some basis for giving you a postponement. If a new specimen is taken from you for testing, it may be evaluated by the lab as "questionable" or "indeterminate" or "atypical" but not "definite", like before. As more time passes for healing to take place, the tests will get even better. Wait for this to happen rather than approving a surgery that could handicap you for life. Yet you must have tangible evidence of improvement. Time is limited and the battle is for your life. Choose wisely.

Stay Clean

Here are a few more facts on where we are getting the human intestinal fluke stages. Since the infective stage in nature is the metacercarial[54] stage, are we eating metacercaria from vegetation like lettuce? I have not seen evidence for this but it must be researched, thoroughly, as a possibility.

You will see in the case histories how some people test YES (positive) for parasites in spite of having completed the parasite killing program and being on the maintenance program. This is possible because a reinfection can occur in as little as one hour! Of course, your own bowel is the most likely source of reinfection. Keep hands sanitary by rinsing with grain alcohol solution. And never, never put fingers in your mouth. Observe the best sanitation rules. Zap daily and stay on the maintenance parasite program and Mop Up. In cases of persistent reinfection the patient either had family members who were infected (although symptom-free), or they had repeatedly indulged in fast foods or delicatessen meats. Parasites can make good progress in two days (eating you up and reproducing in you) if given the chance.

Unfortunately for fast food lovers, the solution is not to make a daily routine out of the maintenance program. Herbs powerful enough to kill parasites probably are not advisable on a daily basis.

You must avoid parasites in daily life!

---

[54] Remember, in nature, the cercaria swim to a plant and attach themselves to a leaf. There they lose their tails and are called *metacercaria*. It is the overwintering stage.

Meat Could Be A Source

Are we getting metacercaria from eating animals that have the parasite[55]? Suppose we eat the raw blood of an animal that has this parasite. The animal's blood has eggs, miracidia, redia, cercaria and metacercaria in it. We swallow those live eggs, miracidia, redia, cercaria and metacercaria.

The metacercaria are meant to attach themselves to our intestine and grow larger, into adults that lay more eggs. But could the eggs, miracidia and redia that we eat also survive and develop in us? The miracidia and cercaria with their tails could simply swim away into our bodies. The eggs could hatch into more miracidia. Isopropyl alcohol will let the stages develop in the liver as well as other tissues that have toxins in them. This causes a population explosion and ortho-phospho-tyrosine production, namely cancer.

ground beef   ground turkey   chicken

Fig. 73 Meat sources?

When would we eat raw blood? In raw beef such as rare hamburger or steak! In raw turkey as in turkey burgers! And in raw chicken as in chicken burgers! Just handling these raw

---

[55] Nobody has checked beef herds in the USA or the imported sources for the presence of *Fasciolopsis buskii*. It is urgent to find out whether cattle, fowl and pets have become a biological reservoir and are transmitting it to some of us. *Fasciola hepatica, Eurytrema* and *Clonorchis* should also be searched for because I find them so frequently.

meats would put the infective stages on your hands! What a terrifying risk this gives us!

Some flukes are large enough to be seen with the naked eye, although their various stages usually need a low powered microscope. Therefore it should be possible to examine any meat sample from the grocery store to verify this source, and I did!

Look at the photos of ground meats. There are objects that look identical to the stages of flukes. Research needs to be done to culture them in order to classify them accurately.

This raises the possibility, in fact, the <u>probability</u>, that our meat animals are the "biological reservoir," namely <u>source of infection</u>, by the cancer causing parasite! The human intestinal fluke was first studied in certain snails in ponds in China. Are our farm ponds similarly infested? If so, our animals have an obvious source of metacercaria.

The best advice is to become a seafood vegetarian immediately.

The second best advice is to cook all meats for at least 20 minutes at the boiling point, as in baking. Roast it until the meat falls off the bone. Don't eat any meat except fish and seafood in a restaurant. Restaurants cannot be entrusted with so important a cooking rule. Don't eat delicatessen meat. Are there other sources of this parasite? We need to search our food supply for other possible sources.

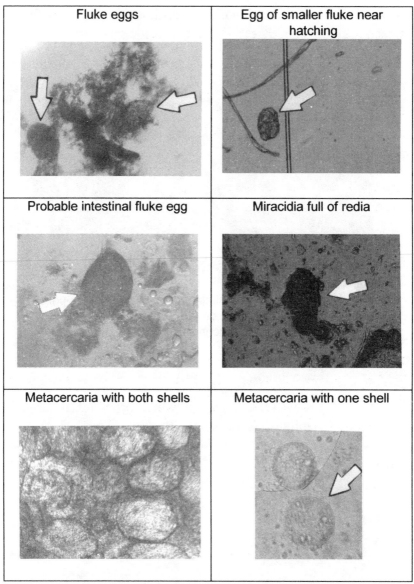

Fig. 74 Likely fluke stages in meat (100x)

Animals could not always have been infested with these fluke parasites. Cows, chickens and turkeys are not the natural hosts of the *human intestinal fluke* (although swine are). And parasite stages, should never be found inside these animals. But

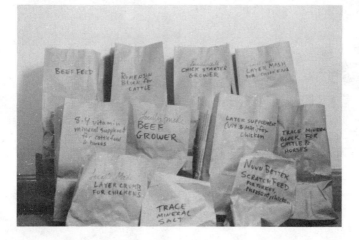

All animal feeds tested, except simple grain mixtures, were polluted with solvents such as benzene, carbon tetrachloride, isopropanol, wood alcohol, etc.
Fig. 75 Some polluted animal feed

their feeds are now full of solvents, which promotes abnormal parasitism in them, just as it does in us.

Even bird feed was found to have benzene and other solvents in it. Buy seed only.

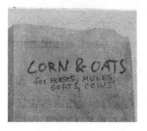

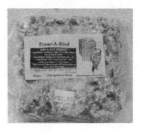

Fig. 77 Solvent free   *Fig. 76 Bad bird feed*

Milk Could Be A Source

Because milk is a body fluid, dairy cows with fluke parasites would be expected to have fluke stages in their milk. Everything made from milk would likewise have fluke stages. This includes butter, cream, and products that contain whey, like acidophilus cultures. Boiling kills them. Pasteurization does not!

Sex Could Be A Source

Since the infective stages of the intestinal fluke are microscopically tiny and can travel throughout the body in the blood, it is possible that some may get into the genital tract and genital fluids. It would be wise to practice protected sex. However, if both parties go through the parasite-killing program, there is no risk of constant reinfection through unprotected sex. See the photos of parasite stages in urine. This is certainly evidence for sexual transmission.

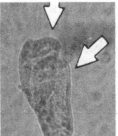

Two overlapped miracidia. (100x)

Fig. 78 Miracidia in urine

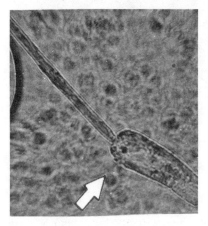 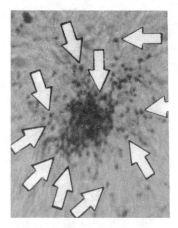

Cercaria seen in urine (400x) Sperm for comparison (400x)
Fig. 79 Cercaria in urine vs. sperm

Cercaria resemble sperm, which you might expect to see in urine from a male. However the size difference makes them easy to distinguish.

Blood Could Be A Source

The blood carries the infective stages of the intestinal fluke. Until the public blood supply can be searched for them[56], it is not safe. If you need surgery, use your own blood or get it from someone who has gone through the parasite-killing program. Of course, without isopropyl alcohol in your body, such an infection could not give you cancer but it is still very undesirable.

Mother's Milk Could Be A Source

If your body is teeming with very tiny fluke stages because of the solvent in your tissues, could they be transmitted through mother's milk? See the photograph of mother's milk. It shows a fluke egg almost ready to hatch. The mother was full of benzene. The baby was full of benzene from drinking the mother's milk. The family was using cooking oil polluted with benzene.

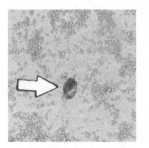
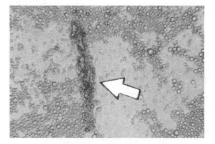

Egg (100x)　　　　　Miracidia developing redia (100x)
Fig. 80 Parasites in human milk

---

[56] Antibodies to the various fluke stages or antigen tests could be used to test the public blood supply for parasite stages. I know of no existing human intestinal fluke test besides my electronic method.

Saliva Could Be A Source

Saliva is another body fluid that carries the tiny developmental stages of the fluke parasites. This means that kissing on the mouth could transmit the cancer parasite. But would you eventually get cancer? Only if you had isopropyl alcohol in you!

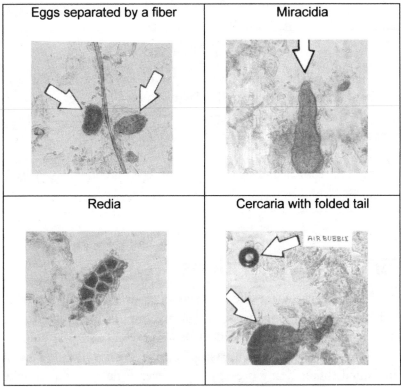

Fig. 81 Parasites in human saliva (100X)

Pets Could Be A Source

Because pet food is heavily polluted with aflatoxins and solvents, including isopropyl alcohol and benzene, is it any wonder that they, too, get the human intestinal fluke? Fluke stages are plentiful in the saliva. <u>Never</u> kiss your pet. Feed your pets home made food as our grandparents did. Keep all your pets on the Pet Parasite Program.

To summarize:

1. We are eating the infective stages of the intestinal fluke in beef, chicken, turkey and dairy products.
2. We then transmit it to each other by kissing on the mouth and sex.
3. Even if we pick it up in these two ways, we would not get cancer from it unless we have isopropyl alcohol in our bodies.

Biological Questions

My tests show me the close association between parasites, solvents and carcinogens. And that mycotoxins and bacteria are also crucially involved in cancer. But many questions remain.

Since there is never a case of cancer without adult human intestinal flukes being present in the liver,[57] do the adults make ortho-phospho-tyrosine, namely cause cancer? Obviously not, because in many of us it is in its normal "home", the intestine, and we do not have cancer. **Only when it is in the liver** do I find ortho-phospho-tyrosine in the body, but usually in a tissue

---

[57] In a few case histories they were not observed.

far away from the liver. It is found where the baby stages and carcinogens (copper, fungus, etc.) are. Do the stages make the ortho-phospho-tyrosine?

Why must there be isopropyl alcohol in the liver and cancerous tissue for cancer to develop? Is isopropyl alcohol part of the chemistry of ortho-phospho-tyrosine formation? Are the eggs and cercaria attracting the isopropyl alcohol or is the isopropyl alcohol damaged tissue attracting the parasite stages? Or is isopropyl alcohol simply force-hatching the eggs or metacercaria?

We have found a bacterium, *Clostridium*, to be present in every tumor. And, indeed, a bacterial theory has been worked on in the past. Dr. Livingstone-Wheeler believed the bacterium to be *Progenitor cryptocides*. A book has been published about her findings.[58]

Could there be a *virus* that is really doing all this instead of the fluke? Again, if the virus belonged to a fluke-bacterium or to the fluke itself, it would be plausible. The virus theory has quite an impressive amount of research behind it.

Why do some people have isopropyl alcohol in their livers, intestine and white blood cells after using shampoo or shaving chemicals while others do not? Evidently, many people can detoxify it quickly so it doesn't build up. Is this a liver problem, caused by the fluke, or a toxin such as aflatoxin B? I never see isopropyl alcohol without aflatoxin B being present. Or do other known carcinogens act by inhibiting isopropyl alcohol detoxification?

If aflatoxin B is the culprit, why does it accumulate in some of us but not others, since we all get plenty of it in our diet? I have evidence indicating vitamin C protects against aflatoxin B.

---

[58] *The Conquest of Cancer* by Virginia Livingston-Wheeler, MD and E.G. Addeo, Franklin Watts 1984.

There are documented cases of large doses of vitamin C being effective against cancer.

Because I always see *Aspergillus* fungus growing in the cancerous tissues, is aflatoxin being produced right then and there? Or are we merely eating too much aflatoxin? I also see *Penicillium* fungus with its mycotoxin, patulin.

What is the role played by human Chorionic Gonadotropin (hCG)? It is always found in the liver, at the same location where the isopropyl alcohol is found, but only <u>after</u> isopropyl alcohol builds up there. And I see hCG <u>before</u> ortho-phospho-tyrosine is made. hCG quickly spreads itself throughout the body (notice how often it is found "everywhere" in the case histories). Does hCG <u>tag</u> the tissue that will become cancerous and begin to make ortho-phospho-tyrosine? Is it being made by a mutant gene?

What is the role played by other growth factors? What about tumor necrosis factor? Why don't cancer patients have this like others do? Are they eating more patulin?

Why does only *Fasciolopsis* cause cancer when many other flukes are also multiplying? Production of ortho-phospho-tyrosine can be stimulated by NMDA receptor activation.[59] Perhaps the intestinal fluke alone possesses a virus, a bacterium, or an antigen epitope that fits in the NMDA receptors.

Fortunately, these questions don't have to be answered before you cure yourself of cancer.

---

[59] Hilmar Bading and Michael E. Greenberg, *Stimulation of Protein Tyrosine Phosphorylation by NMDA Receptor Activation*, Science 1991, vol. 253, pp. 912-914.

A Look On The Bright Side

- Fluke parasites are very easy to kill, much easier than many roundworms or tapeworms (tapeworms survive the parasite herbs).
- Not everything is polluted. Only the processed foods are, and not even all of them. If we eat natural food, we will be safe. (And if we eat malonic-free natural food we will be healthy!)
- I have never seen a case of mercury toxicity from eating fish. It is always amalgam tooth fillings.
- PCB pollution is not in everything (but they are prevalent in detergents).
- I have never seen a case of lead, arsenic or pesticide toxicity from eating fruit or vegetables. Pesticides used on foods haven't penetrated them, as far as my tests show. Simply cut away the blossom and stem end, and wash thoroughly. But don't eat food <u>sprayed to keep it fresh</u>! Such food must be peeled or ozonated, not just washed.
- Municipal water is still the safest source. I found no cases of lead, asbestos, aluminum, or any solvent toxicity due to city water, and only a few cases of arsenic or PCBs. Evidently, the immune system can keep up with this small concentration even with constant use.
- Solvents, PCBs, aflatoxins, and 4,5 benzopyrene leave the body in a few days after you stop getting them into your body, not a few years! Only Freon and copper persist— for weeks.
- Lead is not coming from paint; it is mainly coming from lead solder joints on copper water pipes.
- Asbestos is not coming from municipal water or building materials; it is mostly coming from your own clothes dryer belts (imported varieties) and hair blowers.

- Although milk (or buttermilk) is a much maligned beverage, it is still unpolluted with metals, solvents, or aflatoxins. But it should be bottled in plastic containers to avoid dioxane contamination, and have no dye added. Boil it briefly to rid it of bacteria and parasite stages and have vitamin C added to rid it of malonate. This would protect all the butter and cheeses made from it later.
- Benzene and other solvents are not coming from widespread gasoline pollution. Instead, benzene is coming from our foods and products, due to the mistaken belief that we can use petroleum products in the manufacturing of food. This is an easier problem to correct.

Part Three: Case Histories

The case histories you are about to read are NOT picked out of the files because they got cured, leaving other cases behind who did not get cured. These 138 cases are ALL the cancer cases that walked or were helped into the office over a sixteen month period.

Although not all of them were diagnosed as having cancer by their clinical doctor, I considered them to have cancer if they tested YES (positive) for *ortho-phospho-tyrosine* (the abnormal growth stimulant). See *The Tests* for more information on cancer markers. Similarly I considered them "cured" when they tested NO (negative) to ortho-phospho-tyrosine, even though other symptoms did not immediately abate.

The names have been changed to ones of the same sex picked at random from a telephone directory. Ages have been changed by up to five years. Some personal characteristics have been changed in non-essential ways.

All of them got cured if they carried out the instructions. 35 did not carry out instructions or could not be followed or had special circumstances that prevented them from carrying out the instructions. This leaves 103 who did get cured. As you will read, the method is 100% effective in stopping cancer regardless of the type of cancer or how terminal it may be. It follows that this method must work for you, too, if you are able to carry out the instructions.

Types Of Tests

Cancer We test for ortho-phospho-tyrosine. HCG is tested occasionally as a pre-cancer indicator. As the correlation between cancer, *Fasciolopsis* (human intestinal fluke) in the liver, and isopropyl alcohol became clearer, I often tested those next.

HIV We test for Protein 24 antigen. Remarkably, HIV/AIDS is caused (and cured) very similarly to cancer and is the subject of another book by this author.

Parasites About 120 varieties, including intermediate stages.

Toxic elements About 70 varieties.

Solvents 27 varieties.

Pathogens (bacteria and viruses) About 80 varieties.

Kidney stones Seven varieties.

Blood (which includes urine) This testing is done by a commercial laboratory, and depending on the panels selected, could be 50 or more tests.

Obviously most of these tests are not part of eliminating ortho-phospho-tyrosine and curing cancer. They <u>are</u> essential for learning how to get well, however.

We have the capability of testing each of the above 300 substances in any of the body's 100 tissues for which I have samples. It is unrealistic to even attempt to accomplish these 30,000 possible tests. Typically about 30 tests can be completed in an average office visit, and I select the most useful ones for the client. Only the YES (positive) results and significant NO (negative) results are shown in these case histories.

See *The Tests* chapter for more information about each test.

Not all of the cases are roaring successes, but there are lessons in all of them that can put <u>you</u> on the road to recovery.

| 1 | Lydia Hernandez | Breast Cancer |

Lydia Hernandez is a 62 year old school teacher, developing cataracts and suddenly losing her hearing. She has seen an Ear, Nose and Throat doctor and had a CAT scan and MRI. She is aching all over. The purpose of her visit was her laryngitis which she has had 4 days. Cannot speak at all.

☒ Arsenic (Toxic Element) YES (present in her white blood cells)

We will test home air and school room air for arsenic. She will collect a dust sample in a jar of water. After finding arsenic we did not complete the toxic element test or do other tests because this is not a scheduled visit. She will make an appointment.

Five days later

Both breasts are hot and tender with the nipple affected. Throat still raspy. Ear bothering her.

☒ Ortho-phospho-tyrosine (Cancer) YES

☒ Fasciolopsis (Parasite) YES at liver

She will start on parasite killing program.

☒ Cobalt (Toxic Element) YES at breast

Stop detergent.

☒ Chromate (Toxic Element) YES at breast

Stop cosmetics.

☒ Antimony (Toxic Element) YES at breast

Stop cosmetics.

☒ Copper (Toxic Element) YES at breast

Has no metal tooth fillings but has copper water pipes.

☒ Asbestos (Toxic Element) YES at breast

☒ Bismuth (Toxic Element) YES at breast

Stop cosmetics. She has brought in a sample of school air where she teaches. It was YES (positive) for arsenic and asbestos. She is on antibiotics, cortisone, and sinus medicine from her clinical doctor. She is getting sick leave from teaching.

Four days later

Breasts are feeling better.

☐ **Fasciolopsis (Parasite) NO**

She will continue parasite killing program as on the instruction sheet.

☐ **Asbestos, Bismuth, Antimony, Cobalt (Toxic Elements) NO**

☒ **Copper (Toxic Element) NO at breast, YES at liver**

☒ **Chromate (Toxic Element) YES**

Will disconnect water softener. She went off detergent and cosmetics. She is not in the school building. She has brought water samples from her faucets: hot water is YES (positive) for chromate.

Three weeks later

Throat feels bad. Head is congested. Breasts OK.

☒ **Asbestos (Toxic Element) YES**

From school room air – would like to retire from school teaching rather than go to school office with the news about asbestos.

☒ **Copper (Toxic Element) YES**

From water pipes; husband unwilling to change pipes.

☒ **Fasciolopsis eggs (Parasite) YES**

By some oversight she has not taken cloves in the parasite program, <u>will start immediately</u>. She can find no solution to the copper and asbestos problem.

Two months later

She reports her doctor found a 2½ cm cyst in left ovary. She will repeat parasite treatment.

Two months later

☒ **Arsenic, Copper (Toxic Elements) YES**

She will take 2 thioctic capsules (100 mg) three times a day and change metal glasses to plastic frames to reduce metal absorption.

☐ **Fasciolopsis (Parasite) NO**

☐ **Ortho-phospho-tyrosine (Cancer) NO**

☐ **Solvents (ALL) NO**

She will stay on parasite maintenance program and avoid rare meats in her diet.

Five months later

She had a cavitation cleaned by dentist and two wisdom teeth pulled. Her fibrositis is suddenly gone, groin pain gone, TMJ gone on one side. Arsenic still YES. She will steam clean her carpets, drapes, upholstery. Overall, she feels much better.

Summary: This was a case where cancer was not suspected until she had the breast symptoms. Note how the breast had collected three toxic elements from her cosmetics. The water softener is a toxicity source as well as the copper water pipes. Lydia was fortunate to regain her health but the arsenic is relentless. Hopefully she will get it removed from her home and also retire from school teaching. There are many sources of pesticide (wallpaper, carpet/drape/upholstery treatments, pesticides), but the most likely source at her school would be pesticide in the lunch room and kitchen. Pesticides are generally odorless, so we don't suspect them.

2	Janet Chapman	Carcinoma at thymus and lung

Janet Chapman is a 45 year old pleasant woman whose main problem is carcinoma. At the age of 24 she had hepatitis. It took her several months to get over it. Then, after a few years, she had a partial hysterectomy for numerous cysts in the ovary and uterus. She has one ovary left.

She started having a heavy feeling in her chest and getting tired. Her doctor put her on Premarin™ and Provera™ for energy. She took that for 1½ years. She got some energy out of it. Recently, her doctor took a chest x-ray and found a tumor in the thymus gland. They did a biopsy of the tumor which came back negative to cancer. They did surgery, to remove the tumor, and found it was indeed cancerous with many other "fingers" all over the chest and a couple of spots on the right lower lung. Part of the diaphragm was cut during this surgery; a nerve to the vocal cord was also injured. The thymus gland was removed, but "fingers of thymus" were not.

She also had 36 radiation treatments over a 7-week time period. Then everything showed up OK until about two months ago when she had tightness of chest again.

Last week fluid was taken off [from] her chest. A tumor is in her left chest cavity. Her worst symptom is "terrible tightness over stomach." She got to feeling bad soon after the fluid was taken off her chest.

☒ **Ortho-phospho-tyrosine (Cancer) YES** at thymus, lung

☒ **Fasciolopsis (Parasite) YES at liver, and** unknown location (couldn't find)

☒ **Fasciolopsis redia (Parasite)   YES** at thymus, lungs, bone marrow

☐ **Sheep liver fluke (Parasite) NO**
She will start on parasite program although swallowing is difficult. Her brothers brought her to the office because husband is skeptical of alternative therapies. Janet coughs a lot and holds her mid-abdomen due to pain. But she is interested and willing to try to get well. I suggested they coax her husband to come along next time.

One week later

☐ **Ortho-phospho-tyrosine (Cancer) NO**

☐ **Fasciolopsis and all stages (Parasite) NO**

☒ **Formaldehyde (Toxic Element) YES and very high**
They will test house air and she will sleep out of house, in RV.

Five days later

She is still coughing and very weak. Formaldehyde YES, even higher than last time. The RV has foam and paneling in it. House air tested YES to formaldehyde in one bedroom only. They have a water softener (will ask husband to disconnect). She has lost 5 pounds in the last 3 weeks. They will move the new furniture in the house into the garage so she can safely sleep in the house. Her brothers are planning to take her on vacation.

Three weeks later

Her cough is worse. She has been on vacation with brothers and did OK while away from home but got worse immediately after getting home. Her husband came with her this time.

☐ **Ortho-phospho-tyrosine (Cancer) NO**

☒ **Formaldehyde (Toxic Element) YES and very high**
New foam furniture has not been removed from her bedroom – was a gift; husband didn't want to hurt relatives' feelings.

☒ Dog heartworm (Parasite) YES

Dog heartworm also causes coughing (husband critical of this finding). Note: she is simply dying of heartworm and formaldehyde. The cancer was stopped weeks ago.

Summary: it has been several months and I am afraid we will get a telephone call soon, telling us that Janet died. It would have been so easy to clear the house of formaldehyde just by removing certain pieces of furniture. The heartworm, too, could have been eliminated in a week. But the supportive part of the family lived far away. And the non-supportive part lived with her. Was it because she is a woman, or because she was sick, that kept her from asserting herself enough to follow the treatment she wanted to follow? I fear another wonderful young person has paid the price that dogmatic belief in purely clinical concepts exacts. The husbands, in either this case or the last case, are not to blame. Ignorance is.

3	Ida Birdsall	Cervical Cancer

Ida is middle-aged, recently remarried. She has blood in her urine. She has seen her gynecologist who did a PAP smear. In the hospital she had chest x-ray, blood test, EKG followed by a D & C. One week after D & C, her regular doctor told her the tissue removed from her uterus during D & C showed moderate carcinoma.

☒ Ortho-phospho-tyrosine (Cancer) YES at cervix

☒ Arsenic (Toxic Element) YES at cervix, uterus

☒ Tellurium (Toxic Element) YES at cervix, uterus

Usually from metal in tooth fillings, but she has complete dentures—no metal!

☒ Fasciolopsis (Parasite) YES

Start on parasite program. They have a water softener. Will bypass it immediately. We will test dentures for tellurium by soaking in distilled water overnight and testing the water.

Three days later

☒ Arsenic, Tellurium (Toxic Elements) YES

☒ **Tellurium (Toxic Element) YES in denture water, YES in lower denture white plastic, NO in lower denture pink plastic, NO in upper denture, white or pink.**

The tellurium is apparently in the lower denture, white part. She needs new metal-free dentures. They will steam clean carpets and furniture to get rid of arsenic. They had been commercially cleaned and treated for stain resistance last summer; this is the probable source of arsenic.

Four months later

She has had a complete hysterectomy.

☒ **Ortho-phospho-tyrosine (Cancer) YES**

☒ **Fasciolopsis (Parasite) YES at liver**

☒ **Fasciolopsis cercaria and eggs (Parasite) YES in blood**

Start again on parasite program in spite of loose bowels Note: the hysterectomy did not clear her of cancer.

Two weeks later

☐ **Ortho-phospho-tyrosine (Cancer) NO**

☒ **Fasciolopsis cercaria (Parasite) YES in blood, still!**

Continue parasite program - increase dosage.

Summary: We had been seeing this happy pair of middle-age newlyweds for about a year before the cancer struck. Each time I found arsenic in Ida's white blood cells. They just couldn't seem to get it out of their home. They took such pride in remodeling their home that they just couldn't believe anything like arsenic could be lurking in the carpets. Suddenly it was too late. She had to have a hysterectomy. They were crushed. And they were perplexed when the cancer wasn't gone after the surgery. But they carried out the instructions and took on new living habits and became completely free of it. Maybe they'll live "happily ever after" now with that important lesson behind them.

4	Pamela Charles	Breast Cancer

Pamela Charles is a middle aged woman who had just been discharged from the hospital. She had a lump removed from left breast, also 8 lymph nodes, two of which were cancerous. She is in middle of radiation treatment. The cancer was discovered by mammogram. Three years ago she had a heart attack for which she got angioplasty.

☒ **Ortho-phospho-tyrosine (Cancer) YES at bone, edge of breast**

☐ **Protein 24 (HIV) NO**

☒ **Fasciolopsis (Parasite) YES at liver**

☒ **Isopropyl Alcohol (Solvent) YES**

☐ **Remainder of solvents NO**
> She will search for all sources of "prop" (propyl alcohol, isopropyl, etc.) and remove from her house. She will start parasite program.

Eight weeks later

☐ **Ortho-phospho-tyrosine (Cancer) NO**

☐ **Toxic Elements (All) NO**

☐ **Solvents (All) NO**

☐ **Fasciolopsis and all stages (Parasite) NO**

BLOOD TEST	Result	Comment
phosphate	high	she is dissolving her bones

She will drink three cups 2% milk, reduce phosphate foods, take a magnesium oxide tablet daily (300 mg). Continue parasite program. Client released.

Summary: Note that Pamela still had the cancer in spite of the recent surgery. In fact, it was spreading to the bone. Since she was sandwiched into a 15 minute time slot, I didn't do complete testing. Her finances don't allow her to come back to improve her heart condition.

5	Brenda Rasmussen	Breast Cancer

Brenda Rasmussen is 43, came from three states away for a large, malignant lump (size of hen's egg) over right breast. She has not accepted the doctor's diagnosis, does not wish to talk about cancer. Her friend asked us not to mention cancer! She also has high blood pressure and nervous anxiety. She is using no caffeine, alcohol, nicotine. Her chiropractor is concerned. She gets very little sleep.

☒ **Ortho-phospho-tyrosine (Cancer) YES at breast, with some spreading**

☒ **Antimony (Toxic Element) YES at breast**
Suspect perfume.

☒ **Cobalt (Toxic Element) YES at breast**
Suspect detergent.

☒ **Copper (Toxic Element) YES at breast**
Suspect tooth fillings.

☒ **Aluminum Silicate (Toxic Element) YES at breast**
Suspect salt.

☒ **Nickel (Toxic Element) YES at breast**
Suspect tooth fillings. She will go off salt (buy Hain Sea Salt™ only). She was given ornithine, 4 at bedtime, to sleep. Also thioctic acid, 1 every waking hour to remove heavy metal. She will go off her perfume, lipstick, sunscreen, lip balm, eye cleansing cream, other cosmetics, detergents, and massage oil. She will buy new socks and underwear and use only borax to wash her hair and do laundry.

Next day
We pursued her intestinal problem which she didn't mention yesterday.

PARASITES: No adult flukes found. Didn't test for parasite stages. Giardia and pin worms only. She has been getting colonics. Start parasite program.

☒ **Tungsten (Toxic Element) YES very high at colon!**
Eats no toast, does not use a wok, or drink electrically heated water; suspect water for colonics - will get sample.

Next day
Received sample of colonic water. It was YES (positive) for tungsten (stop colonics). Her urinalysis showed oxalate crystals, blood, etc.

☒ **Asbestos, Cerium, Europium, Tellurium (Toxic Elements) YES in urinary tract**

☐ **Ortho-phospho-tyrosine (Cancer) NO**
Summary: Brenda was one of those fortunate people who can find a friend in time of need. This friend, although older than Brenda by 10 years at least, drove her 800 miles to our office only to hear Brenda

say she couldn't do dental work, couldn't give up cosmetics and could-
n't change detergent. Her friend coaxed her through some of these ob-
stacles and 6 months later called to say she was doing OK but still had
her lump. She had not stopped the colonics nor was she sticking to her
new rules of living. We thanked her kindly and wished her well.

6	Louise McAleer	Colon Cancer

Louise McAleer is a woman in her late 40s who has a number of physical problems: 1) Lower back pain. She went to a neurologist who said pain was caused by scar tissue pressing on a nerve. Pain is unbearable; she can hardly sit or stand. 2) Cannot think straight, trouble concentrating. This is probably due to the pain. 3) Diarrhea, severe for about a year. Colonoscopy did not find anything in the colon. She has not been able to go to church since December. Her legs get numb. They were cold as ice in the office. She shakes inside and gets very sick with diarrhea. 4) Pain syndrome in shoulders and arms. 5) Pain and numbness in her hands and arms. 6). Chest pain. 7) Ulcer. She reported a history of digestive problems. 8) Sleep problems. 9) Pain in left ear, running down left side of her neck.

☒ Dibasic Calcium Phosphate (Kidney Stone) YES

She does not tolerate milk. Carrot juice and vegetable juice, ½ cup/day was recommended. She does not tolerate much of anything now. She was started on kidney herb recipe.

In a brief review of her blood test, her urinalysis showed bacteria, blood, crystals. Her estrogen level was too high. It was suggested that she cut her estrogen replacement (Premarin™) dosage in half. She was also to go off caffeine, tea and benzoate preservative.

12 days later

She felt that her lower back was slightly better. All other pains persisted. She feels nauseous after eating. She reported that she could urinate better. She has a lot of pain at left lower abdomen and says she is very gassy.

☒ Fasciolopsis (Parasite) YES at liver and colon

☒ Fasciolopsis eggs (Parasite) YES at colon

Other parasites not tested.

☒ **Ortho-phospho-tyrosine (Cancer) YES**

Start immediately on parasite program. Digestive program: take Digestive Enzymes (Bronson's) 2 with breakfast, 4 with small meal and 6 with dinner.

One week later

She still has been sick all week with diarrhea, nausea, all the same symptoms. She did not take cloves. She will take them as soon as she is able.

☐ **Fasciolopsis and all stages (Parasite) NO**

☐ **Ortho-phospho-tyrosine (Cancer) NO**

☒ **Platinum (Toxic Element) YES**

Needs metal tooth fillings replaced.

Two weeks later

She is focused on TMJ (pain at hinge of jaw) today. Other pains gone, except for left ear pain and neck pain.

☒ **Clostridium (Pathogen) YES at tooth #21**

See dentist for abscess.

Summary: this youngish woman came in with a long list of severe problems. It came as a shock to her, though, that she actually had colon cancer. In spite of her severe stomach problems, she managed to get down the black walnut tincture and wormwood (in the parasite killing recipe). She didn't take any cloves. But she was lucky and all intestinal fluke stages were gone one week later. This cleared up the colitis and many other pains, too, so in 2 more weeks she was nearly free of the whole list she came with. I hope she completes her dental work and rids herself of her last remaining pains.

7	Mark Pelsuo	Acute Lymphocytic Leukemia

Mark Pelsuo is eight years old. He was diagnosed with acute leukemia, in April 1989. Since then he has been on chemotherapy. He has had radiation. He had testicular involvement and got radiation to testicles. He has responded well and looks and feels good.

His parents installed R.O. (reverse osmosis) water shortly after diagnosis. They got interested in nutrition and added brown rice to their diet. Also lots of soup, macrobiotic diet, also lots of fresh vegetables. Also added vitamins; spirulina, selenium and magnesium. Now on immune pack and vitamin C (powder).

They will bring a copy of his file. He is being monitored with blood test every three weeks.

☒ **Holmium (Toxic Element) YES at all tissues**

☒ **PCB (Toxic Element) YES at all tissues**

☒ **Ytterbium (Toxic Element) YES at all tissues**

They have well water, 25 year old well. They moved into this house 5 years ago. No industry has ever been in their neighborhood. Their pump went out two years ago because lightning hit the house which was grounded to the pump. Pump blew out at that time and was replaced. Well is about 40 feet deep and water was tested after that. Conclusion: I believe PCB source might be the well-pump that blew apart two years ago.

When they first moved into the house, the mother got very sick (in bed). For the next year she had arm numbness, dizziness, could not go up and down stairs. They tested with MRI for multiple sclerosis, brain tumor, and found nothing. She has gradually gotten better. A year later, her oldest daughter got very sick. About six months before diagnosis, Mark fell out of tree and broke both elbows.

☐ **Kidney Stones (ALL) NO**

☒ **Fasciolopsis (Parasite) YES in bone and liver (remainder untested)**

Start on parasite program.

My present theory is that the pump (a submersed type) in their well was damaged by lightning so that it spilled its PCB into the water. Since the PCB would rise to the top, their water would get much more polluted when the water level was low. The pump was replaced with another submersed kind. The father is interested in proving this theory. They agree to not use well water for any purpose and bring sample for testing next time.

Two weeks later

Cough is nearly gone. Right knee pain persists. He is due for a chemo treatment (Vincristine™) next week. They will send results from a previously done blood test and a new one to be done next week. He is on 6 MP™ (1 tab/day, 50 mg tab) daily. No side ef-

215

fects. He is on Methotrate™ 1 time/week. They have brought in water specimen to test for PCBs.

☐ **PCB, Holmium (Toxic Elements) NO**

☒ **PCB (Toxic Element) YES in well water**

☐ **PCB (Toxic Element) NO in reverse osmosis filtered water**

☐ **Ortho-phospho-tyrosine (Cancer) NO**

☒ **Pancreatic fluke (Parasite) YES**

☒ **Fasciolopsis (Parasite) YES in mother**

☒ **Fasciolopsis (Parasite) YES in father**
They need to solve their water problem and finish parasite program for whole family.

Summary: This was a health conscious family. They were intensely interested in how their PCB pollution had come about. They all promised to rid themselves of parasites and stick to some new health rules. Since they were from 2 states away, they did not plan to return unless Mark's health shows signs of deterioration. We have not heard from them for eight months.

8	Nevita Thompson	Hodgkin's Disease

Nevita Thompson is a middle-aged school teacher, very vivacious, lives on handfuls of vitamins, all carefully organized. She spends a lot each month on supplements and is happy with it. She has had Hodgkin's for several years and also has extremely high triglycerides. We saw her April, 1992. Both palms were tender and painful. She had numbness and stinging in various fingers. Her doctor diagnosed it as neuropathy.

☒ **Fasciolopsis (Parasite) YES in kidneys, bladder, colon**

☐ **Fasciolopsis other stages (Parasite) NO**
Start on parasite killing program. We will test toxins next time.

Two months and one week later
Hands are more numb. Her doctor says her Hodgkin's seems to be gone.

☐ **Fasciolopsis and all stages (Parasite) NO**

☐ **Ortho-phospho-tyrosine (Cancer) NO**

☒ **Diplococcus (Pathogen) YES in all tissues**
Must see dentist for abscess.

Four months later

☒ **Acetone (Solvent) YES**
Probable cause of neuropathy, along with bacteria —is planning to
see dentist)
*Summary: Nevita had Hodgkin's disease for about 4 years when
she came to us. She saw her medical doctor regularly throughout that
time. But after ridding herself of the intestinal fluke this spring, her
doctor noted that, for the first time, he saw no evidence of Hodgkin's
anymore. Her spring visit was not a regular visit, nor were her later
ones. She only came in to restock her vitamin supply. That is why her
visits were so short. At her first visit, I told her about the pro-
panol/cancer connection and she took herself off cosmetics. So when
the solvent test was done later on, no isopropyl alcohol was found in
her.*

| 9 | Paula Erickson | Breast Cancer |

Paula Erickson is a healthy looking person, age 58, with metasta-
sized breast cancer to lymph nodes. The lymph node was found in
August, 1987. Mammogram suggested that it was non-malignant. She
has had three mammograms - all non-malignant. Biopsy done in Jan.
1988 showed it <u>was</u> malignant. First breast was removed. Then she
took chemotherapy for six months.

Later that year a doctor put her on Tamoxifen™; it worked for a
while, then it went "haywire." Then she was put on Megace.™ On Oct.
1989 she was started on radiation in right neck and shoulder area. That
did not seem to "do anything." She went to Mayo Clinic and they did
nothing more; said she was on the right course. Then she went to Ellis
Fischel Clinic in Columbia, Missouri, they found a blood clot; they
used heparin in hospital (plus chemo) for eight days. She has had eight
rounds of chemo. End of July 1990, second breast was removed. Finished chemo Nov. 1991. Then she was put on Halotestin™.

Her right arm is very swollen and tight. She has put on 10 pounds
of water in the last month. Soreness in left shoulder since the surgery.
She is not on any morphine yet. She has a cold and is on antibiotic
Erythromycin™. She is still coughing.

217

☒ Fasciolopsis (Parasite) YES at liver

I could not test others because of exceptionally high body resistance, obscuring resonance. Probably due to PCB. Start on parasite program.

Four days later

Can still do only minimal testing.

☒ Antimony (Toxic Element) YES

She is rubbing some kind of ointment into her skin.

☒ Chromate (Toxic Element) YES

They have a water softener. They will bypass it and bring in water sample for testing.

☒ Arsenic (Toxic Element) YES

Living in a new house; no drapes or wallpaper. Baffling.

☒ Silver (Toxic Element) YES

Has dentures; suspect glasses frames.

☒ Rhenium (Toxic Element) YES

Will stop using spray starch.

☒ Thallium (Toxic Element) YES

They are not using well water—has full dentures—knows of no pesticides.

☒ Titanium, Radon (Toxic Elements) YES

This house is built on a slab: no crawl space or basement. They will fill cracks around plumbing. Start on thioctic acid, 100 mg, take 2, 3 times/day. Continue parasite program.

Eight days later

They coated her glasses frames instead of getting plastic frames. Her shoulder pain is much worse, she is back on morphine. Her daughter recalled that the yard was "treated" last fall, this could be her source of arsenic.

☒ Fasciolopsis (Parasite) YES

They had stopped the parasite program because of increased bowel movements (8/day). She must go back on parasite program immediately.

☒ Arsenic, Thallium, Antimony (Toxic Elements) YES

☐ Titanium, silver (Toxic Elements) NO

Not wearing glasses.

☐ **Rhenium (Toxic Element) NO**

☐ **Chromate (Toxic Element) NO**
Disconnected water softener.

☒ **Radon (Toxic Element) YES**
Nobody is now smoking in the house. They have plug-in air fresheners, possible source of antimony. Told her to remove these. They will work on cracks. Thallium is probably in the jaw bone from an old polluted filling.

Four days later
Feeling OK, some pain in shoulder, off morphine.

☐ **Ortho-phospho-tyrosine (Cancer) NO**

☐ **Fasciolopsis and all stages (Parasite) NO**

☒ **Uric Acid, Mono, Di-Calcium Phosphate(Kidney Stones) YES**
Start on kidney herbs.

☒ **Arsenic, Thallium (Toxic Element) YES**

☐ **Antimony (Toxic Element) NO**
Stopped using fragrant tissues.

☐ **Radon (Toxic Element) NO**
Sealed cracks. Note: her cancer is gone; she will probably recover if arsenic source is found.

Ten days later
Telephone call from son - mother in hospital, terminal.
Summary: Paula was very willing to make all the changes necessary to recover. At her last visit, she was planning to go home and live by herself again. She thought this might get her away from the arsenic which must be coming from her son's home (she was staying with her son during this illness). But the son had taken her to her medical doctor for a last follow up before a happy leave-taking. The doctor, seeing her improvement, felt she could tolerate more radiation and chemo. This was a sincere effort on the doctor's part to prolong her life. She never got out of the hospital. No more details were given. How sad it was to see her miss her chance to finish out her life in her own home in a normal way.

| 10 | Ananda Bareno | Cancer At Kidney and Bladder |

Ananda Bareno is a 69 year old woman with a respiratory problem. Her tonsils have been removed three times. Her nose is congested. She also has allergies. She gets allergy treatments often from her doctor. Extreme allergies, asthma - her eyes are itchy, etc. She needs her voice to sing. She is a famous singer.

☒ Scandium, PVC (Toxic Elements) YES at lungs

☐ Kidney Stones (ALL) NO

She will bring in blood test from doctor. We will test house air for PVC.

Two weeks later

She brought in the blood test along with her allergy test and house air samples.

☐ PVC (Toxic Element) NO in air samples

She has lost 7 pounds. She is on Premarin™ and Provera™.

BLOOD TEST	Result	Comment
1. Urinalysis	shows trace of blood	check kidneys
2. Seg/Lymph	is low	virus
3. Eos	very high (10%)	parasites
4. Ferritin	is very high (613)	cancer risk; has been taking iron tablets [Feosol™]
5. FBS	is slightly low (74)	pancreas problem
6. Phosphates	is slightly low	Vitamin D [A and D 1000] take 1 a day for 3 months only
7. Alk phos	is slightly high	
8. GGT	is high	gallstones, needs liver cleanse
9. LDH	is slightly high (180)	check for cancer
10. Iron	is very high	stop taking Iron
11. Triglycerides	is high (225)	kidney

(Blood tests and abbreviations are described more fully in *The Tests*.)

☒ Ortho-phospho-tyrosine (Cancer) YES at kidney, bladder, liver

☒ Fasciolopsis (Parasite) YES at liver

⊠ **Fasciolopsis miracidia (Parasite) YES at kidney, bladder, blood**

Start on parasite program.

One month later

☐ **Ortho-phospho-tyrosine (Cancer) NO**

Has never used the word "cancer"; her friend shields her.

☐ **Fasciolopsis and all stages (Parasite) NO**

She says she feels "like a new person." This is usually the time of year she suffers most and gets shots.

☐ **PVC (Toxic Element) NO**

⊠ **Scandium (Toxic Element) YES**

Probably in tooth fillings. She is not planning on coming back for a while. She will stay on parasite maintenance program.

Summary: This is another one of those cases where it is impossible for the client to discuss cancer. Although I referred to it plainly, her responses were on a different subject as though she didn't hear me. Her friend (who was extremely concerned about her) played this pretend game with her, probably to get her compliance. Fortunately, she did comply with all instructions, and she regained her health in a short time.

11	Ruth Stang	Colon Cancer

Ruth Stang is a young woman in her 20's with lots of pain in neck, right arm, shoulder, chest, ovary. Also tachycardia and mitral valve prolapse. She passes out without a cause. Recurrent kidney infection and blood in urine. Fatigue. Too thin. Can't gain weight. Works in doctor's office.

⊠ **Ortho-phospho-tyrosine (Cancer) YES in colon**

⊠ **Fasciolopsis (Parasite) YES in colon and liver**

⊠ **Fasciolopsis miracidia (Parasite) YES in colon only**

I suspect heart parasites, gallstones and kidney stones. She was to start on parasite program.

Summary: It was heartbreaking to see such a young person so disabled due to no fault of her own. She appreciated the encouragement we could give her that she would be completely well in a few months. A few days later the bank had returned her payment check, saying a "stop-payment" order was given on it. She did not keep her follow-up appointment, and we have heard nothing since. A particularly sad case! Probably her family or friends were angry, in a well-intentioned way, that she was "wasting" her money on alternative therapies.

Six months later

Ruth returned with a friend. She explained her absence and paid her old bill. She has had no more dizziness or passing out since she was last seen. Her whole family has stopped eating beef. She says she feels well and did not need to come back. She was bringing in a friend with cancer; that is why she returned. She wanted to be tested for cancer again, herself.

☐ **Ortho-phospho-tyrosine (Cancer) NO**

☐ **hCG (Pre-Cancer) NO**

☐ **Protein 24 (HIV) NO**

Marilyn Werdick	Pancreatic Cancer and HIV Illness

Marilyn Werdick came with a diagnosis of pancreatic cancer at age 50. It happened suddenly, with stomach trouble two months ago. She thought it was due to her pain medicine for lower back pain. CAT scan showed area of pancreas that was suspicious. Biopsy showed pancreatic cancer. Surgery was begun but they just sewed her back up. She is on morphine. She is still smoking but promised to stop.

☒ **Protein 24 (HIV) YES at thymus, vagina, pancreas**

☒ **Ortho-phospho-tyrosine (Cancer) YES at pancreas**

☒ **Fasciolopsis (Parasite) YES at liver and thymus**

☒ **Fasciolopsis eggs (Parasite) YES at thymus, NO elsewhere**

☐ **Sheep liver fluke (Parasite) NO**

She has no sensations over the breast bone.

☒ **Gardnerella, Flu, Plantar Wart, Strep pn, Trichomonas, Adenovirus, Campylobacter, Alpha Strep, Proteus v, Papilloma 4, Bacillus cereus, Norcardia, Staph aureus (Pathogens) YES**

☐ **Bacteroides fr, Haemophilis inf, Herpes 1, CMV, Borellia, EBV, Shigella, Histoplasma, Chlamydia, Coxsackie B4, Salmonella, Resp Sync V (Pathogens) NO**

Stopped here (this is less than half the test). This shows AIDS-like lost immunity. Too many pathogens are growing in her. Her body must be full of solvent.

☒ **Benzene, Wood Alcohol, Hexane, Pentane, Isopropyl Alcohol (Solvents) YES**

She was started on parasite killing program. She will be off all commercial beverages and cosmetics and benzene sources.

Four days later

She missed her appointment.

Twelve days later

She died (telephone call).

Summary: Marilyn had none of the risk factors associated with HIV. She was just an ordinary middle-age woman who didn't drink alcoholic beverages. If she had acted quickly, she would most certainly have survived and gotten reasonably well again. Perhaps she missed her appointment because of embarrassment over not being able to stop smoking. Maybe I was too hard on her about it. We did not hear any details surrounding her death. Notice the adult fluke in the thymus where T-cells are made. The thymus is a small gland and the fluke is a large parasite; it is like having an elephant in the kitchen. How could the thymus do its work? People often feel strange sensations at the top of their breast bone when flukes are in it, but she didn't. Cancer and HIV illness are first cousin diseases. Cancer results when propanol builds up in the body. HIV develops when benzene builds up.

12	Jean Barish	Cancer At Uterus and Kidneys

Jean Barish is a 31 year old woman. Years ago she had a liver problem: she was throwing up bile. She solved that with herbs. She also had migraines. Now she has these problems: 1) Chronic respiratory problems (a bout of bronchitis every year). 2) Constipation; normal movement only once in two or three days. 3) Chronic fatigue. 4) Colitis for the past ten years, diagnosed by doctor. 5) Uterine polyps in 1986 for which she had a D & C.

☒ **Nickel, Silver (Toxic Elements) YES**

☐ **Toxic Elements (All The Rest) NO**
Needs metal tooth fillings replaced.

☒ **di Calcium Phosphate (Kidney Stones) YES**

☒ **tri Calcium Phosphate (Kidney Stones) YES**

☒ **Oxalate, Uric Acid (Kidney Stones) YES**
Needs kidney herb recipe.

☒ **Ortho-phospho-tyrosine (Cancer) YES at uterus, kidneys; NO at ovaries, breast**

☒ **Fasciolopsis (Parasite) YES at kidney and liver**

☒ **Fasciolopsis cercaria (Parasite) YES at kidney, blood, NO at breast and liver**

☒ **Fasciolopsis miracidia (Parasite) YES at kidney, liver, blood, NO at breast**
The discovery of cancer in Jean came as a surprise. She was put on the parasite killing recipe immediately while the kidney cleansing waited and dental work was to be scheduled. She did not bring a blood test but she will bring a copy since she had a recent one done.

Three weeks later
BLOOD TEST: Thyroid and WBC slightly high. Others OK.

☐ **Ortho-phospho-tyrosine (Cancer) NO**

☐ **Fasciolopsis and all stages (Parasite) NO**

☒ **Cryptocotyl (Parasite) YES**

☒ **E. Hist (Parasite) YES**

☐ **Parasites (remainder of box 1) NO**
Continue parasite program.

Five weeks later

☐ **Ortho-phospho-tyrosine (Cancer) NO**

☐ **Protein 24 (HIV) NO**
Colitis: GONE.

☒ **Onchocerca (Parasite) YES**

☒ **Taenia pis (Parasite) YES**

☐ **Parasites (remainder of box 2) NO**

Continue parasite program.

Summary: Jean did not come into our office because of cancer. She was very shocked but not frightened away, fortunately. She dug right into her tasks. Her finances probably won't allow her to return. So I hope she abides by the meat-avoidance rule and the cosmetics and beverage avoidance rules. Notice that her colitis disappeared as well as the cancer and parasites. She felt very well at the third visit.

Four months later

I was wrong. Happily, Jean came back and brought her husband, too. She has no problems now but wants her husband to get checked out.

Jean

☐ **Ortho-phospho-tyrosine (Cancer) NO**

☐ **Protein 24 (HIV) NO**

☒ **Wood Alcohol, Hexane (Solvents) YES in pancreas**

She has been drinking Celestial Seasonings herb teas.

☐ **Fasciolopsis, Sheep Liver Fluke, Clonorchis (Parasites) NO**

☒ **Pancreatic fluke and stages (Parasite) YES in pancreas**

She will promptly kill these with a 5 day high dose parasite program and stop drinking tea blends or any commercial beverage. Note that only the pancreatic fluke was multiplying in her, although she must be picking up the others at the same time - from rare meat. Only the pancreatic fluke survived and is multiplying - because of the solvents in the pancreas!

13	Sally Corson	Ovarian Cancer

This 70 year old woman had a partial hysterectomy 35 years ago, with the remainder removed 5 years ago. She also reported that she has some urinary tract infection for which she is taking Macrodantin™ at bedtime. Her main problem is ovarian cancer which started about 5 years ago. It was OK until one year ago when it came back. Ca 125[60] test was up to 115; now she is on chemotherapy by mouth, Alkeran™,

---

[60] This is a cancer marker for ovarian cancer.

and Ca 125 is down to 75. Her clinical doctor said that present chemotherapy will not cure, but only "hold it back" for a while.

☐ **Protein 24 (HIV) NO**

☒ **Ortho-phospho-tyrosine (Cancer) YES at liver, ovary (very high), stomach**

>Her clinical doctor had also told her she had cancer in the liver, ovaries, stomach.

☒ **Fasciolopsis (Parasite) YES at liver, colon, ovary, stomach**

☐ **Fasciolopsis other stages (Parasite) NO**

>Chemo is probably killing the stages.

☐ **Sheep liver fluke (Parasite) NO**

☒ **Isopropyl Alcohol (Solvent) YES at liver**

>Remove propanol sources from the house. Start on parasite program.

>*Summary: This woman was given a minimal test at our office, just to remove her cancer. Hopefully she can afford to come back and work on her arthritis, back pain, etc. The cancer had indeed spread as her medical doctor had told her. Fasciolopsis was present in adult form at all these locations. Her chemo seems to be killing the stages which otherwise would be present. Hopefully, she has removed the propanol from her lifestyle and carried out the parasite program. Perhaps we will see her soon, free of cancer.*

Six weeks later

What a joyful occasion. Sally came in for a 20 minute follow-up.

☐ **Ortho-phospho-tyrosine (Cancer) NO**

>She feels "a lot better," her Ca 125 is down further, her stomach is no longer enlarged and hard.

☐ **Fasciolopsis all stages (Parasite) NO**

☐ **Sheep liver fluke all stages (Parasite) NO**

☐ **Pancreatic fluke (Parasite) NO**

☒ **Pentane, Styrene (Solvents) YES**

>The propanol is out of her body. She will stop eating out of styrofoam. And she will stop drinking decaf and switch to 2% milk. She will start on our kidney herb recipe, only half a dose because

of her age, in order to cure her frequent urination and low back pain.

Lenora Wilson	Colon Cancer

Lenora Wilson is a 55 year old woman whose main problem, she said, was ovarian cancer. She had a complete hysterectomy in 1980. After that she was given chemotherapy. In 1991, Ca 125 marker was 60 (should be 0-35); in September Ca 125 was up to 70. She was told to repeat chemotherapy. Instead she went to Ann Wigsmore Foundation for 2 weeks and changed diet to vegetarian. After this her Ca 125 went down to 61. For the last year she has done nothing, not even vitamins.

☒ **Ortho-phospho-tyrosine (Cancer) YES at colon only**

☐ **Protein 24 (HIV) NO**

☒ **Fasciolopsis (Parasite) YES at liver, colon; NO at other sites**

☒ **Fasciolopsis redia (Parasite) YES at liver, blood**

☒ **Isopropyl Alcohol (Solvent) YES**

Start on parasite program. Eliminate commercial cosmetics.

Summary: This woman's cancer history goes back ten years. She had conventional treatment at this time. But it came back recently; her doctor used the cancer marker Ca 125 to monitor it. My test showed it present in the colon, now. There was a Fasciolopsis in the liver and a stage in the liver and blood. There was propanol in her white blood cells. Hopefully, she has eliminated the propanol and cleared up her new cancer. She has not followed up. Her first visit was too brief to do more testing.

14	Mary Emerson	Cervical Cancer

Mary Emerson is a 39 year old woman who described her main problem as follows: In about 1986 a Pap smear showed inflammation of the cervix. Two years later a different doctor found it quite abnormal, and she got cold knife conization. Six months later it was OK. Six months after that it was not normal again. In March 1992, a laser ablation was done. She went financially broke, but saw the doctor anyway. Follow-up showed 5½ on a scale of 6. Doctor wants to do a complete hysterectomy. She began to get hairy, skin greasy; depression hit. Lit-

227

tle warts grew everywhere. She was working in a chemical plant. Allergies began, and she gained 150 pounds!

☒ **Ortho-phospho-tyrosine (Cancer) YES at cervix**

Her regular doctor diagnosed pseudo tumor cerebrii although he couldn't see it. Her cerebral pressure was elevated without visual effects.

☒ **Fasciolopsis (Parasite) YES at liver and colon**

☒ **Fasciolopsis miracidia (Parasite) YES at cervix and pancreas**

☒ **Fasciolopsis redia (Parasite) YES at cervix and blood**

☐ **Fasciolopsis remaining stages (Parasite) NO**

She was put on parasite program.

6 days later

☐ **Ortho-phospho-tyrosine (Cancer) NO**

Cancer cleared! She had a major headache on one day. A joint on right big toe has been hurting.

☐ **Fasciolopsis all stages (Parasite) NO**

☒ **Europium, Silver (Toxic Element) YES**

Root canal, fillings.

☐ **Toxic Elements (Remainder) NO**

Remove metal from mouth. Start on thioctic - 2/day (100 mg capsules).

Five days later

BLOOD TEST	Result	Comment
1. Calcium	slightly low	Drink 2% milk, 3 glasses/day; magnesium (300 mg) 1/day; Vit D (by prescription from dentist 50,000) 1-2/week forever.
2. SGOT, SGPT	very low	B6 500 - 1/day for a while, then 250mg.
3. LDH	high (190)	cancer not yet cleared at the time of test
4. Cholesterol	very low	cancer risk
5. Iron	very low	parasites

6. Urinalysis	shows urinary tract infection and crystals (stones)	Start on kidney program.
7. Platelet count	very high (403)	cancer
8. WBC	slightly high	infection
9. Lymphs	very low	toxin in bone marrow
10. Eos	high	parasites

☒ **Pancreatic fluke (Parasite) YES**

☒ **Cysticercus (Parasite) YES**

☒ **Echinococcus granulosus (Parasite) YES**
Continue parasite program.

5 days later
She has not been able to do dental work yet.

☒ **Cysticercus, Pancreatic fluke (Parasite) YES**

☐ **Echinococcus granulosus all stages (Parasites) NO**
Increase wormwood to 16 for 3 days. Then 16 capsules 2 times a week for 3 months. Then 16 capsules 1 time a week.

☒ **Uric Acid, Phosphate (Kidney Stones) YES**
Continue kidney recipe. Client released.
Summary: Mary came from several states away and had only 16 days to accomplish her goal: to avoid a hysterectomy. After 6 days her cancer had disappeared. We hope she will eventually do a liver cleanse to lose the weight she suddenly gained. She planned to return at her next vacation to get dental work done.

15	Mona Moon	Cancer

Mona Moon, about 70 years old, was worried that she might have cancer and this was her purpose in coming to us. She was not ill. I tested her right away.

☒ **Ortho-phospho-tyrosine (Cancer) YES in her WBCs (cancer location not found)**
I immediately tested for the intestinal fluke.

☒ **Fasciolopsis (Parasite) YES in one side of the liver**

☒ **Fasciolopsis eggs (Parasite) YES in blood and the same side of the liver**

Her husband had died of bone cancer in legs and spine; this made her anxious. I was out of wormwood so I started her on Quassia (see *Recipes*), rather than have her merely wait until it arrived. Note that I did not try to locate cancer. She was to return in 3 days to get wormwood.

Three days later

☐ **Ortho-phospho-tyrosine (Cancer) NO**

☐ **Fasciolopsis and all stages (Parasite) NO**

Wormwood has not arrived yet.

Three weeks later

☒ **Endolimax, Rabbit Fluke, Onchocerca (Parasite) YES**

☐ **Parasites (Remainder) NO**

Note: apparently Quassia is effective in killing all stages of Fasciolopsis, like wormwood. She will switch to wormwood and the usual parasite killing program now that it has arrived.

☒ **Calcium Phosphate (Kidney Stone) YES**

I instructed diet changes: decrease bread, increase fruit and vegetables and milk 2%. Take magnesium oxide (300 mg) one/day.

Three weeks later

☐ **Parasites (ALL) NO**

☐ **Kidney Stones (ALL) NO**

Note: She did not need our kidney stone recipe to dissolve away her phosphate crystals. A change in diet was sufficient.

Summary: This woman did not come in for health problems but only because she was worried about cancer, since her husband had died of it. Indeed, her intuition was right, but very quickly she removed all of the cancer, even though she substituted Quassia for our regular parasite recipe. Even her kidney stones disappeared with a simple change in diet. She has probably not returned for financial reasons (she lives on Social Security). Her good attitude will probably bring her back quickly if she has a health problem.

Dorothy Larson   Breast Cancer

This 56 year old woman reported her main problems as: 1) High blood pressure. She has not been on a blood pressure medication. 2) Ringing in head (more than just in ears).

☐ **Protein 24 (HIV) NO**

☒ **Ortho-phospho-tyrosine (Cancer) YES at breast, colon**

☒ **Isopropyl Alcohol (Solvent) YES at breast, colon**

☐ **Solvents (Remainder) NO**

☒ **Fasciolopsis (Parasite) YES at liver, colon; NO elsewhere**

☒ **Fasciolopsis miracidia (Parasite) YES at breast**

She uses no cosmetics. She will switch shampoo to ours. She will start on parasite program.

Summary: A routine check for cancer and HIV showed the cancer present in the breast and colon. The intestinal fluke was in the liver as usual, with a stage present in the breast. The first priority was to eliminate the cancer, although her purpose in coming to the office was her high blood pressure and ringing in the head. She had propanol in the breast and colon, but the source was not obvious. Hopefully, she will return free of her cancer, so we can pursue her other health problems.

---

16   Andrew Kelly   Lung Cancer

Andrew Kelly is a 49 year old man who reported that his main problems were: 1) tinnitus; 2) respiratory drainage; 3) tendonitis in wrists; 4) kidney stones - he had an attack once.

BLOOD TEST old test he brought with him	Result	Comment
1. FBS	112 slightly high	need to cleanse liver
2. Calcium	(8.8) very low	Drink goat's milk - 3 glasses/day; Magnesium 300mg - 1/day
3. Cholesterol	(148) very low	cancer risk; use butter - no margarine
4. Total protein	(6.3) low	liver problem
5. Platelet count	(449) very high	parasites, cancer?
6. Urinalysis	shows trace of blood and ketone	start on kidney herbs

He drinks about 6 beers/night. He also takes honey + orange juice + bee pollen He does not tolerate cow's milk.

☒ **Gadolinium (Toxic Element) YES at pancreas; NO at lungs**
Glasses frames need to be changed to plastic.

☒ **Holmium (Toxic Element) YES**
We will test hand cleaner.

☒ **Tin (Toxic Element) YES**
He will start on kidney herbs and go off toothpaste (stannous fluoride in toothpaste is a tin compound).

Three weeks later
He has not changed his glasses frames yet.

☒ **mono-Calcium Phosphate (Kidney Stone) YES**
Continue kidney herbs.

☒ **Pancreatic fluke (Parasite) YES**

☒ **Fasciolopsis (Parasite) YES at liver, intestine**
Suspect cancer.

☒ **Fasciolopsis miracidia (Parasite) YES at, liver, intestines, blood**

☒ **Fasciolopsis redia (Parasite) YES at liver, intestines, blood**

☒ **Sheep liver fluke (Parasite) YES at intestines; NO at liver**

☒ **Ortho-phospho-tyrosine (Cancer) YES at lungs**
As suspected.

☒ **Holmium (Toxic Element) YES and in Zepo™ handcleaner**
He will use olive oil to clean hands. He will start parasite program.

Three weeks later
He has cut smoking down to half, or less.

☐ **Ortho-phospho-tyrosine (Cancer) NO**

☐ **Holmium (Toxic Element) NO**
Has stopped using Zepo™ hand cleaner.

BLOOD TEST (new test)	Result	Comments
1. WBC	slightly high	infection

2. Eos	(4%) high	parasites
3. Atyp lymphs	(3%) high	cancer risk
4. Ferritin	(392) very high	cancer risk
5. Uric acid	(5.7) slightly high	kidney
6. SGOT, SGPT	low	take B6 500mg, one a day
7. Iron	(212) very high	liver problem

Two weeks later

He is still smoking.

☒ Dog heartworm (Parasite) YES

Has typical pain over heart occasionally. Increase parasite herbs. Do a 5-day high dose program.

☐ Ortho-phospho-tyrosine (Cancer) NO

His tinnitus persists.

☒ Staph aureus (Pathogen) YES at lung and tooth #1

He should see dentist for cavitation at #1.

Three weeks later

He has had top right wisdom tooth pulled (#1), it had an abscess.

☐ Ortho-phospho-tyrosine (Cancer) NO

☒ Dog heartworm (Parasite) YES

Increase parasite herbs. He is still smoking.

☐ Holmium (Toxic Element) NO

A month later

His tinnitus comes and goes now, much less than before.

☐ Dog heartworm (Parasite) NO

☒ Pneumocystis carnii (Parasite) YES

☐ Ortho-phospho-tyrosine (Cancer) NO

He has good energy now.

Three weeks later

Some return of symptoms.

☒ Fasciolopsis (Parasite) YES in colon only; other stages NO

☐ Solvents (ALL) NO

He picked up intestinal fluke but it stayed in intestine. Should stop eating meat. Go on 5 day high-dose parasite treatment again.

Summary: Andrew came into our office because of a history of kidney stones; he did not want to pass another one. His blood test suggested parasites (high platelet count) and Fasciolopsis was found. Then the cancer test was done and, indeed, he had a cancer started in the lungs. He was a heavy smoker but couldn't quit. But he very promptly cleared himself of parasites. He also had dog heartworm which can cause coughing. He acted quickly to clear up his Staph aureus infection by having a wisdom tooth pulled. This began to help his tinnitus. Later we noticed a common lung infection, Pneumocystis, but he still could not stop smoking. At the last visit he had picked up the intestinal fluke again, probably from eating rare meat but he had no solvents in his body. This explains why the parasite stayed in the intestine and did not move to his liver or lungs. This bout with lung cancer was missed by his medical doctor whom he continues to see regularly. Perhaps if his medical doctor had also seen the cancer, he would have quit smoking. Maybe not!

Four months later

Andrew is still smoking.

☐ **Protein 24 (HIV) NO**

☐ **hCG, Ortho-phospho-tyrosine (Cancer) NO**

He is very relieved. He and his wife have been neglectful of the parasite program and other restrictions.

☒ **Mothballs, Carbon Tetrachloride, Benzene (Solvent) YES (others not tested)**

He will go back onto parasite maintenance program, go off the benzene list, and try to stop smoking.

Richard England	Lymphoma In Bone

Richard England has 2 preschool children and a wife who brought him here. He is not really interested in my approach. He was diagnosed two years ago.

☒ **Strontium (Toxic Element) YES at bone marrow**

Off toothpaste.

☒ **Scandium (Toxic Element) YES at bone marrow**

Tooth metal.

☒ **Beryllium (Toxic Element) YES at bone marrow**

Gasoline ?

☒ **Radon (Toxic Element) YES at bone marrow**

☐ **Toxic Elements (Remainder) NO**

☒ **Oxalate (Kidney Stones) YES**
He will stop drinking tea. They will fill cracks around plumbing. He will stop toothpaste. They will bring in an air sample from home to test for beryllium.

One week later

☐ **Strontium, Radon (Toxic Elements) NO**

☒ **Beryllium, Scandium (Toxic Elements) YES**

☒ **Beryllium (Toxic Element) YES in home air sample, garage air sample**
Conclusions: He is getting beryllium from garage. The furnace is built into garage. They must IMMEDIATELY change this furnace setup or move. His wife is willing, he is not. He has utmost confidence in bone marrow transplant scheduled soon.

Nine months later

He had his transplant and did OK for a while. His wife is very anxious but he is not very concerned. He lost 30 pounds since last fall but regained 10. Now he weighs 162 pounds. He is getting 10 units irradiated platelets every 4th day, 3 units of packed RBC's every 12-14 days. He has a strep infection in the blood. He has been on heavy antibiotics for several months. Due to his resentment at being "dragged" in by his wife, I tested only for *Fasciolopsis* and Sheep liver fluke.

☒ **Fasciolopsis (Parasite) YES**

☒ **Fasciolopsis miracidia (Parasite) YES in bones**

☐ **Sheep liver fluke (Parasite) NO**
I explained to him that this infestation could be eliminated rather quickly and gave him the parasite killing items and recipe.

Five days later

He missed his follow-up appointment. We called his home. His wife said the herbs nauseated him so he didn't take them.

Ten days later

His wife called to say he had passed away. She and the children would take a vacation with a friend.

Summary: This was a particularly tragic case. His young children sat quietly in their chairs during the appointment, sensing the grave danger their father was in. But he made jokes about my technical competence and devices instead of listening. A friend who had gone through our cancer program successfully tried to encourage him at home. He could have saved himself even at the last visit. He had such great hopes for the bone transplant. He was always talking about his exceptional oncologist and the great rapport and team work in the hospital. It was as if he couldn't see that he was dying, although his preschool children saw it clearly. His wife would have gladly moved from their fossil fuel contaminated home or turned the furnace off and put in an electric space heater till they could sell the home. But she had no influence over him.

17	Margaret Barnes	Multiple Myeloma

Upon arrival at the office, the husband explained that due to her pain, we should discuss as much as possible with her seated in the car. So I began with a conversation with her husband in the office instead of with her.

The chronology of her illness was: 6 months ago she had arthritis; 3 months ago it became more serious; 1½ months ago walking was very painful; 1¼ months ago she needed a walker; 4 weeks ago she could not walk. Her clinical doctor diagnosed rheumatoid arthritis and treated her with a steroid. Her pain did not alleviate.

On January 2, 1992, she was rediagnosed and confirmed with an MRI as having multiple myeloma. On January 6, 1992, she had surgery. They put steel reinforcement in one leg and cut out the cancerous part in the other leg. Radiation was begun one week ago. She will have another week of this but her doctor let him know they could only expect a short remission, if any. They are thinking of going to a doctor in Philadelphia who does megadose chemo IV. I discussed my approach with her husband, reassuring him that I did not controvert any clinical treatment. I persuaded him to bring her in briefly to verify existence of parasites. She was using a walker and had visible pain, but she was interested in my approach.

☒ Fasciolopsis (Parasite) YES at liver and colon

I did not search further. She will start on parasite killing program. They took a blood test form with them.

Four days later

☒ **Tin (Toxic Element) YES at bone marrow**
Off toothpaste

☒ **Lanthanum (Toxic Element) YES at bone marrow**
Suspect using a copy machine We will test house air. They have a lot of electronic equipment in house, but no copier; computer is on porch.

☒ **Zirconium (Toxic Element) YES at bone marrow**
She will be off deodorant, toothpaste, all lotions and body products. She purchased a plastic watch. She will go off cosmetics.

☒ **Kidney Stones (ALL) YES**
Start on kidney herbs.

Six days later

☐ **Oxalate, Urate, Dibasic Calcium Phosphate(Kidney Stone) NO**

☒ **Tribasic Calcium Phosphate (Kidney Stones) YES**
Continue kidney herbs.

☐ **Lanthanum, Tin, Zirconium (Toxic Elements) NO**

☒ **Fasciolopsis (Parasite) YES in liver**

☒ **Ortho-phospho-tyrosine (Cancer) YES bone, bone marrow**
Continue on parasite program.

Three days later

She says she is feeling much better. She is coming in with a walker, rather laboriously. She is sitting on 1 pillow plus 1 behind her back.

☐ **Tribasic Calcium Phosphate (Kidney Stone) NO**
She will continue on kidney herbs at half dose for 3 months.

☒ **Ortho-phospho-tyrosine (Cancer) YES at bone, NO at bone marrow**
It is receding. She is wearing a metal partial denture; she will not wear it at night and change this to plastic soon. She will wrap her walker with masking tape to avoid touching aluminum. "It's a whole new way of life," she sighed. She has been using Efferdent™ for cleaning her teeth; she will switch to grain alcohol. She

likes our shampoo very well and will start using citric acid instead of hair conditioner. She is not on any supplements except magnesium (300 mg) 1/day and Vitamin B6 (500 mg) 1/day. We will start her on dairy food (2%). Aim at 3 cups milk or plain yogurt a day. She has no appetite. Her friend who is cooking for her said she would eat only noodles with any enjoyment. She is rubbing her thigh more or less constantly for pain. She will make her own hair spray. We are adding Vitamin D, prescribed by dentist (50,000 u) 1/day for 30 days for pain and to help healing.

Three days later

Legs are not as painful. She saw her surgeon yesterday. She thinks the kidney herbs were instrumental in her suddenly feeling "like my old self."

☒ Fasciolopsis (Parasite) YES but not in liver

☒ Ortho-phospho-tyrosine (Cancer) YES at only a small area of bone

She is still sitting on a pillow and using a walker. She dressed herself this morning, she says. She usually needed help. She is going on vacation since she feels up to it.

Three weeks later

She is back from vacation. She is walking better. She has tried walking with a cane "but it's not as secure as the walker." She can take a shower by herself now.

☐ Fasciolopsis (Parasite) NO

☒ Fasciolopsis cercaria (Parasite) YES in liver

☒ Fasciolopsis miracidia (Parasite) YES in colon

☒ Ortho-phospho-tyrosine (Cancer) YES at same location in bone

Continue on parasite program. Start thioctic acid (100 mg capsules) 3 a day. She has been on 20 days of Vitamin D (50,000) once a day. We are now starting a regimen of: 6 caps per week only; then 5 days/week; then 4 days/week; then 2 caps per week indefinitely. Thioctic acid is a metal chelator, acting where the cancer is at work.

One month later

She has been traveling. Seems rather well. She is not using any assistance with walking and sits down easily on a chair by herself without discomfort. No walker or cane or cushion!

☐ **Ortho-phospho-tyrosine (Cancer) NO**

☐ **Fasciolopsis (Parasite) NO**

☒ **Fasciolopsis redia (Parasite) YES, remaining stages NO**

Increase wormwood from 8 to 12 capsules a day, then 12 wormwood twice a week plus 30 drops of black walnut tincture once a day.

☐ **Zirconium, Lanthanum (Toxic Elements) NO**

☒ **Tin (Toxic Element) YES**

She is using a health brand deodorant; will stop. She is using 2 tablets of Tylenol™ about once a week only; she's not using any other drug.

One week later

She is not using her cane and is sitting comfortably on a chair without a cushion. Seems to have normal energy and health.

☐ **Fasciolopsis (Parasite) NO all stages**

☒ **Fischoedrius, Eimeria, Echinococcus granulosus (Parasites) YES**

Increase wormwood to 14 capsules once a day for 3 days.

☒ **Tin, PCB (Toxic Element) YES**

☒ **Tin, PCB (Toxic Element) YES in NuSkin™ products**

She will go off these. Continue on Thioctic - 3 a day.

☐ **Ortho-phospho-tyrosine (Cancer) NO**

Next: liver cleanse. Start on 07 (a commercial preparation of chlorine dioxide) and peroxy (17½ % hydrogen peroxide).

Three weeks later

She says she feels wonderful. She has been to a week-long convention. Her regular doctor says her hemoglobin is up to 11 and she is "doing great." All CBC counts are correct.

☐ **Fasciolopsis (Parasite) NO**

☒ Nickel (Toxic Element) YES

Probably coming from a rod implant from hip prosthesis on both sides.

BLOOD TEST	Result	Comment
1. WBC	5.7	
2. RBC	2.88 - low	
3. Hemoglobin	11.0	
4. MCV	105.2 - high	add B12 500mg, use as lozenge
5. Platelet count	244	
6. Lymphs	18.5 - low	toxin in bone marrow: Tin, PCBs, Nickel

Increase calcium, magnesium, zinc (she is on iron), manganese. Increase salmon or sardines in diet. Add zinc 60 mg 1/day.

One month later

She says she feels "wonderful." Her oncologist appointment is in a few days. She has felt "great." She has had energy, feels much better than even before surgery (for a year she had not had energy).

☐ Ortho-phospho-tyrosine (Cancer) NO

☒ Nickel, Vanadium (Toxic Element) YES

Has no gas appliances, but has candles - will remove candles from house.

One week later

She says she is "great." She has been vacationing on a houseboat for two weeks. She is due for a check-up and blood test soon.

☒ Silver (Toxic Element) YES

She is using her retainer again and it needs to be changed to plastic. She will use her spare plastic retainer. All her utilities are electrical. Her candles are in closed containers.

☐ Ortho-phospho-tyrosine (Cancer) NO

☐ Fasciolopsis (Parasite) NO

She had a spasm in her upper back that frightened her. We need to clean the liver. She will go back on 07 and Peroxy. She will clean the liver. She says she feels better than she has in years. She will go on Bronson's Vitamin C 500 mg.

Summary: Margaret was considered terminal at first. Fortunately for her she did not go East for more clinical treatment. She was only in her early 50's and had been a dynamic, active person. She had friends willing to help her husband with transportation to the office. She did everything promptly without complaining. Her husband and friends supported her and were not negative about alternative therapy. She had a particularly difficult time killing all the parasite stages but pursued the program diligently without being discouraged and quitting. She seemed to enjoy life enough to make the effort worthwhile. She was an inspiration for all of us in the office. At the last visit she was her former busy self.

| 18 | Martha Zendel | Ovarian and Bone Cancer |

This is a very pleasant middle-aged woman from a neighboring state who was diagnosed with ovarian cancer about ten years ago. However, she did not do any treatments except wheat grass, herbs, etc. on her own. She now has a pain syndrome over most of her body, especially her lower body. She has a lot of dizziness. She had a PAP smear recently, but she did not go back to the doctor to learn the results.

☒ **Ortho-phospho-tyrosine (Cancer) YES at ovary and bone**
She aches through whole lower half of her body.

☒ **Fasciolopsis (Parasite) YES at liver**

☒ **Fasciolopsis eggs (Parasite) YES at bone, liver, blood**

☒ **Fasciolopsis miracidia, redia (Parasite) YES at bone, liver**
She will start on parasite program.

Nineteen days later

☐ **Fasciolopsis (Parasite) NO, all other stages NO**

☐ **Ortho-phospho-tyrosine (Cancer) NO**
Cancer is gone.

☒ **Molybdenum (Toxic Element) YES**
She will be cautious about automotive chemicals in the house. She will bring wheat grass sample for me to see. She is enthusiastic about doing a liver cleanse.

☐ **Kidney Stones (ALL) NO (remarkable)**
Her joints are stiffening up. Terrific pain in her arms. She has had kidney infections (pain over kidney, frequency of very yellow urine, dizziness, ears are shut). She was started on our kidney

herbs in spite of absence of stones. This is probably a dental problem.

☒ **Babesia, Capillaria, Dipylidium (eggs and adult) (Parasites) YES**

☒ **Sheep liver fluke (Parasite) YES at liver**

☒ **Sheep liver fluke cercaria (Parasite) YES at liver, blood**

☒ **Sheep liver fluke miracidia (Parasite) YES at blood**
She will continue the parasite program.

Two months later
She is not feeling well today. Itching. Poor bowel movements. She has problems breathing all the time. Heart palpitations scare her (probably dental).

☐ **Babesia, Capillaria, Sheep liver fluke (Parasites) NO**

☒ **Moniezia tape worm, Notocotylus (Parasites) YES**

☐ **Parasites (Remainder) NO**
Continue parasite program.

☒ **Histoplasma (Pathogen) YES**

☐ **Molybdenum (Toxic Element) NO**

Three months later
She feels much better.

☐ **Ortho-phospho-tyrosine (Cancer) NO**
Summary: This super-intelligent woman could see that current clinical treatment of her cancer would give her very little chance of survival. She studied alternative treatments and was doing fairly well after 9 years. Hopefully, she will continue to work on her health and clear her remaining parasites. She might not be here today if she had gone the clinical route.

Half a year later
She had all metal removed from her mouth but got a severe infection afterward. She is still not completely healed. She neglected to take Vitamin D (50,000), 2 a week and has not drunk milk. She will get back to it.

☐ **Ortho-phospho-tyrosine, hCG (Cancer) NO**

☐ **Protein 24 (HIV) NO**

☒ **Haemophilus infl, Gardnerella vag, Eikenella, Lepto inter, Diplo pne, Klebsiella pn, Histomonas mel (Pathogens) YES**
She is obviously not well; has low immunity.

☒ **Pancreatic fluke stages (Parasite) YES**

☒ **PCB (Toxic Element) YES**
She will stay off detergents.

☒ **Benzene (Solvent) YES in thymus**

☒ **Isopropyl Alcohol (Solvent) YES**
These solvents would explain Martha's low immunity. Her cancer has not returned but it is only a hair's breadth away. She will avoid eating solvent-polluted food and products and using solvent-polluted products and go back on the parasite program.

19	Anna Stewart	Colon Cancer

Anna Stewart is 83 years old, a charming intelligent person, interested in how everything worked and quite conversational. She is living alone in an apartment although her son brought her to see us. Her complaint is bloating and gas, loss of bowel control, and pain across the mid-abdomen. She had bone cancer 40 years ago and was treated at the Hoxsey Clinic for it. This clinic was shut down soon after her visit. It was considered quackery. She has stayed on their herb recommendations and been health conscious ever since.

☐ **Kidney Stones (ALL) NO**
Most unusual.

☒ **Eimeria (Parasite) YES**

☒ **Fasciolopsis (Parasite) YES at liver**

☒ **Fasciolopsis miracidia (Parasite) YES at liver and blood**

☒ **Ortho-phospho-tyrosine (Cancer) YES at colon, NO at bone**
Has colon cancer. She will start parasite program.

One week later

☐ **Fasciolopsis and all stages (Parasite) NO**

☐ **Eimeria(Parasite) NO**

☐ **Ortho-phospho-tyrosine (Cancer) NO**

Her pain is gone; her diarrhea is gone.

☒ **Radon (Toxic Element) YES**

She will continue the parasite program to completion. Her son will fix cracks around plumbing pipes. She asked about a safe deodorant! She asked whether she should risk expanding her food list now that her pain and diarrhea are gone.

One week later

She can eat cheese and applesauce again, her favorite foods, without pain.

☒ **Radon (Toxic Element) YES**

☐ **Ortho-phospho-tyrosine (Cancer) NO**

BLOOD TEST	Result	Comment
1. WBC	4.5 low	probably due to radon in bone marrow
2. RBC	Low	probably due to radon in bone marrow
3. Total protein	slightly low	liver problem
4. Potassium	very low	radon in adrenals

She will live with son for a while to clear radon from her body. She is interested in doing a liver cleanse to gain some energy. She will start on our readiness program for the cleanse.

Summary: This very pleasant woman apparently recovered from bone cancer decades ago! A case like this should have been followed by the National Cancer Institute to verify all the facts and not miss finding out what was responsible for her survival. She seemed at least 10 years younger than her real age - even needing deodorant! Could this be due to the herbs she was taking, too? She has no kidney stones and only one additional parasite: possibly the herbs, whose names she had forgotten after she threw them out recently, kept her free of parasites and also kept her youthful!

20	**Debbie Lai**	**Breast Cancer**

This 56 year old female reported that her main problems were: 1) Cancer of the breast (R. side). Diagnosed 4 weeks ago via mammogram. She will be scanned tomorrow. They called it an inflammatory "invasive" inoperable cancer. 2) Lower back. She has had chiropractic treatment for 25-30 years. 3) Sleep problems. 4) Headaches. 5) Weight problem - of recent origin.

☐ **Protein 24 (HIV) NO**

☒ **Ortho-phospho-tyrosine (Cancer) YES at liver, side of breast**

☒ **Isopropyl Alcohol (Solvent) YES at liver, side of breast**

☒ **Fasciolopsis (Parasite) YES at liver, intestine**

☐ **Fasciolopsis other stages (Parasite) NO**
Start on parasite program. Go off caffeine and onto milk, 2 pints of water/day, citrus juice, freshly squeezed or fresh squeezed frozen.

Five days later

☐ **Ortho-phospho-tyrosine (Cancer) NO**

☐ **Fasciolopsis and all stages (Parasite) NO**

☐ **Isopropyl Alcohol (Solvent) NO**
Has gone off cosmetics.

☒ **Beryllium (Toxic Element) YES**
Bedroom is over their garage

☒ **Lanthanum (Toxic Element) YES**
Has been doing computer work, keep printer covered, don't touch ink on pages.

☒ **Vanadium(Toxic Element) YES**
Gas leak in home; had been staying with family in last few days - will test home air.

Twenty days later
She is feeling OK. There is still some pain on mid-sternum and under left breast but not at nipple.

☐ **Beryllium, Lanthanum, Vanadium (Toxic Element) NO**
2 gas leaks were found. The breast biopsy done by regular doctor came back YES (positive). She brought reports.

☒ **Loa Loa (Parasite) YES**
Probable cause of sternal pain. She will go on 5 day high dose parasite program.

☐ **Dirofilaria (Parasite) NO**

Twelve days later
Still a small pain under R. breast.

245

⊠ **Wood Alcohol (Solvent) YES**

She will go off commercial beverages. Her body current level seemed low, suggestive of PCB's.

⊠ **PCB (Toxic Element) YES**

She will switch to using borax for everything.

⊠ **Loa Loa (Parasite) YES**

Repeat 5 day high dose parasite program.

Three weeks later

She is feeling much better. Pain over mid-chest is all gone. Still a little pain under R breast coming in from the side. The coloration of breast is back to normal. Some low back pain persists.

⊠ **Dibasic Calcium Phosphate (Kidney Stone) YES**

Continue kidney herbs.

☐ **Ortho-phospho-tyrosine (Cancer) NO**

☐ **Loa Loa (Parasite) NO**

Stay on maintenance parasite program.

☐ **Solvents (ALL) NO**

⊠ **PCB (Toxic Element) YES**

☐ **PCB (Toxic Element) NO in drinking water sample**

Source still not found - has switched off detergents.

⊠ **Zirconium (Toxic Element) YES**

Probable cause of breast pain. She is using no body products that could have zirconium. She uses contact lens cleaner, however. Will make her own.

Summary: Debbie and her elderly mother who came with her were radiating joy at her last visit. She had cancer in the liver as well as breast, although her regular doctor's diagnosis was breast cancer. Five days after starting the parasite-killing program all the malignancy was gone. She moved her bed to the other end of the house and the computer-room door was kept closed. Her husband was supportive. She complied immediately with all the changes recommended. She is interested now in learning to make home-made cosmetics. She was so happy to have her life returned to her, she feels radiant and full of plans for the future.

One month later
She is free of cancer, headache, and low back pain.

| 21 | Susana Clausson | Skin Cancer |

The main problems reported were: eyes - developing cataracts at the young age of 66; skin rash - for about 6 years, especially after showering. It does not itch. Respiratory problem comes and goes. She chokes and coughs, especially in damp weather, asthma-like; a lot of laryngitis. Lower back pain; knee pain. Sleep problems. Nervousness.

☒ **Ortho-phospho-tyrosine (Cancer) YES found at skin only**

☒ **Fasciolopsis (Parasite) YES at liver and colon**

☐ **Fasciolopsis eggs (Parasite) NO**

☒ **Fasciolopsis redia (Parasite) YES in blood**

☒ **Ancylostoma, Dipylidium caninum (eggs and adult), Endolimax nana, Taenia pisiformis, Haemonchus contortus, Heterophyes, Macracanthorhynchus (Parasite) YES**
Has lived with dogs entire life. Start on parasite killing program.

☐ **Kidney Stones (ALL) NO**
No kidney stones - has been using herbs of various kinds a long time; maybe this accounts for no kidney stones. Her dad died of prostate cancer. She said she had skin biopsies done by a dermatologist in Illinois about one year ago, taken from the red big blotches on her skin. They came back negative for cancer.

Two weeks later

☐ **Ortho-phospho-tyrosine (Cancer) NO**
The pinching in the skin has stopped.

☒ **Lanthanum (Toxic Element) YES**
Will test her dentures.

☒ **Lanthanum (Toxic Element) YES, pink side of dentures; NO, white side of dentures.**

☒ **PVC (Toxic Element) YES**
We will test carpets, they have indoor/outdoor carpet.

☒ **Thulium (Toxic Element) YES**
She is using a brand of vitamin C which I always find polluted with thulium. She will go off it. She will take thioctic - 2 a day. She will arrange for new dentures.

Two weeks later

☐ **Ortho-phospho-tyrosine (Cancer) NO**

☒ **Fasciolopsis (Parasite) YES at one side of liver only**

☒ **Fasciolopsis cercaria (Parasite) YES at one side of liver and blood**
Note: Cancer is already gone, although one part of liver still has the fluke parasite and stage. Continue parasite program.

☐ **Lanthanum (Toxic Element) NO**

☐ **PVC (Toxic Element) NO**
Was away from home most of the time.

☐ **Thulium (Toxic Element) NO**
Went off all supplements.
Summary: This is a happy story where Susana came in for a simple skin rash. Then she got terribly shocked and frightened to hear it was cancerous, in spite of her clinical doctor's negative results. She was rid of all of it in just over 2 weeks. We did not see her again but trust that she would hurry back if a new problem occurred.

Dale Austin	**Lung Cancer**

Diagnosed lung cancer a few months ago. It started with bronchitis last fall. X-ray showed abnormality. Pleural biopsy showed adenocarcinoma (scattered malignant clear cell carcinoma). Right side was clear. Several CAT scans have been done. He had 36 radiation treatments. He is now having pleural fluid accumulation for the third time. The first 2 times he was drained. They do not want to drain again.

☒ **Titanium (Toxic Element) YES at lung and bronchioles**
Has a bridge.

☒ **Tantalum (Toxic Element) YES at lung and bronchioles**
Tooth metal.

☒ **Zirconium (Toxic Element) YES at lung and bronchioles**
He will go off deodorant and toothpaste (onto grain alcohol and baking soda).

☒ **Scandium, Hafnium, PVC (Toxic Elements) YES at lung and bronchioles**

☒ **Europium, Cerium, Iridium(Toxic Element) YES at lungs**
Dental alloy.

☒ **Gold (Toxic Element) YES at lungs**
Teeth.

☒ **Asbestos (Toxic Element) YES at lung**
Clothes dryer and hair dryer.

☒ **Oxalate (Kidney Stones) YES**
He is to take metal bridge out of mouth. Get all metal tooth fillings replaced with plastic immediately. They will take their laundry to a commercial laundry to dry and not use clothes dryer nor hair dryer. Start thioctic, 100 mg, 2 every waking hour the first day, then 10/day.

10 days later
A person called on the telephone saying they had decided "not to go this route."

Summary: This man had 4 obvious problems: 1) his dental ware; 2) his deodorant; 3) asbestos source in his house; 4) PVC somewhere in his house. I made the mistake of thinking he would certainly return in a few days for his appointment and we would get him started on his parasite program then. It was not to be. I can't help wondering who made the choice: his wife, his children, or himself? I often do see a family member making the choice for the sick person. Often it's the sick person's fault for not stating his or her wishes; they are afraid of inconveniencing the family and being a burden and costing money. He was an alert, intelligent man at age 67; he still had a lot to live for.

| 22 | Joyce Stegeman | Breast Cancer, Colon Cancer, HIV |

Joyce has been going to a clinical doctor for 2 months, but no diagnosis has been reached. She reported the following problems: 1) fatigue; 2) hunger and nausea both; 3) warmth in head (mild fever?), occasional chills; 4) sounds like wind tunnel inside the head (roaring); 5) loose bowels, 3 to 4 times daily; 6) weight loss; 7) weakness; 8) tired and restless at same time; 9) some numbness. Slight inflammation of the liver was seen by one doctor.

⊠ **Fasciolopsis (Parasite) YES at gallbladder, liver, thymus; NO at intestine**

⊠ **Fasciolopsis redia (Parasite) YES**

⊠ **Ortho-phospho-tyrosine (Cancer) YES at colon and breast**
She had intense stinging in her colon and in both her breasts and under armpits 2 months ago, but it went away.

⊠ **Protein 24 (HIV) YES**
This came as a surprise. She was tested clinically for HIV a few months ago; it was NO (negative). She seemed relieved to hear these findings; that is, that she was HIV positive; she thought she'd had it for some time.

⊠ **Dipetalonema, Echinococcus granulosus, Fischoedrius, Haemoproteus, Toxoplasma (Parasite) YES**
Start on parasite program.

Four days later

☐ **Fasciolopsis (Parasite) NO**

☐ **Ortho-phospho-tyrosine (Cancer) NO**

⊠ **Benzene (Solvent) YES at muscle, bone, thyroid, thymus**
She is using Tom's™ fennel toothpaste. Will go off.

⊠ **Tin (Toxic Element) YES at muscle, bone, thyroid, thymus**
Toothpaste.

Three days later

☐ **Tin (Toxic Element) NO**

⊠ **Benzene (Solvent) YES**
She has been off toothpaste. She will go off the whole benzene list. She is too fatigued to go to work.

Six days later
She is feeling more like herself. No hot spells, but she is not well.

☐ **Benzene (Solvent) NO**

☐ **Protein 24 (HIV) NO**

☒ Dipetalonema, Pancreatic fluke (Parasite) YES; remainder of box 1 NO

Summary: Joyce had both cancer and the HIV virus. Small wonder that her symptoms were too confusing for clinical doctors to reach a diagnosis. By the time I saw her I was routinely testing everybody for Protein 24 in their white blood cells (immune system); P24 is a small chip off the core of the virus. When the intestinal fluke was gone, both cancer <u>and HIV</u> were gone! She had the solvent benzene accumulated in her; propanol was not tested at the first visit so it can't be ruled out of the picture. Joyce got her health back. Her illness had made her financially broke, so she did not come back. She was only in her early 30's. We hope she is staying off benzene and propanol sources.

Edna Kennedy	Breast Cancer, Lung Cancer

Edna Kennedy is a vivacious, middle-aged woman with a slightly stocky frame, age 59. She communicates readily about all the issues involved in her health problem. She came with her daughter who had her toddler with her. She is currently undergoing chemotherapy for recurrence of breast cancer. Her breast cancer started just 5 years ago. She had a mastectomy and chemo at that time.

Five months ago the cancer recurred in the lung. It was treated to completion, showing no presence of cancer. But now it has broken out again and is present in her lung, liver, and brain, as well as other sites. Her history of previous surgeries are: breast lump - benign, hysterectomy - parotid tumor, benign. She is currently on four drugs.

She has been on the Birth Control Pill in the past. She has a minor vision problem. She has overall weakness in her arms, elbows, shoulders, wrist and hands. Some back ache, legs and knees are very weak. Energy is very low. She will go off caffeine. She does not smoke or use alcohol. She will also be off mustard, nitrites and artificial sweeteners in her food.

☒ Nickel (Toxic Element) YES at lungs, liver, breast, brain

This high level of nickel in her tissues, including brain locations, suggests tooth metal. She has a rather small amount of visible tooth metal. She says she also has a crown. I recommended immediate removal with no replacement except Duralon™ sealer for 1 or more months until the cancer is gone. We discussed this at length, since she has a preference for her own dentist at home (several states away).

⊠ Beryllium (Toxic Element) YES at lungs, liver, breast, brain

She has none of the usual sources of beryllium. She has no attached garage, no hurricane lamps or containers with fuel or solvent in the house. Nobody is a smoker in the house. (I believe she lives alone.) She works in a doctor's office. She has gas heat at home. We will test her home air by getting a dust sample sent to us by overnight mail taken from various rooms and her basement.

⊠ Scandium, Mercury (Toxic Elements) YES at lungs, liver, breast, brain; remainder NO

The scandium, mercury, and nickel are quite probably all coming from tooth metal. I started her on a moderate amount of thioctic acid, 100 mg, 6/day. She had not been on vitamin C, so I started her on 3000 mg/day (with meals). Start on parasite program.

She brought her blood test with her, done one month ago:

BLOOD TEST	Result	Comments
1. FBS	slightly high (117)	pancreas problem, needs to cleanse liver
2. BUN	high (23)	kidney disease
3. Creatinine	slightly high (1.1)	kidney
4. Triglycerides	very high (260)	kidney disease
5. Alk phos	very high (221)	cancer
6. GGT, SGPT (103), SGOT (69)	All very high	reflecting a liver problem
7. LDH	very high at 277	reflecting the cancerous cells product of lactic acid. Her CBC showed lymphs only 9.7% (toxin in lymphocytes).
8. RBC	3.78	anemic, parasites

Weight 150, temperature 97.9, blood pressure 120/80, pulse 80.
We agreed to cleanse liver as soon as possible after parasite program.

Three weeks later

She is looking pale and fatigued. She will have dental work done this week. Her daughter found container of lamp oil and solvent, etc. in the basement, and she threw it out 1 week ago. She was in the hospital Monday through Saturday (5 days). She got platelets, potassium and nourishment through IV. They got her blood normal. She is resting her head on her right hand and breathing fast. *She did not get started on parasite program* (didn't find the time).

☐ **Beryllium (Toxic Element) NO**

☒ **Oxalate, Uric Acid (Kidney Stones) YES**
She will start on kidney herbs. She is scheduled for chemo for a week.

☒ **Fasciolopsis, Endolimax, Loa Loa, Naegleria (Parasites) YES at colon, lung, liver, breast (massive infestation)**
She agreed again to start on parasite program.

Summary: What a terrible way to die: being eaten alive by a horde of hungry mouths. Maybe she just didn't believe what I was telling her. So she gave the parasite program last priority. I will never know because her daughter called to say she died before her next appointment. She could have easily recovered. What a loss to society as well as her family.

| 23 | Janice Crooks | Liver Cancer |

Janice Crooks is a middle aged, slightly overweight woman with a pleasant disposition. She appears healthy. She is on Halcion™ for sleep and has been on it for three years. Her whole family has a lot of sleep problems. She has extreme sweats during the night; she gets wet all over with feeling hot. She agreed to shower off her sweat each time to get rid of the toxins in sweat. She is on morphine for pain. Her dosage is 30 mg taken at 9 am, 2 PM, and 9 PM daily. She has pain from her right upper abdomen across the front to the left side. It is more like soreness, when moving. She was on Percocet™ for pain before morphine until it failed. She is on Hytrin™ for high blood pressure and has been on it for eight years. It keeps her blood pressure at 140-150/70-80. She is on stool softener each night.

Many years ago she went to the doctor to say that she had pain to the right of her gallbladder. They never found anything. In the early 70's, she had malignant melanoma on her forehead. The doctor froze it and it has not returned.

In the 70's she had a bowel obstruction and needed surgery. About three years ago the bowels bled a little. Her doctor found a tumor. They proceeded with chemotherapy and radiation therapy. The tumor was biopsied and labeled "oat germ," a very rare tumor. The surgeon said it was inoperable because it was on the spinal bone - too dangerous. It was sent to the Mayo Clinic. The oncologist said it was hopeless. The liver showed holes where the cancer had eaten it away.

Some months ago she took radiation for the tumor. They said it would only shrink it slightly, so her bowels would move better.

☒ **Ortho-phospho-tyrosine (Cancer) YES**

☒ **Oxalate, Uric Acid (Kidney Stones) YES**
Start on kidney herbs.

☒ **Fasciolopsis (Parasite) YES at liver and adrenals**

☒ **Ascaris (Parasite) YES at liver and adrenals**

☒ **Cat Liver Fluke (Parasite) YES at liver**
Start on parasite program also.

Four days later
Yesterday morning her heart pounded for about an hour, then it cleared. She will reduce her blood pressure pill.

☒ **Asbestos (Toxic Element) YES at liver**
She does not use a hair dryer. They will sample their clothes dryer exhaust and bring it in to test for asbestos. They have city gas heat. Temporarily they will not use their electric heater which may have asbestos.

☒ **Mercury (Toxic Element) YES at liver**
Very high reading. She will get her fillings removed and not replaced except with Duralon™ sealer for one month or until cancer is gone.

☒ **Palladium, Thorium (Toxic Elements) YES**
They need to put plastic sheet under trailer to keep out thorium and radon.

☒ **Rhodium, Cadmium (Toxic Elements) YES**
Assume this is tooth metal. They have plastic water pipes so suspect old tooth fillings. They will save drillings to test for cadmium.

☒ **Tungsten (Toxic Element) YES**
She uses an electric percolator, but will stop. They have a gas stove and electric oven. We will test the oven for tungsten with a piece of toast done in the oven.

Three days later
She had a blood test done yesterday. She had metal teeth (3) removed this morning. Radon problem will be worked on Friday.

☐ **Oxalate, Uric Acid (Kidney Stones) NO**
Continue kidney program for several months. We will now speed up the parasite program.

☒ **Fasciolopsis (Parasite) YES at liver and gallbladder**

☒ **Tungsten (Toxic Element) YES; electric oven NO; toaster YES**
She never uses the toaster (has not used in a few months). We have not positively identified the source of her tungsten yet.

☒ **Asbestos (Toxic Element) YES at liver and lungs; clothes dryer NO; electric heater YES; hair dryer NO**
This is a 3-4 year old electric oil heater shaped like a radiator. It was washed first. Then they placed a damp paper towel on top and over the air vent to make the sample for testing. They are fond of it but will turn it off.

☒ **Cadmium (Toxic Element) YES**
She is off caffeine now. We tested hot water from Hardees™ where they often eat. It had tungsten in it. She will buy milk there instead. They have an electric water heater which may be putting out tungsten. They will bring in a sample of the hot water to test for tungsten.

Six days later
They have had plastic sheet put under their trailer two days ago for radon protection. She is removing her earrings that have metal posts. She can get polyethylene posts.

☒ **Tungsten (Toxic Element) YES at liver and lungs**
Toast: YES (positive), but she has not eaten toast for 2+ days.

☒ **Tungsten(Toxic Element) YES hot water from kitchen faucet**
It is an 8 year old electric water heater. They will drain it and replace heater element to see if this clears up the tungsten problem. If not, they will get a gas water heater. They will also bring in a cold water sample next time.

☒ **Fasciolopsis (Parasite) YES at colon, gallbladder and liver**

☒ **Onchocerca (Parasite) YES**

☐ **Parasites (remainder of box 2) NO**

Her cyst used to impede a bowel movement - had to have laxative each time. Now she does not need laxative, it seems easier to pass. She would like to be released from Hospice. Her regular doctor sent her home to die and gave her over to Hospice. "They only check my blood pressure and temperature and listen to my heart", she said. She is completely released from her doctor. She will not use any hot water. She will shower at her sister's or heat her cold water to take a shower to get away from tungsten.

Five days later

The pain is beginning to subside. She is off all morphine.

☒ **Tungsten (Toxic Element) YES at liver, and hot water**

Putting in the new element didn't help.) Suggest switching to gas water heater.

☐ **Mercury, Radon, Cadmium, Palladium, Rhodium, Asbestos (Toxic Elements) NO**

☐ **Fasciolopsis (Parasite) NO everywhere**

☐ **Ortho-phospho-tyrosine (Cancer) NO**

Her cancer is completely gone. She is very pleased. Only problem remaining is tungsten.

Five days later

She has laundered clothes in cold water and is in newly washed clothes. The hot water line has not been used. This was an effort to avoid the tungsten.

☐ **Tungsten (Toxic Element) NO**

Due to being off hot water - will put in a gas water heater.

Pain is starting to go down all over. We will next clean the liver. She has been on 10 drops of 07 and peroxy 3 times a day. She will start on liver cleanse.

Summary: This was a very pleasant couple to work with. They always came together. She had more than her share of toxic elements in her liver. Flukes in her adrenals may have caused her high blood pressure for the last 8 years. She was obviously a terminal patient, put on morphine to ease dying. But she conquered every problem with her husband's help. All except one: tungsten in her water supply, from a faulty rod that is meant to prevent metal loading of water in the elec-

tric heater. Then, just as she was bounding with joy at her miraculous recovery, her husband was diagnosed with prostate cancer! (He was also cured.)

| 24 | Jerry Crooks | Prostate Cancer |

He is having difficult urination. His regular doctor put him on a pill to ease urination, but he is worried about it. His gallbladder was taken out 10 years ago. He had a stroke one year after that. He used to smoke, but he quit two years after his stroke. He has paralysis since his stroke.

Prostate was trimmed when he had prostate cancer six years ago. Radiation treatments were given at that time. Since the stroke he developed seizures and has been on Tegretol™ for this from about four years ago.

☒ **Oxalate (Kidney Stones) YES; remainder NO**

☒ **Fasciolopsis (Parasite) YES at liver**

☒ **Ortho-phospho-tyrosine (Cancer) YES at prostate**

He will start on parasite program.

Two months later

He has skipped all earlier appointments. He has been on maintenance parasite program and done everything correctly. His urination improved right away so he didn't think it was important to come in so soon. (I had not told him he had cancer again, since a return to his clinical doctor would have had serious consequences for him. He was only recently remarried.)

☐ **Ortho-phospho-tyrosine (Cancer) NO**

☐ **Fasciolopsis all stages (Parasite) NO**

BLOOD TEST	Result	Comment
1. WBC	has been very low in the past few years	bone marrow
2. RBC	low and has been frequently low over the past few years	probably parasites
3. Platelet count	high (408)	search for cancer, parasites
4. Eos	very high (7%)	parasites
5. Potassium	very low (3.7) and has been low over the years	adrenal problems

6. CO2	very high	He explains this as "heavy air." I think toxin in lungs
7. Creatinine	high, and it has been moderately high over the years	Toxin in kidneys
8. BUN	high	toxin in kidneys
9. Urinalysis	shows chronic urinary tract infection	

Start on kidney herbs. He had a check-up recently. The prostate was checked. The doctors felt he was merely suffering from stroke effects. They found no cause for frequent urination problems and merely put him on a pill.

His body current is very low. I have to raise the calibration setting. His current only goes to 40 microamps with 5 volts across his hands, instead of 60.

☒ Tungsten (Toxic Element) YES

He has an electric water heater. We will test water.

☒ Asbestos (Toxic Element) YES at prostate

☒ Niobium (Toxic Element) YES throughout body

Probably a pill - will go off.

☒ Holmium (Toxic Element) YES throughout body

Search for PCB.

☒ PCB (Toxic Element) YES

Wife also PCB positive - have been using regular laundry detergent and hand soap. Switch to borax for laundry, dishes and shampoo. Start on thioctic 100 mg 6/day. He will be off caffeine.

Summary: Jerry had me quite concerned during his long absence. It was a great relief to see him walk in briskly 2 months later, stating he was fine. Hopefully he has also cleared up his asbestos and PCB problem. He was heard from a month ago and was doing fine. Holmium and PCB are often found together.

25	Phylis Petrie	Lung Cancer

This is a pleasant woman, age 56, who was first seen by us two years ago. Her reasons for coming were: 1) Arthritis everywhere (arms, elbows, shoulders, wrist, hands, legs, knees, feet) even her ears hurt; 2) gas in stomach; 3) high blood pressure for which she was on Tenormin™; 4) appetite down; she lost about 15 pounds in the last 6 months.

She was on Voltaren™, codeine, Tylenol™, Niferex™. She smokes, and her son has came to live with her. He is a builder. By early 1990, she had cleared a lot of her problems. She was gaining some weight. We encouraged her to get dental work done and stop smoking. (Needs metal out of mouth.)

She did not come back for six months and is still smoking. Toxic element test showed PVC and cesium in her immune system. They were doing some remodeling. We also found bismuth, antimony, vanadium. She was using Vick's Vaporub™. They searched for a gas leak (vanadium source) and found it. She resented being told to stop smoking. Her son was intimidated by her; he bought cigarettes for her since she wasn't strong enough to shop herself. We begged her to stop after our ortho-phospho-tyrosine (cancer) test was YES (positive).

We did not see her again until four months after that. She had seen a clinical doctor who "tested her for cancer and gave her a clean bill of health." Still smoking.

☒ Ortho-phospho-tyrosine (Cancer) YES

☒ Radon, Asbestos (Toxic Element) YES

They will stop home remodeling and seal cracks but don't wish to do anything else since they feel I am wrong about the cancer.

Three months later

Doctor found mass in lung at a routine checkup and diagnosed it as Large Cell Carcinoma. She stopped smoking and wants to get well. They will use commercial clothes dryer and seal cracks to get rid of asbestos and radon. Down to 75 pounds. Her regular doctor gives no hope. Family is arriving. They will do the complete parasite program.

One month later

She has gained 6 pounds. Son is enthusiastic. She misses "her" cigarettes!

☐ Ortho-phospho-tyrosine (Cancer) NO

Three months later

She has missed her earlier appointments, but she is doing OK. Her regular doctor is amazed at her survival. Toxic Element test showed cerium in her lungs. They refuse to do dental work. They are going on vacation. She will stay with other relatives.

Eleven months later

Telephone call from her son. Phylis Petrie died 2 weeks ago.

Summary: This was a particularly tragic case because the children all wanted their mother to stop smoking. But she was so strong a personality that she just "snapped their heads off if they even brought up the subject." Even when she was bedridden and coughing without stopping, the children still brought her cigarettes. The asbestos probably came from the clothes dryer. She rallied after she stopped using it. They had vented it <u>into</u> the house to save heat! We detected the cancer originally with the hCG marker, not ortho-phospho-tyrosine; at that time I was still searching for the best cancer marker, one that wouldn't miss a single case of early malignancy. I have no doubt that Phylis would have recovered if she had continued on the parasite program while she was away with relatives. Without a maintenance program it is too easy to become reinfected.

| 26 | **Norman Jones** | **Prostate Cancer** |

Prostate cancer was diagnosed one month ago. He had surgery two weeks ago - reamed it out (TUR) and analyzed it. Eight days ago his other testicle was removed. The first testicle was removed 11 years ago for Lymphoma (non-Hodgkin's). They will follow-up clinically in three months. No chemo or radiation is scheduled at this time.

☒ Ortho-phospho-tyrosine (Cancer) YES at the prostate

☒ Nickel (Toxic Element) YES at prostate and throughout body

Suspect tooth fillings.

☒ Thorium (Toxic Element) YES at prostate

They live in a condominium on a slab. Suspect uranium in construction fill underneath. Uranium decays into thorium, then into radon.

☒ Radon (Toxic Element) YES at lungs

They will repair cracks and test the air by dust collection.

☒ Cadmium (Toxic Element) YES throughout body

They will bring in water samples, hot and cold, from the kitchen, bathroom, and shower to test for cadmium. They will see dentist, seal basement and do air test for radon. He has a mouthful of tooth fillings. Will get all metal out.

☒ Oxalate, Dibasic Calcium Phosphate (Kidney Stone) YES

☐ **Kidney Stones (remainder) NO**
Start kidney herbs. They will bring in copies of recent blood test.

Three days later
He is enjoying kidney herbs. They have brought in water samples to test for cadmium.

☒ **Cadmium (Toxic Element) YES in shower hot and cold, kitchen hot and cold, NO in master bedroom hot and cold**
They will get new socks and underwear so that their clothing is free of cadmium until plumbing is changed to PVC. He feels the repairs needed may be under the slab they live on.

☒ **Fasciolopsis (Parasite) YES at colon and liver**
We have not tested other parasites. He will start on parasite program.

One week later

☐ **Oxalate, Dibasic Calcium Phosphate (Kidney Stones) NO**
Continue on ½ dose herbs for 2 to 3 months.

☐ **Fasciolopsis (Parasite) NO**
Continue parasite program.

☐ **Ortho-phospho-tyrosine (Cancer) NO**

☒ **Cadmium (Toxic Element) YES at genital tract**

☒ **Thorium, Radon, Nickel (Toxic Element) YES**
They have not sealed cracks around plumbing pipes yet.

Summary: Norman still had the cancer after his surgeries but in 7 days it was all gone after killing the intestinal fluke. He did not return after hearing this happy news, hoping that the dental problem and plumbing and radon problems would go away by themselves. However, he continued to have pain which was interpreted by his clinical doctors as ongoing cancer and was given anti-male hormone. This made his wife angry; she insisted on the dental work and radon work. After this, the genital pain went away: we learned this from one of the children. Also, they stopped using water from the cadmium-polluted faucets. Norman had a jolly nature; hopefully he is doing fine.

27	Joan Matlock	Lymphoma

Joan Matlock was diagnosed as having lymphoma several months ago. Her only symptom was swelling of lymph node in neck and arm. She has 6 children.

She went to the doctor when she noticed her spleen was enlarged and hard. She has had chelation since then but spleen is still swollen. She has been on Hoxsey herb concentrate from Mexico. She is using chaparral, sweet clover, white oak bark, Immunoplex, potassium iodide, goldenseal, and Echinacea. She is on parsley and mullein tea in the morning. Also, hawthorn at lunch, violet leaf tea at supper, milk and ½ cup coffee. Lymphoma is common around her home. She knows 3 others with it! She is from 2 states away

Her chelator doctor recommends that she drink two 10-12 ounce glasses of vegetable juice each day made from: carrots, apples, grapes, ¼ beet, 1 ounce raw liver, and alfalfa sprouts. (I suggested omitting the raw liver.)

☒ **Fasciolopsis and miracidia, cercaria (Parasite and stages) YES at gallbladder, liver**

☒ **Iodamoeba, Schistosoma, Pigeon tapeworm, Chilomastix, Sheep liver fluke, Pancreatic fluke, Dientameoba, Notocotylus (Parasites) YES, remainder of box 1 and 2 NO**

She is having 3 bowel movements a day. Start on parasite program.

☒ **Uric Acid (Kidney Stone) YES**

She will go on kidney herb recipe also.

Two weeks later

☒ **Fasciolopsis miracidia (Parasite) YES at colon**

☒ **Fasciolopsis eggs (Parasite) YES at colon, blood**

☒ **Fasciolopsis cercaria (Parasite) YES at colon**

Continue parasite program.

☒ **Ortho-phospho-tyrosine (Cancer) YES at spleen**

☒ **Indium (Toxic Element) YES**

Metal tooth fillings.

☒ **Mercury (Toxic Element) YES**

Tooth fillings.

☒ **Titanium (Toxic Element) YES**
Tooth fillings? powder?

☒ **Thallium (Toxic Element) YES**
Pollutant in Mercury fillings?

☒ **Vanadium(Toxic Element) YES**
Check for gas leak in home.

☒ **Niobium (Toxic Element) YES**
Pill?

☒ **Ytterbium (Toxic Element) YES**
Pills she is taking.

☒ **Ytterbium (Toxic Element) YES in supplements Twin Lab™ Vitamin E, KAL™ Calcium Magnesium (fast acting), Mayumi Shark Oil™ caps (Japan Health Products), Kwai™**
She needs to get metal teeth replaced. Go off all supplements except from Bronson's Pharm.

One month later
All her tooth metal is out. Spleen is still enlarged and she is experiencing lower back pain. She has to take cortisone two times a week. The gas company found no gas leaks. She will put out jars for air samples. She has lost 5 more pounds.

☐ **Fasciolopsis all stages (Parasite) NO**

☒ **Bismuth (Toxic Element) YES**
Off fragrances.

☒ **Ytterbium (Toxic Element) YES**
Off all supplements.

☒ **Ytterbium (Toxic Element) YES in her digestive enzymes**
She will switch to Bronson's Digestive Enzymes.

Eleven days later
Spleen has not gone down. She has to take ACTH shots twice a week to keep it under control.

☐ **Ortho-phospho-tyrosine (Cancer) NO**

☐ **Fasciolopsis all stages (Parasite) NO**

☒ **Schistosoma (Parasite) YES at spleen**
Continue parasite program. There are numerous pets. She is treating all animals with black walnut tincture. She will bring saliva sample from dog. It is possible she is picking it up from her pets.

☐ **Bismuth (Toxic Element) NO**

☐ **Ytterbium (Toxic Element) NO**

☒ **Haemophilus infl (Pathogen) YES at spleen and wisdom tooth**
In teeth - needs cavitations cleaned.

Two weeks later
She had a cavitation cleaned followed by penicillin.

☐ **Ortho-phospho-tyrosine (Cancer) NO**

☒ **Salmonella, Strep pneum, Gardnerella, Campyl, Resp Syncytial virus (Pathogens) YES at spleen**
She is still drinking a juice of carrots, beets, apple, grape, plus raw beef liver non-medicated source. Stop beef liver.

Two weeks later
One front tooth (with a root canal) has been pulled about 2 hours ago.

☐ **Haemophilus infl (Pathogen) NO**

Four days later
Spleen not down. She has been on Amoxicillin™ from Thursday evening. It is a one-week prescription. Her pulse is down from 115 to 90 beats per minute (this is an improvement).
Summary: The cancer was stopped for Joan but her spleen has not returned to normal size. It looks like more dental work is needed but she did not return. She was strong enough to return to work again, so she did not come back.

| 28 | Jane Elliot | Lung Cancer |

Chronic bronchitis. Smoker.

☒ **Ortho-phospho-tyrosine (Cancer) YES at lungs**

☒ **Fasciolopsis (Parasite) YES at liver, lungs**

☒ **Fasciolopsis eggs (Parasite) YES at liver and blood**

☒ **Fasciolopsis cercaria (Parasite) YES at kidney, bladder, liver, lungs, and blood**

☒ **Mercury (Toxic Element) YES at brain and liver**

☒ **Mercury (Toxic Element) YES in cigarettes, Marlboro 100's™**

Switch cigarette brands.

☒ **Vanadium(Toxic Element) YES**

Search for gas leak.

☒ **Uric Acid (Kidney Stone) YES**

Start on parasite killing program.

Eight days later

☒ **Fasciolopsis cercaria (Parasite) YES at lungs, skin, blood, cervix, intestine**

She has had skin cancers removed in the past.

☒ **Ortho-phospho-tyrosine (Cancer) YES at lungs**

☐ **Mercury (Toxic Element) NO**

Switched cigarette brands. Continue parasite program.

Three weeks later

Bronchitis gone.

☒ **Histoplasma, Proteus (Pathogen) YES at lung**

☒ **Mercury (Toxic Element) YES**

Went back to her old cigarettes.

☐ **Fasciolopsis, Dog heartworm (Parasite) NO**

☐ **Ortho-phospho-tyrosine (Cancer) NO**

Summary: Although Jane had had several bouts of skin cancer, this was not enough to stop her from smoking. Not even the news of lung cancer could stop her addiction. But she switched her cosmetics to propanol-free varieties and carefully stayed on a parasite maintenance program. This was enough to stop her cancer. Perhaps she will some day find the strength to stop smoking.

29	Jennifer Carver	Ovarian Cancer

Jennifer Carver is a vivacious young person, a university student, and accustomed to high achievement. Her high pitched voice suggested high estrogen levels. This would increase her risk of breast cancer. Indeed, it was 150 pg/ml. She stated her mother had breast cancer. But her reason for coming to the office was a digestive problem. Her other problems were: upper back pain, insomnia, and frequent yeast infections. She would like to lose weight.

Urinalysis showed trace of protein. She empties bladder only 2 or 3 times in 24 hours. She will drink a lot more water and stop eating salted popcorn. We will test for toxic elements next time. She did not keep her next appointment.

Two and one half years later

She has a sore throat. Feels tired and must take a midday nap even though she's only in her mid-20's.

☐ Kidney Stones (ALL) NO

No evidence of crystal deposits (has been drinking a lot of water since her first visit).

☒ Ortho-phospho-tyrosine (Cancer) YES at ovary

☒ Fasciolopsis (Parasite) YES at liver and intestine

☒ Fasciolopsis redia (Parasite) YES at ovary, kidneys, bladder, and blood

Start on parasite program.

☒ Benzalkonium, Hafnium, Zirconium (Toxic Elements) YES

Nail polish, hair spray, and most of her cosmetics tested YES (positive). She will discontinue them.

Five weeks later

☐ Ortho-phospho-tyrosine (Cancer) NO

☐ Fasciolopsis (Parasite) NO

☐ Protein 24 (HIV) NO

☒ Isopropyl Alcohol, Mineral Oil (Solvents) YES

She will remove all "prop" from her lifestyle. She will stop using "bag balm" and commercial cosmetics.

Five weeks later

(10 weeks after visit which indicated cancer.) A minor complexion problem has returned. She has normal energy again.

☐ Ortho-phospho-tyrosine (Cancer) NO

☐ **Fasciolopsis and all stages (Parasite) NO**

☐ **Protein 24 (HIV) NO**

☐ **Sheep liver fluke and all stages (Parasite) NO**
She did a 5 day high dose parasite program, followed by maintenance. Boyfriend will get cleared of parasites also.

☐ **Solvents (ALL) NO**
She wants to do a liver cleanse next.
Summary: Cases like Jennifer's are inspirational. Two years earlier, in her early 20's, she sensed her cancer risk because of her mother's and aunts' cancer history. But she felt better as soon as she drank a lot more water and did not follow up. Notice how drinking more water washed away any beginning stone formation without having to take the kidney herb recipe! She might have had a small cancer started then already. How fortunate that she returned for a simple sore throat. Her cancer was already going strong and would have overwhelmed her soon. But she complied in every detail and got her radiant health back, although giving up her favorite cosmetics was hard.

30	David Whitman	Acute Lymphocytic Leukemia

Dave is a 9 year old boy, in good health, by appearance, with normal energy and good mood. Two months ago he was diagnosed with acute lymphocytic leukemia for which he has been treated continuously. He is on Methotrexate™ once a week, Mercaptopurine™ every day, Vincristine™ once in 3 weeks, Prednisone™ after the Vincristine.™ He gained 20 pounds.

☒ **Benzalkonium (Toxic Element) YES at lungs**

☒ **Asbestos (Toxic Element) YES at lungs**

☒ **Cobalt (Toxic Element) YES at skin**

☐ **Toxic Elements (Remainder) NO**
Testing the mother for asbestos: she is YES (positive). It must be in their home which is new. Note: at this time I did not have a separate set of solvents for testing. I assume that he would have tested YES for isopropyl alcohol. As I came to realize the importance of solvents I expanded my test set and discovered the correlation.

☒ **Oxalate (Kidney Stones) YES**
Start on kidney herbs.

One day later
They have brought air samples with them to test for asbestos.

☒ **Asbestos (Toxic Element) YES in master bedroom, family room, laundry room, and dining room**

☐ **Asbestos (Toxic Element) NO in den, basement, sister's bedroom, mother's bedroom, brother's bedroom, upstairs bathroom, master bathroom, kitchen, and half bath**
Conclusion: The clothes dryer in the laundry room may be shedding asbestos and getting into a few rooms but Dave's bedroom is not contaminated; this does not seem sufficient to give Dave such high levels. We will check school air. His 2 classrooms will be dust checked for asbestos. They will send air samples since they live 2 states away. The school has been removing asbestos during summer vacation. They will check into asbestos tests done at school. They will switch off detergent to stop getting cobalt. They will stop using paper cups and napkins and plates to reduce getting benzalkonium; also switch to goat milk to reduce benzalkonium in udder wash used for cows, also switch off toothpaste to baking soda.

☒ **Fasciolopsis (Parasite) YES at WBCs, lungs and intestine**

☒ **Pneumocystis carnii (Parasite) YES**

☒ **Giardia (Parasite) YES at intestine**
Start on parasite program. Keep Dave out of school until air can be tested for asbestos. Do blood test every week to avoid over treatment with chemo as Dave's condition improves.

☒ **Ortho-phospho-tyrosine (Cancer) YES**

Six days later
Testing air sample sent by mail.

☒ **Asbestos (Toxic Element) YES Church schoolrooms A and B, hair blower B (they have two)**

☐ **Asbestos (Toxic Element) NO Hair blower A, clothes dryer vent**
Conclusion: the source of asbestos in Dave's home is not the clothes dryer; it is a single hair blower. There is a limited amount

of asbestos coming from Dave's home (all due to one hair dryer; she will stop using it). He is getting asbestos all day at school. He must stay out of school.

☐ **Oxalate (Kidney Stone) NO**

He can go off kidney herbs.

Seven days later

Clinical doctors have reduced his chemo.

☒ **Asbestos (Toxic Element) YES**

☐ **Benzalkonium (Toxic Element) NO**

☒ **Cobalt (Toxic Element) YES**

They switched off detergent. Cobalt must be coming from water softener. Bypass immediately. Testing mother for asbestos: NO. She stopped using hair blower so Dave must be getting all of it from school. She did not keep him out of school because she feels intimidated by school authorities. She will try again.

Two weeks later

☐ **Asbestos (Toxic Element) NO**

Moved to different classroom.

☐ **Benzalkonium (Toxic Element) NO**

☐ **Cobalt (Toxic Element) NO**

☒ **Fasciolopsis (Parasite) YES**

Continue parasite program.

☐ **Ortho-phospho-tyrosine (Cancer) NO**

Note: the cancer is gone and *Fasciolopsis* is still present, <u>but not in the liver</u>.

Summary: This was a happy story. The parents openly stated that they did not believe my explanations or test results but would carry out my instructions anyway due to their simplicity. At the last visit, Dave's chemo had been reduced further, showing that his clinical doctors were watching him closely. I believe this all began with the school asbestos-removal program. Although a building is tested for asbestos at the end of a job, the test equipment isn't good enough to pick up the smallest fibers. One can't help wonder if other children in this school developed illness.

Cynthia Broadhurst	Retinoblastoma

Cynthia is a beautiful 19 year old girl, blind due to cancers dating back to infancy. They brought a description summary with them. A recent return of the cancer is threatening the loss of most of her face. Her parents are professional, highly trained people. They could discuss all the kinds of cancer Cynthia has had from retinoblastoma after birth to rhabdomyosarcoma at age 14 to fibrous histiocytoma earlier this year. They are using well water. They will get her latest blood test.

☒ **Toxoplasma (Parasite) YES at the eye**

Toxoplasma is a parasite that comes from a cat box, this is the reason pregnant women are told not to change their cat boxes. Cynthia is allergic to cats, and doesn't have one.

☒ **E. hist, Trichinella (Parasites) YES at the eye**

☒ **Ancylostoma, Human liver fluke (Parasite) YES at part of eye only**

The *human liver fluke* is not the same as *Fasciolopsis*, the human INTESTINAL fluke, which starts a cancer when it moves its "home" from the intestine to the liver.

☒ **Fasciolopsis (Parasite) YES at retina and same part of eye**

Very unusual.

☒ **Oxalate (Kidney Stones) YES**

She will stop drinking tea and start vitamin B6 and magnesium oxide 300 mg/day. They are suspicious of herbs, so won't start on kidney herb recipe.

☒ **Cadmium (Toxic Element) YES at kidneys**

Corroded water pipes.

Summary: The parents left abruptly at this point. I could not persuade them to start on anything. She was scheduled to have half her face, including part of the jaw, removed by surgery in a few weeks. Yet a harmless herbal treatment did not tempt them to try it. I'm sure they loved their daughter as much as life itself. Yet, my methods seemed to arouse anger instead of joy at finding a fresh approach to a hopeless situation. They took no supplies and did not return. I believe this must be a case where Fasciolopsis stages crossed the placenta into the unborn child. The mother may have had high levels of a solvent causing them to disperse from the mother's intestine. I must also wonder whether this solvent was fed to the baby through the mother's milk so that the fluke stages would quickly multiply in the baby. Wood alcohol is a solvent that might do this because it accumulates in the eye (as well as pancreas).

31	John Knowles	Prostate Cancer

This 67 year old man reported the following main problems: history of stomach problems, history of lower back pain, occasional numbness of feet; some sinus problems, history of prostate problems, hemorrhoids. Recently, he has been getting sleepy during the daytime, which was the reason for coming to our office.

☒ **Eimeria (Parasite) YES**

☒ **Fasciolopsis (Parasite) YES at liver and colon**

☒ **Fasciolopsis eggs, cercaria (Parasite) YES at liver, colon, blood, and prostate**

☒ **Ascaris, Cat liver fluke, Diphyllobothrium, Plasmodium vivax (Parasites) YES**

Seeing the intestinal fluke in the liver, I suspect cancer.

☒ **Ortho-phospho-tyrosine (Cancer) YES**

Start on parasite program.

Two weeks later

Not as sleepy as he used to be.

☐ **Ortho-phospho-tyrosine (Cancer) NO**

☐ **Fasciolopsis and all stages (Parasite) NO**

☒ **Cesium (Toxic Element) YES**

Drinks distilled water in plastic jug.

☒ **Vanadium(Toxic Element) YES**

Has a gas hot water heater, furnace, stove and clothes dryer but does not believe there is a leak anywhere. Continue parasite program.

Three weeks later

He still gets occasional sleepy attacks.

☐ **Cesium (Toxic Element) NO**

Stopped drinking distilled water.

271

☒ **Vanadium(Toxic Element) YES**

He did nothing about gas pipes. They will do an air test in their home and bring it next time to test for gas.

☒ **Human liver fluke, Cysticercus, Echinococcus granulosus cyst, Endolimax (Parasites) YES**

☐ **Parasites (Remainder) NO**

Continue parasite program.

Summary: This strong, tall man came in for a minor problem - just needing to nap in the middle of the day. But his intuition told him there was something wrong about that. The prostate cancer shocked him, but he attacked the problem immediately. In 2 weeks the cancer was gone, but his fatigue spells weren't. We have not seen him since his last visit; hopefully his wife will smell the gas in time to prevent a tragedy in their home.

32	Anne Brill	Breast Cancer

Anne Brill is a physically active 61 year old woman with few health complaints. She is a former home economics teacher who has traveled extensively and is now retired. She has pain in her lower back, knees, and feet; a rash on her face periodically; and considers herself to have a weight problem. She has a history of breast cancer, starting over twenty five years ago. She has had radical surgery. Now, for about two months, she has had pain in the left breast area under the left armpit, midline with the nipple.

☒ **Ortho-phospho-tyrosine (Cancer) YES**

☒ **Fasciolopsis (Parasite) YES at liver**

☒ **Fasciolopsis redia (Parasite) YES at breast, liver, blood**

☒ **Fasciolopsis eggs (Parasite) YES at gallbladder, liver, blood**

☒ **Chilomastix (Parasite) YES**

☒ **Pancreatic fluke (Parasite) YES**

Gets waves of nausea - doctor gave medicine for it.

☒ **Echinococcus granulosus, Echinococcus granulosus eggs, Gyrodactylus, Human hookworm (Parasites) YES**

⊠ **Oxalate, all types Calcium Phosphate (Kidney Stones) YES**

Start on parasite program and kidney herb recipe.

Three days later

She reported that she had followed the parasite and kidney programs as recommended. Her lower back, knee, and foot pain is gone, and she is back playing golf this morning. Left breast is no longer sore in old spot, but there is still a little soreness in another place on breast.

☐ **Fasciolopsis and all stages (Parasite) NO**

☐ **Echinococcus granulosus all stages (Parasite) NO**

☐ **Pancreatic fluke, Chilomastix, Gyrodactylus, Necator (Parasites) NO**

☐ **Ortho-phospho-tyrosine (Cancer) NO**

Continue parasite program and kidney herbs. The cause of remaining soreness is not determined yet.

Six days later

She reported no new symptoms. Feet and knees continue to be much better, and the breast pain is all gone.

BLOOD TEST	Result	Comment
1. FBS	slightly high	prediabetic, need to clean liver
2. Total Protein	slightly low	liver problem
3. Alk Phos	high	start on vitamin A&D, magnesium, milk
4. GGT, SGOT, SGPT	high	gallstones and liver problem
5. Iron	low	parasites

⊠ **Asbestos (Toxic Element) YES**

We will test her hair blower.

⊠ **PCB (Toxic Element) YES**

Probable cause of rash on face. She is to go off detergents and use borax only for all purposes.

One week later

Her feet are still painful sometimes, but better. Rash is still on her face. She has continued with parasite and kidney programs.

☐ **Asbestos (Toxic Element) NO**

Must have been coming from her hair blower - stopped using it but used clothes dryer yesterday.

☒ **PCB (Toxic Element) YES**

Is still using detergent for dishwasher, will stop.

☐ **Ortho-phospho-tyrosine (Cancer) NO**

Summary: It only took Anna 3 days to rid herself of cancer and a little over a week to be rid of her pains. The pain under the armpit is typical of a cancer development in the breast. Since she was back to playing golf again and free of pain, she did not follow-up to be sure the PCBs were gone.

33	Claudia Stein	Breast Cancer

Claudia Stein is a 27 year old woman with exposure to contaminated well water. The whole family got sick. The baby does not nurse well. Claudia has pain at lower back, neck, and below both breasts.

☐ **Kidney Stones (ALL) NO**

☒ **Ortho-phospho-tyrosine (Cancer) YES**

☒ **Fasciolopsis (Parasite) YES at liver**

☒ **Fasciolopsis miracidia (Parasite) YES at liver, breast, and blood**

☒ **Fasciolopsis redia (Parasite) YES at breast**

☒ **Fasciolopsis cercaria (Parasite) YES at breast and blood**

She and her husband will start on parasite program. She will start the children (but not the baby) on vermifuge syrup.

Two weeks later

All pain is gone. She has been on parasite program. There is some burning or ache in middle of right groin and both sides of upper chest.

☐ **Ortho-phospho-tyrosine (Cancer) NO**

☒ **Fasciolopsis (Parasite) YES at colon only**

☒ **Fasciolopsis redia (Parasite) YES at colon and breast**

The baby is breast feeding OK now.

☒ **Fluoride (Toxic Element) YES at breast**
Stop toothpaste.

☒ **Scandium (Toxic Element) YES**
Tooth metal.

☒ **PVC (Toxic Element) YES, high**
Husband is a painter - will test air at home and work. She will continue parasite program.

One week later

☐ **Fasciolopsis (Parasite) NO all stages, all locations**

☐ **Ortho-phospho-tyrosine (Cancer) NO**

☐ **Fluoride (Toxic Element) NO**

☒ **Scandium (Toxic Element) YES**

☒ **PVC (Toxic Element) YES**

☒ **PVC (Toxic Element) YES in bedroom, TV room; NO in other rooms**
There is old carpet backing in the PVC YES rooms. They will remove it and do new air tests 3 days later.

Summary: This young mother of 4 was concerned when her baby did not nurse well, thinking that the contaminated well water experience might still be having bad effects. She was not very shocked, though, to hear she had cancer because her sisters had it. She was delighted that the baby was feeding well again after 2 weeks. Their limited finances prevented her from coming back to solve the PVC problem. I should have gotten a milk sample to see if Fasciolopsis stages are in her milk. This question has been on my mind for some time, since it is a body fluid where parasite stages could be transmitted.

| 34 | **Marlene Broad** | **Hodgkin's Disease** |

Marlene Broad, a 32 year old woman, began having shoulder pain about 2 years ago. It was treated as bursitis, but the pain became worse. She lived with it. A few months ago, a varicose vein was noted on her right arm, as well as swelling on the right side of her neck. Her WBC (white blood cell count) had been rising. A venogram and CAT scan showed lymphoma. They also saw 2 tumors, 6-7 cm, believed to be behind the sternum. Numbness of arm has occurred in the past. She will have a biopsy at the hospital soon.

☒ **Fasciolopsis (Parasite) YES at liver and intestine**

She will stop smoking today and get a patch of nicotine. She has only one kidney. The other one was removed due to congenital deformity.

☒ **Oxalate, Uric Acid, Tribasic Calcium Phosphate (Kidney Stones) YES**

☐ **Kidney Stones (remainder) NO**

Start on kidney herbs. Start on parasite program. Go off margarine onto real unsalted butter (and salt it herself with aluminum-free salt).

Six days later

She is on Darvocet Plus™ for pain. She is scheduled for a CAT scan on Monday and will be on Prednisone™. She is now smoking under 1 pack/day but got a Habitrol Patch™ and put it on today (23 mg). She is feeling fine and will stop smoking today. She slept all night for the first time in 6 months (no bathroom visits).

☒ **Fasciolopsis (Parasite) YES but not at liver or intestine**

☒ **Ortho-phospho-tyrosine (Cancer) YES**

☒ **Palladium, Mercury (Toxic Element) YES**

☐ **Toxic Elements (remainder) NO**

See dentist immediately to remove metal tooth fillings.

Four days later

Pain is out of shoulder today. She received a diagnosis of Hodgkin's disease by her clinical doctor yesterday. Dentist took out a root canal from her upper left incisor and removed all metal fillings except lower left side.

☐ **Fasciolopsis (Parasite) NO**

☒ **Fasciolopsis eggs (Parasite) YES at liver**

☐ **Fasciolopsis (other stages) NO**

She is scheduled for a CAT scan of her abdomen.

☐ **Kidney Stones (ALL) NO**

Continue kidney herbs for 1 month.

□ **Ortho-phospho-tyrosine (Cancer) NO**

She is scheduled for chemo and x-ray in about 1 week - after seeing her oncologist. Of course, this is unnecessary now.

Three days later

□ **Fasciolopsis (Parasite) NO**

☒ **Fasciolopsis cercaria (Parasite) YES**

□ **Fasciolopsis (other stages) NO**

She needs one more quadrant of dental work.

Summary: This young woman started out with a handicap at the location of the kidney that was inherited, plus surgery at the kidney. The remaining kidney was clogged with mercury and palladium from her tooth fillings; this gave her 3 kinds of kidney stones. In addition, she smoked. But 7 days later the cancer was gone. She had reduced smoking, removed the metal fillings and a root canal, removed the kidney stones with herbs, and killed the parasites in her liver. Parasite stages hung on, but she will have those eradicated soon. She seemed committed to improving her life style and beat-out the scheduled x-ray and chemo. We have not seen her since, but we have no reason to think she was unsuccessful. Notice that the pain and swelling in her shoulder and arm was gone the day after the dental work was done.

35	Lisa Lindley	Colon Cancer

Lisa Lindley is an 82 year old woman whose main problem is: she spends 20 hours a day in bed because she is so fatigued. Two years ago, she had colon cancer surgery (14 feet of her colon was removed). She had 17 radiation treatments. She also has high blood pressure.

☒ **Ortho-phospho-tyrosine (Cancer) YES at colon**

☒ **Fasciolopsis (Parasite) YES at liver and colon**

☒ **Fasciolopsis redia (Parasite) YES at colon and blood, other stages NO**

She was started on parasite program. However, we were out of wormwood capsules, so we substituted Quassia herb. She was to drink 1/8 cup of a strong tea of quassia 4 times/day.

Seven days later

She had taken everything as directed.

□ **Ortho-phospho-tyrosine (Cancer) NO everywhere**

☐ **Fasciolopsis (Parasite) NO everywhere**

☒ **Fasciolopsis redia (Parasite) YES at blood, NO at colon**
She was to continue on parasite killing program and start on our kidney herb recipe for the high blood pressure (kidneys and adrenal glands are responsible for water and salt regulation, which in turn determines blood pressure). Note that cancer is gone but a stage of the fluke remains in the blood.

Three months later
She is still fatigued.

☐ **Ortho-phospho-tyrosine (Cancer) NO**

☐ **Protein 24 (HIV) NO**

☐ **Fasciolopsis (Parasite) NO**

☒ **Fasciolopsis redia (Parasite) YES at colon and blood**
She has extensive fluid around the eyes and is on B12 shots from her clinical doctor twice a week. Swollen eyelids are usually due to *Ascaris*, the common roundworm of cats and dogs.

☒ **Ascaris (Parasite) YES**
She has a cat and will treat it with our pet parasite program.

Three weeks later

☐ **Fasciolopsis (Parasite) NO**

☐ **Solvents (ALL) NO**

☒ **Antimony (Toxic Element) YES**
Will stop using Noxzema™.

☒ **Formaldehyde (Toxic Element) YES**
She will replace the foam mattress they got from the hospital (free of charge) for a common cloth one.

☒ **Mercury (Toxic Element) YES very high in tissues**
She will see dentist to remove metal tooth fillings. She is not fatigued and can work around the house.
Summary: This intelligent elderly woman got rid of her cancer in 7 days. Swelling of the eyelids always implicates common roundworm of cats and dogs, Ascaris. The eggs are always on their fur so petting them transfers it to human hands. I encouraged her to keep her pet in top health, as well as herself.

Four months later (eight months after the first visit)
She is still very tired, napping 2 hours a day.

☐ **Ortho-phospho-tyrosine, hCG (Cancer) NO**

☒ **Benzene (Solvent) YES in all her organs**
She is still using Noxzema™ daily, liberally on herself. She will stop.

☒ **Acetone, Methyl Butyl Ketone, Methylene Chloride (Solvents) YES**
She will go off commercial beverages. She has not done dental work yet.

☒ **Antimony (Toxic Element) YES**
Probably in Noxzema™

☐ **Formaldehyde (Toxic Element) NO**
Threw out the foam furniture. She will get dental work done.

36	Josefine Flores	Cancer Of Genital Tract

This 46 year old woman reported her main problems as: hands and ankles swelling (probably a kidney condition); coughing (I suspect a respiratory toxin), fatigue, irregular periods, often lasting 3 to 4 weeks, migraine headaches, especially with period (most likely Strongyloides parasites), and a weight problem. Her clinical doctor did a bone density test and found osteoporosis.

We told her to take the following: 3 glasses of 2% milk/day; magnesium oxide tablets from Bronson's, 300 mg, 1/day; vitamin D 1/day any size.

☒ **Isopropyl Alcohol, Xylene (Solvents) YES, remainder NO**
She will go off shampoo and use borax for all purposes. She uses no cosmetics.

☐ **Protein 24 (HIV) NO**

☒ **Ortho-phospho-tyrosine (Cancer) YES throughout genital tract**

☒ **Fasciolopsis (Parasite) YES at colon only**
Note: Absent in liver!!

279

☒ **Fasciolopsis redia (Parasite) YES, other stages NO**
Start parasite program. This is a strong, healthy-looking woman. She has a disseminated cancer of the genital area, including her vagina and uterus. This news was shocking to her. She will go off commercial beverages to get rid of solvents.

Six days later

☐ **Ortho-phospho-tyrosine (Cancer) NO**

☐ **Fasciolopsis (Parasite) NO all stages**
Cancer is gone. Continue on parasite program at maintenance levels.

☒ **Hexane (Solvent) YES**
She is drinking Folger's™ decaffeinated instant coffee. She will go off it and drink water.

☒ **Cysteine, Phosphates (Kidney Stones) YES, high**
The numerous phosphate crystals are probably the result of drinking so much carbonated beverages. She will stop. Her diet will change as follows: Decrease animal food, grains, carbonated beverages (phosphates), increase milk, fruits and vegetables. Start kidney herbs.

One month later

Her period is normal. Her swelling is down, her headaches are better, she has more energy. She is still coughing. She is off caffeine.

☒ **Fluoride (Toxic Element) YES**
Uses no toothpaste.

☐ **Toxic Elements (remainder) NO**
She is preparing to do a liver cleanse.

One month later

She is still coughing. She has a slight swelling in her hands and ankles. She is feeling very well.

☒ **Cysteine (Kidney Stone) YES, remainder NO**
Continue kidney herbs.

☐ **Fasciolopsis and all stages (Parasite) NO**

☐ **Pancreatic fluke and all stages (Parasite) NO**

☒ **Sheep liver fluke (Parasite) YES**

Remainder of parasites not tested. Continue parasite program. Avoid undercooked meats. Eat no meat in restaurants.

One month later

She is no longer coughing, but her left hand is hot and swollen.

☐ **Protein 24 (HIV) NO**

☐ **Ortho-phospho-tyrosine (Cancer) NO**

☒ **Xylene (Solvent) YES**

☒ **Uric Acid (Kidney Stone) YES**

Go back on kidney herbs. Drink milk instead of soda pop.

Summary: This was such a friendly, pleasant woman it would have been a tragedy to lose her to massive genital cancer. She saved herself from this dreadful fate in 6 days. She knew intuitively she was drinking too much pop and was rather glad to be told to be off pop and caffeine both. She may have had the liver fluke from the start since I had not done the complete parasite test. Her visits had to be very brief since they were shared by other family members.

37	Peter Smith	Cancer At Colon

This is a 41 year old man with psoriasis for over 10 years. It began behind his calf. He has large patches about 4 inches in diameter on his elbow and right side and all over him, including his scalp. He is using a non-prescription drug. He has used cortisone. His scalp is also very bad, and it is getting worse. He has spent a lot of money on the problem over the years. He also has arthritis in his elbows, feet, wrist, shoulders, hands, and back. He developed a stomach ulcer about 1 year ago. He has a minor sleep problem as well as depression and a weight problem. He is a building contractor.

☒ **Oxalate, mono-Calcium Phosphate (Kidney Stones) YES**

Start on kidney herb recipe.

Four days later

He is feeling better and has lost about 6 pounds.

☒ **Dipylidium caninum (Parasite) YES at skin**

Dog tapeworm.

☒ **Echinococcus granulosus (Parasite) YES**

Has always had dogs.

⊠ **Fasciolopsis (Parasite) YES at one side of liver**
Suspect cancer.

⊠ **Fasciolopsis redia (Parasite) YES at skin, liver, blood, and colon, other locations NO**

⊠ **Ortho-phospho-tyrosine (Cancer) YES at colon**
Start on parasite program.

Nine days later

BLOOD TEST	Result	Comment
1. Cholesterol	is low (177)	liver problem
2. Phosphate Calcium	high very low	He is dissolving bone and making calcium phosphate deposits. He will change his diet: less phosphate, more Calcium and Magnesium: 3 glasses of 2% milk/day. Vitamin D (50,000) 2/week, by prescription from dentist. Magnesium oxide, 300 mg, one/day.]
3. Potassium	low	due to adrenal/kidney problem
4. SGPT	slightly high	needs to clean liver
5. Iron	very low	parasites
6. Platelet count	slightly high	parasites

☐ **Ortho-phospho-tyrosine (Cancer) NO**

☐ **Fasciolopsis (Parasite) NO**

⊠ **Fasciolopsis eggs (Parasite) YES in blood**
Continue parasite program. Skin is starting to improve.
Summary: Skin eruptions of all kinds are always due to parasites. But I gave his pain a higher priority than his skin, so I started him with the kidney treatment at his first visit. Consequently, I did not find the cancer until his second visit. Since his pains were lessening, he was not too angered by the bad news. His income did not allow him to return after his third visit.

Stella Rowley	**HIV and Cancer**

This 23 year old woman came in because of her chronic yeast infection, cramps she has suffered from "all her life," migraines, bunions, and heart arrhythmia. She also noted that she has sinus problems during the fall and spring. Her right wrist is sore. She has occasional constipation and diarrhea; her right knee is sometimes sore. She is on several medications for her various ailments, way too many for her age.

☒ **Ortho-phospho-tyrosine (Cancer) YES**

☒ **Protein 24 (HIV) YES**

She has both cancer and HIV illness unbeknownst to her, but she is not too surprised. I am surprised at her calmness.

☒ **Isopropyl Alcohol (Solvent) YES high**

Eliminate propanol polluted products like cold cereal and shampoo.

☒ **Benzene (Solvent) YES high**

Off benzene list.

☐ **PCB (Toxic Element) NO**

Summary: She arrived with HIV test results that were NEGATIVE. Apparently, however, she had the intuition that something was quite wrong with her but could not get it established clinically. We recommended a vegetarian diet for her, which appealed to her anyway. She has not returned, and three months have passed. Hopefully, she has followed some of the advice we gave her. Her finances may not have been adequate for her to return for follow-up.

38	Earl Grad	Prostate Cancer

Earl Grad, age 72, came in for prostate cancer. His clinical doctor had found a high PSA (prostate cancer marker). He also found a small nodule on the left side of Earl's prostate. Earl has diabetes and high blood pressure. He is on Lopid™ to lower triglyceride; a diuretic, Hytrin™, to lower his blood pressure and Lanoxin™ to strengthen his heart.

He will start on parasite program. Since he could barely sit because of pain, I only took 5 minutes to get him started and let him leave the office. I had to assume the ortho-phospho-tyrosine and Fasciolopsis tests would be YES.

Twenty days later

His blood test with his clinical doctor showed PSA is very high (45). He also has to get up every hour in the night to urinate.

☐ **Ortho-phospho-tyrosine (Cancer) NO**

His cancer is now gone. He will continue with parasite program. He will start on kidney herbs to cleanse prostate.

☒ **Niobium (Toxic Element) YES**
Probably polluted pills.

☒ **Platinum (Toxic Element) YES**
He has full dentures so this is not coming from metal tooth fillings. He will change to wearing a plastic watch.

☒ **Tin (Toxic Element) YES**
He will switch to salt water to clean his dentures and stop commercial tooth cleaners that have stannous (tin) compounds.

☒ **PCB (Toxic Element) YES, high**
He will switch off detergent to borax.

BLOOD TEST	Result	Comment
1. FBS	very high (209)	needs to cleanse liver
2. Potassium	very low	take kidney herbs, drink vegetable juice
3. Triglycerides	very high	clean kidneys
4. LDH	very high	heart stress, recent cancer
5. PSA	very high	prostate cancer

Six weeks later
There is no pain in his prostate. He still has frequent urination (3 to 4 times/night, which is much better than before). He has dizziness. He stopped his parasite treatment.

☒ **Acanthocephala (Parasite) YES**
He will continue parasite treatment.

Nine days later

☒ **Heterakis (Parasite) YES**
Stay on parasite treatment.

☐ **Ortho-phospho-tyrosine (Cancer) NO**

☒ **Tin, Platinum (Toxic Elements) YES**

☒ **Prescription drugs (in WBC) YES**
He will try ginseng and stop caffeine to keep down blood pressure.

Two weeks later
He is off all drugs. His blood pressure is 128/76 (normal). He is getting up less at night.

☐ **Toxic Elements (ALL) NO**
He will get ready to clean liver for his diabetes.

Four months later

He feels fine, has good elimination, still urinates 3 to 4 times at night, has sexual function back.

☐ **Ortho-phospho-tyrosine (Cancer) NO**

☐ **Protein 24 (HIV) NO**

☐ **Fasciolopsis and all stages, Sheep liver fluke and all stages, Pancreatic fluke (Parasites) NO**

☒ **Ascaris (Parasite) YES**

Probable cause of remaining prostate problem. He has been on maintenance parasite program twice a week. He has a cat. This is probably a source of daily reinfection. He will give his cat the parasite program. He will give himself 5 days of the high dose parasite treatment. He would like an aphrodisiac.

Summary: Earl was at the turning point in his life, from general good health to invalidism. Fortunately, he chose to work on his health instead of settling for a handful of prescription drugs. I encouraged him to follow up his PSA test with his clinical doctor so his clinical doctor wouldn't worry about him. He should tell his clinical doctor what he is doing. He still needs to clear his diabetes. He is strong and healthy again, able to work.

| 39 | Lynn Mercer | Cancer Of The Uterus and Colon |

Lynn came into the office for menstruation problems; she was experiencing excessive bleeding. Provera™ got it stopped once before but not now. Recently, she has been having severe diarrhea that she thinks is stress related. She will go off caffeine. She is very fatigued.

☒ **mono-Calcium Phosphate, Oxalate (Kidney Stones) YES**

She will start on kidney herbs.

☒ **Ortho-phospho-tyrosine (Cancer) YES at colon, uterus**

She had a polyp removed from the outside of her uterus during her last pregnancy.

☒ **Fasciolopsis (Parasite) YES at liver**

☒ **Fasciolopsis eggs (Parasite) YES at uterus and in blood**

Start parasite program and postpone kidney herb recipe until later. She has had a colonoscopy in the past, she was diagnosed with spastic colon. Her father had colon cancer. Her child has abdominal pain.

Five weeks later

She has had a normal period.

- ☐ **Ortho-phospho-tyrosine (Cancer) NO**

- ☐ **Protein 24 (HIV) NO**

- ☐ **Fasciolopsis and all stages (Parasite) NO**

- ☒ **Echinoporypheum, Pancreatic fluke, Entamoeba histolytica (Parasites) YES**

Continue parasite program.

One month later

She is concerned mainly about her hip and knee pain.

- ☒ **B strep, Histoplasma, Adenovirus (Pathogens) YES**

- ☒ **A strep (Pathogen) YES at tooth #17**

Stay on maintenance parasite program. Start on kidney herb recipe. See dentist for cavitation at lower left wisdom tooth.

- ☒ **Isopropyl Alcohol (Solvent) YES**

Remove from home and everywhere.

- ☒ **Hexane (Solvent) YES**

Is drinking Folger's™ decaf - off commercial beverages.

Two months later

A cyst was seen on the top of her pelvis on an x-ray given by her clinical doctor.

- ☐ **Protein 24 (HIV) NO**

- ☐ **Ortho-phospho-tyrosine (Cancer) NO**

- ☒ **Fasciolopsis (Parasite) YES at colon**

- ☐ **Fasciolopsis stages (Parasite) NO**

- ☐ **Sheep liver fluke and all stages (Parasite) NO**

- ☐ **Pancreatic fluke and all stages (Parasite) NO**

- ☒ **Xylene (Solvent) YES**

Off commercial beverages.

Summary: Lynn's period problem of long standing cleared up after taking the kidney herbs and doing the parasite program. What was diagnosed as a spastic colon was actually the beginning of cancer. Her hip and knee pain were eliminated by cleaning an old tooth cavity. But she allowed herself a cosmetic and got her parasite back. She caught it, though, before it established itself in the liver and avoided getting cancer again.

Six weeks later (5½ months after the first visit)

☐ **Protein 24 (HIV) NO**

☒ **Ortho-phospho-tyrosine (Cancer) YES**
Has cancer back, this time at uterus and not colon - has been eating home fried chicken, using regular shampoo and commercial hair spray.

☒ **hCG (Pre-Cancer) YES everywhere in her body**
She will go on a 5 day high dose parasite program.

☒ **Isopropyl Alcohol (Solvent) YES**
Will make her own hair spray.

☒ **Benzene (Solvent) YES**
Has been using Vaseline products and hand creams.

☒ **Cobalt (Toxic Element) YES**
Off detergent.

☒ **Silver, Mercury (Toxic Elements) YES**
Tooth fillings. Lynn needs all the metal in her mouth replaced with metal-free plastics.

☒ **Antimony (Toxic Element) YES**
She will stop using fragranced household products.

☒ **Formaldehyde (Toxic Element) YES**
Has a new couch and chair - will move them into one room and lock it to see if this clears up the problem.
Second summary: Lynn's body is continuing to drain mercury and silver from her tooth fillings into the old cancer site, the uterus. Hopefully, she will get the dental work done soon.

40   Heidi Mertens   Lung Cancer

At a routine X-ray and mammogram, the x-ray showed a "marble size" item on the left lung. The radiologist suspected a calcium deposit. The CAT scan showed the lesion was contained, not spreading. Bronchoscopy is scheduled. She is stopping smoking today. She also has a pain at the left lower abdomen.

☒ **Chromate (Toxic Element) YES at lungs and colon**
Off cosmetics.

☒ **Barium (Toxic Element) YES**
Off lipstick.

☒ **Titanium (Toxic Element) YES at colon**
Probably due to cosmetics.

☒ **Tin (Toxic Element) YES at colon**
She will go off toothpaste; start on 17½% food grade hydrogen peroxide to brush.

☒ **Tungsten (Toxic Element) YES**
She is using an electric coffee percolator. She will use nothing coming from electrically heated devices. She is in her friend's home temporarily where there is electrically heated hot water. She will move to another friend's home.

☒ **PVC (Toxic Element) YES at colon**
Her bedroom may have been painted in the last 3 weeks. Also, she used a lot of household cleaners 3 weeks ago. She is away from it now. We will see if PVC goes away.

☒ **Fasciolopsis (Parasite) YES at liver and colon**

☒ **Ortho-phospho-tyrosine (Cancer) YES in many organs, not only the lungs**
She will go off all cosmetics. Start parasite program.

Two days later

She jumped the parasite treatment to twice the doses to speed things up; she's feeling fine. She is not smoking. She is using no makeup. She has moved to a friend's house where they have a heat pump.

☒ **Fasciolopsis (Parasite) YES at liver only**

☐ **PVC, Barium, Tin, Tungsten (Toxic Elements) NO**

☒ Chromate (Toxic Element) YES at lungs

She will stop wearing a metal watch and will get plastic glasses (hers were metal rimmed). There is no metal in her mouth. She does not wear a metal bra support.

☒ Titanium (Toxic Element) YES at lungs and breast

She is scheduled for a bronchoscopy later today and will take the parasite medicine if not too nauseated after she gets home.

Three days later

She had a bronchoscopy yesterday and will get the results tomorrow. She started thioctic acid (100 mg) this morning, taking 2 every 2 hours. Since her bronchoscopy showed bleeding in the lung, start Ginger capsules, 2 per day.

☒ Fasciolopsis (Parasite) YES at unknown location, NO at liver

☐ Tungsten, PVC, Titanium, Samarium, Chromium (Toxic Elements) NO

I presume the chromium, samarium, and titanium were in her glasses or cosmetics. She taped up her glasses.

☒ Ortho-phospho-tyrosine (Cancer) YES at lung only

Apparently she has gotten rid of all the other cancerous areas. She has not had a cigarette in 75 hours.

Two days later

She has not smoked for 5 days (at 1 PM today). She has made a substitute cosmetic for herself.

☐ Fasciolopsis (Parasite) NO

Reduce ginger to 1/day with meal.

☐ Ortho-phospho-tyrosine (Cancer) NO

The cancer is stopped. We can expect to see the tumor begin to shrink on the x-ray in three weeks.

Four days later

She has not smoked for 8 days now. She is trying to avoid having surgery. She will try to shrink the tumor.

⊠ **Copper, Benzalkonium, Nicorette™ gum (Toxic Elements) YES**

She has picked up 2 new metals. She has started using decaf coffee packs; will go off. She is craving nicotine and needs the nicorette gum; I recommended a patch plus herbs.

☐ **Fasciolopsis (Parasite) NO**

We will increase thioctic to 10/day for 2 days to remove the copper and benzalkonium. Then she will go back to 4/day. Start on mullein and lung herbs (she is on comfrey already).

Three days later

She has not smoked for 12 days (as of 1 PM today).

⊠ **Copper (Toxic Element) YES at lungs, kidney, colon**

⊠ **Toxoplasma (Parasite) YES at lungs, kidney, and colon**

Copper and Toxoplasma in the lungs and colon will prevent tumors from shrinking.

Ten days later

⊠ **PCB (Toxic Element) YES at lungs**

☐ **Copper (Toxic Element) NO**

Stopped coffee. She must stop PCB's immediately since this makes cysts in her body. Probably from detergent. Will switch to borax.

Eight days later

☐ **PCB (Toxic Element) NO**

She has had about 6 cigarettes in the last week. She will check into the nicotine patch.

Summary: Heidi made an excellent beginning but her craving for nicotine overwhelmed her. She took up smoking again and returned to the clinical methods for dealing with tumors; she is now unable to drive a car and is a permanent invalid.

| 41 | Jane Stepenuck | Lymphoma |

Jane and her husband, Scott, are missionaries. They had to return from the Far East because of her cancer. She first got lymphoma two years ago, lumps were removed from her left shoulder and left cheek. She finished all her treatments a year later and returned to her missionary work. Half a year after that, a sudden severe pain in her lower back

290

occurred in the night. The clinical doctor said it was a collapsed verte-
bra due to radiation or chemo. Pain continued. She came home to the
USA since she couldn't work. A new lump is growing under the jaw.
She decided to try some health routines, cutting out a lot of poor foods,
starting on Echinacea, vitamin E, and various cleansing routines. She
has not gone back to the clinical doctor.

☒ **Fasciolopsis, and eggs, miracidia, cercaria (Parasite) YES
at liver**

☒ **Sheep liver fluke redia, miracidia (Parasite) YES at liver**

☒ **Echinococcus multilocularis, Strongyloides, Ancylostoma
d., Trichinella, Ascaris, Dipylidium can, Taenia pis, Onchocerca, Dipetalonema, Endolimax, Fischoedrius
(Parasites) YES**
Note large number of serious parasites. Start on parasite program.

☒ **Oxalate (Kidney Stones) YES**
Probable cause of lower back pain - start on kidney herbs.

Five days later

☐ **Oxalate (Kidney Stone) NO**
Lower back much better.

☒ **Chromate (Toxic Element) YES**
Hair spray?

☒ **Antimony (Toxic Element) YES**
Cosmetics.

☒ **Neodymium (Toxic Element) YES**
Probably a pill.

☒ **Germanium, Thallium (Toxic Elements) YES**
When germanium and thallium are seen together, it is coming
from tooth fillings. Thallium, more toxic than arsenic or lead, is
used as an alloy of mercury to make outdoor thermometers for use
in the Arctic or Antarctica. Could the mercury being shipped to
the dentist sometimes be contaminated with thallium? Is the same
company that ships mercury to dentists also making the thal-
lium/mercury alloy for thermometers? Thallium affects the legs
first, climbing higher to reach the lower back and then makes it
difficult to walk. 90% of the wheelchair cases seen in this office
are actually full of thallium. Thallium was used as a rat poison

291

until it was banned! It is simply too toxic to set out as poison! Yet it has found its way into some people's mouths! She will see a dentist to remove all mercury fillings and save the drillings for me to analyze for thallium.

☒ PVC (Toxic Element) YES

They had new carpeting installed plus linoleum in the kitchen (glued down). We will test the house air for PVC.

☒ Cadmium (Toxic Element) YES, high

Will test hot and cold water.

Eight days later

Slight nausea returned this morning but is now gone. She feels much better. Back pain OK.

☐ Antimony (Toxic Element) NO

☒ Chromate, Neodymium, Cadmium (Toxic Elements) YES

☒ Cadmium (Toxic Element) YES in kitchen cold, kitchen hot, and distilled water

They have their own distiller.

☒ PVC (Toxic Element) YES, and in bedroom air, kitchen air

☒ Twin Labs Multi Mineral Caps™, Solgar™ Rose Hips Vitamin C (Undetermined Elements) YES

There is something toxic in them. Go off.

☒ Neodymium (Toxic Element) YES in Provera™

She will go off all supplements and pills. She will switch to borax from detergents. She will drink store bought spring water and rotate brands even though they may be polluted too. They will change water pipes to plastic for kitchen and bathroom. It is a very old house and they are living in it cheaply. Their income is low. The kitchen and bedroom are the rooms where carpet and linoleum were installed. They will keep fan on and window open to blow out the PVC. She is breaking out in a rash on the thigh. They cannot afford to come back; we will do remainder gratis.

One week later

☐ Fasciolopsis (Parasite) NO at liver

☒ Fasciolopsis eggs (Parasite) YES at blood only

☒ **Fasciolopsis cercaria (Parasite) YES**

She is nearly rid of her parasites. I did not do cancer test so she will not stop coming. (If I found the cancer to be gone, she might stop coming.)

☒ **Chromate, Cadmium, PVC (Toxic Element) YES all very high**

☐ **Germanium, Thallium (Toxic Element) NO**

Her own dentist removed the mercury fillings; she brought me the drillings. Her thallium is gone. She appears healthier. Her leg rash is better.

One week later

Her leg rash is worse. Probably PCB. She will switch dish soap to borax, too. Her energy is good now.

☐ **Fasciolopsis and all stages (Parasite) NO**

☐ **Ortho-phospho-tyrosine (Cancer) NO**

☒ **Chromate (Toxic Element) YES**

She will go off hair spray.

☒ **PVC (Toxic Element) YES**

They are trying to get their carpets changed. She will stay on maintenance parasite program. She is to eat butter (3 pats a day), not margarine.

Summary: We saw no more of her after this last happy visit, when she heard the cancer was gone. I had tested her husband for intestinal fluke earlier, and he was rid of it, too, by the last visit. They are a happy couple. There were no lumps anywhere, she was free of pain, and she had enough energy to bring up the idea of going back to Taiwan. Her husband deserves a medal for all the work he did to get Jane well.

42	Charlene Neely	Breast Cancer

This 50 year old woman reported that her main problems are: fibrocystic breast disease; lower back pain; headaches; bloating (she's on Lasix™ for this); sinus problems (she's on Actifed™ for this); pain over liver at right side.

☒ **Ortho-phospho-tyrosine (Cancer) YES at breast**

☒ **Fasciolopsis (Parasite) YES at liver and colon**
Gets loose bowels after eating.

☒ **Fasciolopsis miracidia (Parasite) YES at liver, breast, cervix, blood, and colon**

☒ **Fasciolopsis cercaria (Parasite) YES**
Her mother died of liver cancer.

☒ **Isopropyl Alcohol (Solvent) YES at liver, breast, cervix, and colon; NO at blood**
She will go off cosmetics with "PROP" on the label. Start on parasite program.

One month later

☐ **Ortho-phospho-tyrosine (Cancer) NO**

☐ **Protein 24 (HIV) NO**

☐ **Fasciolopsis (Parasite) NO**

☒ **Fasciolopsis miracidia (Parasite) YES at breast only**

☒ **Sheep liver fluke eggs (Parasite) YES**
She has been eating hamburger. She will eat only overcooked meat, done only at home. Start on 5-day high dose parasite program, then maintenance.

☒ **Isopropyl Alcohol (Solvent) YES**
She will go off commercial shampoo and hair spray.

☒ **Aluminum (Toxic Element) YES**
Off deodorant.

☒ **Copper (Toxic Element) YES**
Replace metal tooth fillings.

☒ **Formaldehyde (Toxic Element) YES**
Sleeps on foam pillow - will change to dacron or cotton.

Three weeks later

☐ **Fasciolopsis and all stages (Parasite) NO**

☒ **Sheep liver fluke redia, eggs (Parasite) YES**

☒ **Pancreatic fluke (Parasite) YES**
She is still eating hamburgers but will stop. Will order only fish and seafood in restaurants. She will start a 5-day high dose parasite program again.

☒ **Isopropyl Alcohol (Solvent) YES**
Will switch to homemade hair spray this time.

☒ **TCE, Benzene, Xylene, Hexane, TC-Ethylene, Methyl Ethyl Ketone (Solvents) YES**
She is eating ice cream and drinking carbonated beverages. She will make her own.

☐ **Formaldehyde (Toxic Element) NO**
Changed her pillow.

One month later

☐ **Protein 24 (HIV) NO**

☐ **Ortho-phospho-tyrosine (Cancer) NO**

☐ **Fasciolopsis and all stages (Parasite) NO**

☒ **Sheep liver fluke and miracidia (Parasite) YES**
Probable cause of liver pain.

☐ **Pancreatic fluke and stages (Parasite) NO**

☒ **Acetone, TCE (Solvent) YES**
Drinking tea - will stop commercial beverages.

☒ **Oxalate, Uric Acid, Cysteine, Phosphate (Kidney Stones) YES**
Start on kidney herbs.
Summary: The cancer news must have surprised her since she came in only for fibrocystic disease. But she started her program eagerly. The hardest change for her was changing her hamburger and pop habit. She had 4 kinds of kidney stones causing her low back pain. But she wants to improve and is making progress.

One month later (4 months after the first visit)
She still has pain over the gallbladder region. She still has soreness in her breasts. Her lower back pain is gone, but she will continue on kidney herbs.

☐ **Protein 24 (HIV) NO**

☐ hCG, Ortho-phospho-tyrosine (Cancer) NO

☐ Fasciolopsis and all stages (Parasite) NO

☐ Sheep liver fluke and all stages (Parasite) NO

☐ Pancreatic fluke and stages (Parasite) NO

☐ Human liver fluke and stages (Parasite) NO
   She is staying on parasite maintenance program.

☒ Methylene, Carbon Tetrachloride (Solvents) YES
   She is drinking Nestea™ and using Sweet N' Lo™; she will stop.
   Our next goal is to cleanse the liver to clear the gallstones. Prepare
   by starting on 07 and peroxy.

43	Andrew Elmer	Lung Cancer

Andrew Elmer is a 58 year old man who, just this week, finished lung cancer therapy - both chemotherapy and radiation. Lung cancer was diagnosed several months ago, and they first operated on the right lung, removing the top lobe. Then he noticed he was spitting up blood. They went down and found cancer in the bottom of the left lung. But his lump was inoperable. So therapy was started. He had 34 radiation treatments and 5 chemotherapy treatments (originally scheduled to have 6). He is experiencing fatigue with exertion, and his energy has not returned yet from the last "blast." He was on Cisplaten™ and VP (Carboplatin™) also. He is a recovering alcoholic of 20 years. He quit smoking about 4 years ago when he had two angioplasties. He is presently on drugs for his heart: Cardizem™, Delatrate™, Coumadin™ and Mevacor™ for blockage. He has no appetite and needs to gain weight.

☒ Fischoedrius, Dientameoba (Parasites) YES

☒ Fasciolopsis (Parasite) YES at liver and colon

☒ Fasciolopsis eggs (Parasite) YES at blood and lungs

☒ Prosthogonimus eggs, Hypodereum, Paragonimus, Plasmodium vivax (Parasites) YES at lungs

☒ Sarcocystis (Parasite) YES at muscle
   Remaining 70 parasites were negative

⊠ Ortho-phospho-tyrosine (Cancer) YES

He will start on a parasite killing program, using an aqueous black walnut tincture to avoid the alcohol. We are out of wormwood presently, so he will do without.

He is getting freshly made carrot juice with celery, ginger root and other vegetables, and 1 apple and sometimes beet or cabbage. He is also eating Meritene™ and Carnation Instant Breakfast™ and papaya. He got some blood tests done yesterday.

He did not seem enthusiastic and asked how many times he would have to come back. I said "six," and he looked dismayed. I tried to encourage him. His wife seemed more receptive, and she took all the notes during the visit.

Six days later

He has followed the parasite program.

☐ Ortho-phospho-tyrosine (Cancer) NO

☐ Fasciolopsis adults, miracidia, redia, eggs, cercaria, Fischeodrius, Dientameoba, Prosthogonimus, Hypodereum (Parasites) NO

⊠ Sarcocystis (Parasite) YES

All parasites were NO except Sarcocystis. We will add Quassia to the program since our wormwood is not in yet.

⊠ Calcium Phosphate, all types (Kidney Stones) YES

This is the probable cause of deposits in heart blood vessels for which he needed angioplasties. He needs to decrease phosphate (reduce meats, grains, eggs, and cheese). He needs to increase his mineral consumption by consuming the following: whole milk to 3+ glasses a day; magnesium (300 mg) 2/day; zinc (50 mg Bronson's) 1/day; manganese (50 mg) 1/day for one bottle only; increase fruits and vegetables.

Start on kidney herb recipe. Stop using aluminum pots and use of aluminum.

For sweetening use: glycerin (pure vegetable); Stevia powder; honey (3 kinds), pure maple syrup, molasses, sorghum. He has been using Sweet-n-Low™ and other chemical sugars. He is to throw it all out. He is a big meat-eater. He will have 4 cans of sardines per week, seafood and salmon for two days, and one vegetarian day per week.

He brought two recent blood tests with him:

BLOOD TEST	Result	Comment
1. Chloride	slightly high (107)	adrenal
2. Platelet count	very high (402, 417)	parasites
3. RBC	very low (3.4, 3.5)	parasites
4. WBC	low (4.6, 4.7)	toxin in bone marrow
5. Lymphs	low (12, 14%)	toxin in bone marrow
6. Monocytes	high	due to illness
7. Calcium	very low	needs more milk, fruit, vegetables to offset phosphate
8. FBS	slightly high	probably due to nonfasted state at test time
9. BUN and Creatinine	slightly high	kidney
10. Total protein	very low	liver problem
11. LDH	slightly low	muscle fatigue
12. SGOT	low	needs 1/day Vit. B6 [500 mg] from Bronson

Also needs B-50 complex, 2/day; vitamin C (1000-3000 mg/day); vitamin E (100 mg/day, all before meals); beta carotene (25,000 mg, 2/day).

Seven days later

Energy is better. Appetite still poor. No weight gain yet. For breakfast he should eat cooked cereal (buy salt-free variety and add own salt - aluminum-free salt) with cream and sweeteners. Add Vitamin. D (50,000 - 1/day) for three weeks, then move to 2/week; get Rx from dentist. Still has shortness of breath but is playing golf now.

☐ **Sarcocystis (Parasite) NO**

One month later

We have received his hospital records but not x-rays yet. Appetite better. Energy better. Low back pain gone. Breathing unchanged. Add comfrey to kidney herb recipe. Add fresh garlic to diet (1 clove/day), both are for lungs.

☐ **Kidney Stones (ALL) NO**

☒ **Neodymium (Toxic Element) YES**
Possibly a pill.

☒ **Radon (Toxic Element) YES**
Will test air at home and at office.

298

Two weeks later

He has gone back to work at his office.

☐ **Neodymium (Toxic Element) NO**
Changed brands of medicine.

☒ **Radon (Toxic Element) YES, high**

☐ **Ortho-phospho-tyrosine (Cancer) NO**

☐ **Fasciolopsis and all stages (Parasite) NO**
His voice is very weak. This problem is probably due to radon. Home air sample shows it is NO (negative). Office air is YES (positive). He will move his office to other end of hall.

One month later

No improvement in breathing capacity. He has gained 2 lbs. He wants to go off garlic and comfrey. Pathogen test showed *Clostridium* botulinum in lungs and in 2 teeth (teeth #10 and #28). He needs to see the dentist.

One month later (3 months and 2 weeks since first visit)

Teeth numbers 10 and 28 were extracted. His breathing is better, and his voice is stronger. No weight gain. He is on penicillin from his dental work. He is on parasite maintenance program. He feels fine and is back to work. His appetite is better. He is very happy to be off garlic and comfrey. He needs to start on 07 and peroxy to prepare for liver cleanse.

Summary: This was an exemplary couple; they wasted no time in carrying out every instruction. We heard from them recently; they wanted to tell all their friends and especially their clinical doctor about this treatment program. My attorney advised against this, so we asked them not to. Note that Quassia is a rather good parasiticide. At the end he began to prepare for a liver cleanse.

During the following year

He looks rather well; has gained weight. He has not yet done a liver cleanse. He has had all the metal removed from his mouth. Andrew went to the hospital for clogged arteries. X-ray and CT scan showed no trace of cancer in lungs or anywhere, according to his wife. Doctors are surprised.

| 44 | Edward Steinman | Prostate Cancer |

Edward Steinman is a 64 year old man who has beginning diabetes. He is not on medication for it. He states his main problem is his eyes. He also has a respiratory problem, pain in the upper arm, aching hands, and lower back pain. Possible neuropathy in left leg. Numbness of 2 middle toes. History of scrotal problem and skin cancer (a new spot is forming). History of prostate problem. Frequent urination. Family members died of diabetes and cancer. His aunt died of cancer. His father had colon cancer and Parkinson's disease. He has osteoarthritis in his neck.

☒ Oxalate and others (Kidney Stones) YES very high

Start on kidney stone removal with herb recipe.

One week later

He has not started on kidney herbs yet.

BLOOD TEST	Result	Comment
1. Urinalysis	very good	probably due to recent antibiotics
2. WBC	very low	bone marrow toxin
3. RBC	slightly low	minor bleeding, needs to follow up with CBC in March/April 1992. He has had polyps removed in the past.
4. Platelet count	low	possibly due to bone marrow problem
5. CO2	slightly high	toxin in air
6. BUN	slightly elevated and Creatinine is high	kidney
7. Total protein	slightly low	liver problem
8. LDH	slightly high	liver or heart, possibly due to pain syndrome, muscle cramps at night, or cancer
9. Iron	high	

Three weeks later

☒ Uric Acid (Kidney Stone) YES

Had not obtained black cherry concentrate for kidney herb recipe.

☒ Antimony, Palladium, Rhenium (Toxic Elements) YES at bone marrow, lung, prostate

☐ Toxic Elements (Remainder) NO

He will stop using Vaseline products and Vicks™. He needs metal tooth fillings out.

Two weeks later

☐ **Kidney Stones (ALL) NO**

☒ **Antimony (Toxic Element) YES**
Stop after-shave

☒ **Thulium (Toxic Element) YES at prostate and stomach**
Go off her brand of vitamin C.

☒ **Cat liver fluke, Ascaris (Parasites) YES**

☒ **Fasciolopsis (Parasite) YES at liver and colon**
Must check for cancer. Start parasite program. He will stop hand lotion (has antimony) and use ours.

☒ **Ortho-phospho-tyrosine (Cancer) YES at prostate**

Two months later

☐ **Fasciolopsis (Parasite) NO**
Onto maintenance parasite program, 2 times/week.

☒ **Thulium, Palladium, Rhenium (Toxic Elements) YES at bone marrow and prostate**
Palladium and rhenium possibly in gold crowns. He did not get crowns replaced. He will go off his vitamin C and switch to Bronson's brand.

Five weeks later

☒ **Loa Loa, Strongyloides, Chilomastix, Trichinella (Parasites) YES**

☒ **Fasciolopsis cercaria (Parasite) YES**

☐ **Antimony, Thulium (Toxic Elements) NO**
Will stay on parasite maintenance program.

One week later
He had a medical check-up 2 weeks ago. Dermatologist says he is OK, doesn't have skin cancer.

☒ **Calcium Phosphate (Kidney Stone) YES**
Increase milk consumption. Take vitamin. D (1000 u, 3/day). Decrease phosphate (breads, meat).

☒ **Asbestos (Toxic Element) YES, high**
Will test house air and water.

☒ **Sheep liver fluke, Pancreatic fluke (Parasites) YES**

He is eating rare-cooked beef, but will stop. He will eat only fish and seafood in restaurants. He is still using commercial shaving products with propanol. He will switch to an electric shaver.

One month later

☒ **Fasciolopsis (Parasite) YES at one side of liver**

☒ **Fasciolopsis eggs (Parasite) YES at blood and prostate**

☐ **Ortho-phospho-tyrosine (Cancer) NO**

Note: He is just beginning to develop adult flukes in the liver but O.P.T. (cancer test) is not yet positive. He will stay on parasite program and not eat beef.

☒ **Silver, Uranium, Palladium, Platinum (Toxic Elements) YES**

Needs crowns out.

Five weeks later (six months one week after first visit)

☐ **Fasciolopsis and all stages (Parasite) NO**

He is strictly on maintenance parasite program.

Summary: Edward took many risks and one could say that he had poor compliance, but due to his wife's persistence, he returned many times, making a little progress each time. After his pains were gone and his clinical doctor said he was free of skin cancer, he lost interest in improving his health. Hopefully, his wife is keeping a watch over his shampoo and shaving products to avoid propanol. She can do nothing about his eating habits in restaurants. Edward is one of the rare cases where the fluke adult is already present in the liver, and yet there is no cancer marker, ortho-phospho-tyrosine, being produced. Perhaps an additional stage, besides eggs, is necessary, since reproduction is the parasites' objective.

Loreen Pennell	Lymphoma

This 60 year old woman reported 3 main problems: 1) She had cancer (lymphoma) 3½ years ago. Recently, she developed a lump in the neck at her left lymph node. She had 12 chemotherapies. The lump was removed and tested POSITIVE to lymphoma. Her last test three months ago appeared normal. She had a CAT scan yesterday. 2) She has a sleep problem. 3) She has had arthritis in her right hip for 1 to 2 years.

☒ **Ortho-phospho-tyrosine (Cancer) YES**

☐ **Protein 24 (HIV) NO**

☒ **Fasciolopsis (Parasite) YES at liver and colon**

☒ **Fasciolopsis miracidia (Parasite) YES at liver and colon**
Start on parasite program.

BLOOD TEST recent one she brought with her	Result	Comment
1. RBC	very low (3.95)	parasites
2. Platelet count	very low (109)	bone marrow
3. WBC	low (4.4)	bone marrow
4. Urinalysis	shows urobilino-gen	liver
5. FBS	slightly high (107)	needs to clean liver
6. Iron	very low	parasites
7. Cholesterol	very low	cancer risk, clean liver

Summary: Loreen has not returned. We can see that the cancer was not gone as she had hoped after her clinical therapy. The adult fluke was alive in her liver. The solvent test was not recorded, but I generally discuss propanol at the first visit. Hopefully, she has removed all propanol-containing body products from her life-style and has taken the parasite program.

45	**Kirk Gunderson**	**Colon Cancer**

He reported that his main problems were: 1) Colostomy for colon cancer in mid-70s. 2) Two years later he went to Tijuana, Mexico for bladder cancer. They took the cancer off the bladder wall with a laser. He then had laetrile treatment. Since then several more have been removed at local hospital. 3) Minor sleep problem due to getting up 5 to 6 times a night. His clinical doctor said that within 3 months they would need to remove a testicle. Prostate test showed bad pathology. He has lost about 10 lbs in 3 months, and now weights 140.

☒ **Ortho-phospho-tyrosine (Cancer) YES**

☒ **Fasciolopsis (Parasite) YES**
Note: No fluke stages anywhere; only adults. Start parasite program.

☐ **Kidney Stones (ALL) NO**

Note: He has no kidney crystals! He says he has always drunk 2 quarts water/day! I cut short his testing since he was in the office under pressure of his family, not willingly.

Four days later

☐ **Ortho-phospho-tyrosine (Cancer) NO**

☒ **Mercury (Toxic Element) YES**

☐ **Toxic Elements (Remainder) NO**

Continue parasite program. Get all metal fillings replaced with plastic. Start on thioctic, 4/day.

One week later

He has a very sore seat, he can hardly sit. He seems very sick.

☐ **Mercury (Toxic Element) NO**

He has not done any dental work! He said he went to a kinesiologist who did a special routine and said it would get rid of his mercury without dental work.

☐ **Ortho-phospho-tyrosine (Cancer) NO**

☐ **Fasciolopsis and all stages (Parasite) NO**

☒ **Borellia (Pathogen) YES at prostate, lungs, penis and teeth**

☒ **Clostridium (Pathogen) YES at lungs and teeth**

Recommend cavitation cleaning by dentist.

☒ **Diplococcus (Pathogen) YES high at teeth**

☒ **Histomonas, Mycobacterium (Pathogens) YES**

☒ **Salmonella (Pathogen) YES at penis**

Needs dental work.

☐ **Pathogens (Remainder) NO**

Six weeks later

He has had both testicles removed by surgery. He looks terminally ill. His family has arrived. Family members are pushing him in different directions.

☐ **Ortho-phospho-tyrosine (Cancer) NO**

☐ **Protein 24 (HIV) NO**

☒ **Strep pneumonia (Pathogen) YES and very high throughout his body**

He was in the hospital for dehydration. He did not get his mercury-filled teeth out. He now is septic with bacteria throughout his body. He still resists getting his teeth pulled in spite of his terminal condition. He raised the issue of cost. Due to the systemic infection, the remaining bacteria and virus were not tested. Possibly no dentist would take him in this condition. Note: he will die of sepsis, not cancer.

Another 4½ months later (6½ months after first visit)

His family reported that he is well and active, doing the farm work with horses, as before his illness.

Summary: Mr. Gunderson has surprised me with his survival. I had given up hope. If the family found a health practitioner using a special method, I will try to find out. He is staying on a maintenance parasite program, according to his family.

Dan Johnson	Leukemia (AML)

Dan Johnson is a thin young man, age 37, with a sallow complexion and hair loss from chemotherapy. He has had leukemia for 8 years. His clinical doctors told him this would be his last remission, and it would only last 4 months. His first remission lasted 4 years and 2 months. Last year he got a hard dose of chemo; they also took out his gallbladder. He got candidiasis in the liver, spleen, and kidneys. He has been on Diflucain™ (400 mg/day) since then. He still has a temperature of 101-102 nightly. In the hospital it was called "fever of unknown origin." The present remission began two months ago.

☒ **Fasciolopsis (Parasite) YES at liver, intestine**

☒ **Fasciolopsis redia (Parasite) YES at intestine, testicles**

☒ **Ortho-phospho-tyrosine (Cancer) YES at testicles and bone marrow**

He was started on parasite killing program.

BLOOD TEST	Result	Comment
1. FBS	very high	due to chemotherapy

2. Phosphates	high	dissolving bone. Change diet: reduce phosphate (grains, animal food, carbonated beverages - increase milk (2%) and fruits and vegetables)
3. Uric acid	very high (8.1 mg/dl)	kidney problem
4. Alk. phos	very high (368)	bone disease and cancer
5. WBC	low	bone marrrow toxin
6. Lymphs	very low (15%)	toxin in bone marrow
7. Blasts	high (4%)	typical of leukemia

Summary: Dan seemed quite enthusiastic but never returned. We have not heard about him since this first visit. He could have corrected his problems by changing the products he used in daily life. I hope we will hear from him eventually.

---

46 Joel Neal   **Prostate Cancer**

This 71 year old man reported that his main problems were: cataract developing in the right eye (he already has a lens replacement in his left eye); ear pain close in behind his right ear; shoulder pain and bursitis in shoulder; minor pain under rib cage on both sides; gastritis (he is on medication for it); spastic colon; lower back pain; migraines; recent UTI; prostate enlarged. He is on numerous medications. He will start on digestive enzymes from Bronson's Pharm. and charcoal capsules.

☒ **Uric Acid (Kidney Stone) YES**
Start on kidney herb recipe.

☒ **Ortho-phospho-tyrosine (Cancer) YES at prostate**

☒ **Fasciolopsis (Parasite) YES at liver and colon**

☒ **Fasciolopsis miracidia (Parasite) YES at prostate, colon, blood. Other stages NO**
Due to presence of cancer, he was started on parasite program instead of kidney herbs.

Seven days later
He has had some spells of dizziness.

☐ **Ortho-phospho-tyrosine (Cancer) NO**
Cancer is gone.

☐ **Fasciolopsis and all stages (Parasite) NO**
Continue parasite program.

☒ **Cobalt, Zirconium (Toxic Elements) YES at prostate**
He will go off denture cleaner (Efferdent™) and use grain alcohol (50%).

☒ **Strontium (Toxic Element) YES at prostate**
Efferdent™? water softener? doesn't use toothpaste.
Start kidney herbs.

Eight days later

☐ **Cobalt, Zirconium, Strontium (Toxic Elements) NO**

☒ **Calcium Phosphate (Kidney Stone) YES**
Continue kidney herbs, correct diet.

☐ **Ortho-phospho-tyrosine (Cancer) NO**

☒ **Chilomastix, Taenia pisiformis (Parasites) YES**
Daughter also has Taenia pisiformis.

☒ **Dog heartworm (Parasite) YES at heart**
Pain over top of heart occasionally.

☒ **Strongyloides (Parasite) YES**
Cause of migraines.

☒ **Schistosoma mansoni (Parasite) YES**
Continue on parasite program. (had gone off for a while).

One week later
He shows a drop in body current, hard to get my measurements. PCB?

☐ **Zirconium, Strontium (Toxic Elements) NO**

☒ **Cobalt, PCB (Toxic Elements) YES**
Off detergent.

☒ **Coxsackie B #4, Haemophilus inf (Pathogens) YES at 2 teeth, remainder were NO**
Needs cavitations cleaned, see dentist.

BLOOD TEST done 2 months previously	Result	Comment
1. PSA	high (16)	cancer marker for prostate
2. Creatinine	slightly high	kidney

3. Calcium	low (9.0)	Drink 2% milk - 3 glasses/day; take Magnesium 300 mg 1/day.
4. Triglycerides	high (198)	kidney. Take Vit. D (50,000 2 times per week.
5. SGPT	slightly high	needs liver cleanse
6. FBS	slightly high (116)	prediabetic - clean liver
7. Potassium	very low (3.6)	adrenal problem, clean kidney
8. WBC	high (9.3)	infection somewhere
9. Platelet count	very high (513)	had cancer at the time
10. Lymphs	very low (17.6)	toxin in bone marrow

Take vitamin C - 1000 mg each meal, from Bronson's Pharm only. Try going off Bentyl™ and muscle relaxant. Still having dizziness and mid-abdomen pain.

Three weeks later

He is working at the office again and around the house. Energy is up, big improvement. Disposition is better according to his wife.

Eight weeks later

He is feeling quite well. He had cavitations cleaned on left side (7 or 8 teeth). He will get Vitamin D from dentist (50,000 units 2/week).

Bone healing program:
1. Milk - 3 glasses/day, 2%
2. Magnesium oxide - 300 mg 2/day
3. Zinc - 60 mg once a day for 100 days from Bronson's Pharm.
4. Vitamin D - 50,000 2/week

Three months later

Prostate is fine, urination is fine. Still has occasional pain across chest (needs to clean liver). He still has daily headache (uses pain killer).

☒ Dog heartworm (Parasite) YES

Go back on high dose parasite program followed by maintenance.

Summary: Joel became a well, productive person in the course of a few months by working at cleaning his kidneys, killing parasites and changing his daily habits. Notice how dog heartworm easily comes back; it takes about ½ year on maintenance program to completely kill it. He was a very happy man at his last visit and was preparing for a liver cleanse.

| 47 | Deanna Kaiser | Colon Cancer |

Deanna, age 40, came in for pain in her right leg, thigh, and foot. Hot flushes disturb her sleep. She has very low energy in the afternoon. Two years ago she had a lump removed from her left breast; she found it herself; it was cancerous. Her menstrual periods stopped after chemotherapy for this cancer.

BLOOD TEST	Result	Comment
1. Uric acid	high (6.7)	clean kidneys
2. Phosphates	high (4.4)	dissolving bone. Change diet: decrease phosphates in diet (decrease meats, grains, carbonated drinks). Increase calcium, magnesium, potassium (increase milk, fruits and vegetables). She is intolerant of milk. Will use a tablet until she is tolerant. Oyster shell calcium 2/day. Magnesium oxide 300 mg, 1/day.
3. LDH	slightly high	check for cancer
4. Iron	low	parasites
5. Triglycerides	high (151)	clean kidneys
6. Urinalysis	shows low level infection	clean kidneys

☒ **Ortho-phospho-tyrosine (Cancer) YES**

☒ **Fasciolopsis (Parasite) YES at liver and colon**

☒ **Fasciolopsis redia (Parasite) YES at blood**

☒ **all phosphates, Cystine (Kidney Stones) YES**

Start on kidney herbs and start parasite program.

One month later.

☐ **Ortho-phospho-tyrosine (Cancer) NO**

☐ **Fasciolopsis (Parasite) NO**

☒ **Fasciolopsis cercaria (Parasite) YES at blood and colon**

☒ **Fasciolopsis miracidia (Parasite) YES at breast and blood**

Notice that she still has some fluke stages, although no adults remain. She used grocery store ground cloves instead of ours to save money, but they were not as effective. She will switch to fresh ground cloves and add quassia (see *Recipes*).

☒ **Arsenic (Toxic Element) YES at breast**
Will test home air.

Three weeks later

☐ **Kidney Stones (ALL) NO**
Do kidney cleanse twice a year.

☐ **Ortho-phospho-tyrosine (Cancer) NO**
She is concerned about pains persisting.

☒ **Nickel (Toxic Element) YES at breast**
She has had tooth problems recently. This is probable cause of pains at hip, leg, and foot. She needs to replace all metals in her mouth.

☒ **Thulium (Toxic Element) YES**
Will not use vitamin. C except from Bronson's.

☒ **Campylobacter, Salmonella (Pathogens) YES**

☒ **Besnoitia at tooth #12, Anaplasma at tooth #31, Diplococcus diph. at tooth #12 (Pathogens) YES**
She will reduce Nickel intake, cook and eat with non-metal ware.
Mouth program:
1. Baking soda from box (dissolve in water) to brush teeth.
2. Potassium iodide (white iodine) drops on toothbrush from dentist.
Brush at bedtime. Use no toothpaste, nor peroxide (it reacts with metal).
Mouthwash: flush mouth with water at the faucet after each meal. Floss once a day, before brushing, with Osco Unwaxed Floss™.

Two months later
She is feeling well. Pains are gone. Hot flushes gone. Sleeping fine. Energy is back up.

☐ **Fasciolopsis and all stages (Parasite) NO**
Parasite maintenance twice a week.

☐ **Arsenic (Toxic Element) NO**
Removed pesticide from house.

☒ **Nickel (Toxic Element) YES**
Has not done dental work.

☒ **Thulium (Toxic Element) YES**
Stopped vitamin C so source is probably a different supplement.

☒ **Wood Alcohol (Solvent) YES**
Off commercial beverages.

☒ **Isopropyl Alcohol (Solvent) YES**
Will eliminate it.

☒ **Influenza (Pathogen) YES**
Use homeopathic Oscillococcinum.

☒ **Borellia, Strep pneu, Coryne dip, Clostridium tet, Bacill anth, Clost sept, Clost bot (Pathogens) YES at teeth**
Needs to do dental work.

Summary: Deanna got rid of the problems she came in for and her cancer, too, in 3 visits, but she is choosing the unwise path. The bacteria under her metal teeth will continue to infect her body and let others grow as well. Hopefully, she will get the metal out soon. Notice how the breast was next in line for the cancer and how the breast had been accumulating arsenic and nickel. Toxic substances from the top of the body are collected by lymph nodes and passed into the breast for storage when there is too much for the kidneys to eliminate.

Sherry Wu	Cervical Cancer

Sherry had a hysterectomy for endometrial cancer in 1965. A year ago her PAP test came back with suspicious results. She had pain from her left hip down her left leg. She had a hip replacement a few years ago, but her clinical doctor said this was not the cause of her pain. She also saw the dentist, Dr. J., who found no problem with her dentures.

BLOOD TEST	Result	Comment
1. WBC	low (4.9)	bone marrow toxin
2. Seg/lymph	low	chronic virus
3. Eos	high (5%)	parasites
4. Phosphates	high	dissolving bones She will drink 3 glasses of 2% milk and take Magnesium oxide (300 mg) one a day. She will reduce phosphate foods and increase fruit and vegetables. She will get Vitamin D, (50,000 u) from Dr. J. and take 3/week.
5. LDH	slightly high	cancer

6. Cholesterol	low	cancer risk. She will use butter, not margarine, and olive oil for cooking.

☒ **Ortho-phospho-tyrosine (Cancer) YES at cervix**

☒ **Fasciolopsis (Parasite) YES at liver**

☒ **Fasciolopsis redia (Parasite) YES at liver**

☒ **Acetone (Solvent) YES**

☒ **Isopropyl Alcohol (Solvent) YES**

☐ **Protein 24 (HIV) NO**

Start on parasite program. She will search for "PROP" on labels and eliminate these items. She does not use carbonated beverages. She will have a follow-up PAP by her clinical doctor next week.

Summary: Sherry is a very active person; it would break her heart to be forced to stop her gymnastics class. This is what drove her 2000 miles to see us for a mere pain in the leg. But it turned out to be cancer. Since she is an old client who had seen us over the years for any major problem, I do not doubt she carried out our instructions precisely. She has probably saved herself surgery, and without any interruption of her gymnastics class.

48	Maria Perez	Skin Cancer

This 44 year old woman reported that her main problems are: 1) A lesion on her right lower leg which appeared about a year ago. It has been surgically removed but has returned. It tested negative to cancer, but it isn't healing. It heals temporarily if cortisones are used on it. 2) Six months ago a small "cyst" was removed from her lip, diagnosed cancerous. (At the time, she had recently switched to a new lipstick.)

☐ **Protein 24 (HIV) NO**

☒ **Ortho-phospho-tyrosine (Cancer) YES at skin and colon**

☒ **Fasciolopsis (Parasite) YES at colon and liver**

☒ **Fasciolopsis miracidia (Parasite) YES at blood, liver, skin**

☐ **Sheep liver fluke (Parasite) NO**

☒ **Isopropyl Alcohol (Solvent) YES at liver and skin**

Start on parasite program.

Sixteen days later

- ☐ **Ortho-phospho-tyrosine (Cancer) NO**

- ☐ **Fasciolopsis and all stages (Parasite) NO**

- ☒ **Sheep liver fluke cercaria (Parasite) YES**
  Ate filet mignon yesterday.

- ☒ **Pancreatic fluke (Parasite) YES**

- ☒ **Isopropyl Alcohol (Solvent) YES**
  Will stop using her regular cosmetics.

- ☒ **Wood Alcohol, Hexanedione, TCEthylene, Toluene (Solvents) YES**
  She was told to go off all commercial beverages except fresh orange juice made in the store. She is to drink milk (2%), water, herb tea (not Celestial Seasoning™), homemade vegetable juice, and fruit juice only. Start on kidney herb recipe.
  Summary: Maria got rid of her cancer in 16 days when the intestinal fluke was gone. But she still had other flukes that were multiplying in her, due to a variety of solvents accumulated in her body. Hopefully she will try to eliminate them.

49	Gladys Jackson	Cervical and Breast Cancer

Gladys is a young, vivacious person, only 39, complaining of chronic fatigue. Her arms and legs are especially weak. She was diagnosed with tendonitis and CMV virus a year ago. She also has a complexion problem (not significant to my mind), breathing problem, and insomnia. She has thumb pain and frequent urination.

BLOOD TEST	Result	Comment
1. Calcium	very low (8.7)	She will drink 2% milk, 3 glasses/day and take Magnesium oxide from Bronson Pharm. (300 mg), 1/day and a Vitamin A and D perle, any size, one/day.
2. SGOT, SGPT	very low (14, 11) showing low serum B6 levels	She will take B6 (250 mg) from Bronson's, two/day.
3. LDH	high (182)	We will test for cancer.

☒ **Ortho-phospho-tyrosine (Cancer) YES at breast, genital tract**

This came as a bad surprise. She had just had a mammogram and it was NEGATIVE. We explained that it was probably very early, too small for the mammogram to detect.

☒ **Fasciolopsis (Parasite) YES at liver, NO at colon**

☒ **Fasciolopsis redia (Parasite) YES at genital tract and breast**

Start on parasite program.

Nine days later

☐ **Ortho-phospho-tyrosine (Cancer) NO**

☐ **Fasciolopsis and all stages (Parasite) NO**

With the cancer out of the way we can pursue the problems she came in for but with priority given to toxic elements due to their cancer connection.

☒ **Cadmium (Toxic Element) YES**

Probably her plumbing, we will check water.

☒ **Gallium, Nickel (Toxic Elements) YES**

Tooth fillings.

☒ **Thorium (Toxic Element) YES**

Reduce dust in the house, repair cracks, open crawl space vents regardless of fuel cost.

☒ **Silver (Toxic Element) YES**

Metal teeth. She needs to replace all metal in her mouth.

☒ **Oxalate (Kidney Stones) YES, remainder NO**

Since oxalate is the main pain-causing kidney stone, Gladys should get considerable improvement from taking our kidney herb recipe. Continue parasite program. She should make an appointment with us after she gets her dental work done.

Summary: Gladys did not come back after her second visit. She did well, considering that she was barely able to believe she had cancer after her negative mammogram. Perhaps the diet improvement made her feel so much better that she didn't think the dental work was needed at this time. Perhaps her husband could not accept the need for plumbing improvement. But I hope she stayed with the parasite program to protect herself from cancer, at least.

| 50 | Debra Ells | Colon, Stomach, Liver Cancer and HIV |

This is a 41 year old woman who came in for a long list of problems: 1) Cysts and rashes on skin. She has had them removed from back of neck, ears, chin, breast and even fingers. (My guess is these are PCB caused.) 2) Swelling at joints all over body. 3) Pain everywhere: elbows, shoulders, wrists, hands, chest, lower back, legs, knees, feet, and headaches. This suggests gallstones and rheumatoid arthritis but the chest pain doesn't fit into this picture. I will test for HIV (She is using Advil™ as a pain killer. It doesn't help much.) 4) Stomach problem.

She had a hysterectomy for excessive bleeding in her early 20's and her ovaries were removed 5 years ago. A total mastectomy was done 8 years ago for multiple cysts and she got breast implants but had to have them removed for leakage later.

I discussed with her the need to do all 5 of our routines and that she would probably be much better in 3 months. These would be: 1) Kidney cleanse; 2) Parasite killing; 3) Toxic element removal; 4) Bacteria and virus elimination; and 5) Liver cleanse.

Since her urinalysis showed crystals in the urine, we would start with a kidney cleanse.

☒ Ortho-phospho-tyrosine (Cancer) YES at colon, liver, and stomach

I explained to Debra that this unexpected result would change the order of our program; we would kill parasites first. She said her brother had died of cirrhosis of the liver; she was not too surprised she had liver cancer!

☒ Fasciolopsis (Parasite) YES at thymus, blood, colon, stomach; NOT IN LIVER!

☒ Fasciolopsis cercaria (Parasite) YES at thymus and stomach only

☐ Fasciolopsis remaining stages (Parasite) NO

This picture suggests HIV/AIDS illness together with cancer. There are probably other flukes, like the liver fluke and pancreatic fluke at the extra locations. But I did not test since she had enough shock from hearing about the cancer. I postponed the tests for 2 days. She will start on parasite killing program.

Two days later

☐ Ortho-phospho-tyrosine (Cancer) NO

☐ **Fasciolopsis and all stages (Parasite) NO**

When I gave her this exceptionally good news, she was not happy since she did not feel any differently; she had no pain relief and she expressed her disappointment.

☒ **Arsenic (Toxic Element) YES**

☒ **Europium, Lutetium, Yttrium, Ytterbium (Toxic Elements) YES**

☐ **Toxic Elements (Remainder) NO**

Since health supplements and drug tablets were implicated, plus her carpets, she could not believe my explanations. I decided to postpone this part of her corrective programs and go directly to HIV testing.

☒ **Protein 24 (HIV) YES at genital tract and thymus**

She did not believe this result, nor was she willing to go for a conventional HIV test at the Health Department. I could see she was very angry and would not come back to see me. I emphasized the primary importance of staying on a parasite killing maintenance program. I did not manage to warn her of the solvents benzene and isopropyl alcohol, or of the danger of eating undercooked beef, chicken and turkey.

Summary: It is understandable when a sick person finds our methods and results too strange to believe. Hopefully, as illness worsens, she will get tested and find her way back here. Note: In HIV cases, the adult fluke has developed from a cercaria in the THYMUS, not in the LIVER.

51	Leona Taylor	Cancer Of Cervix

Leona was referred to us by a recovered cancer client. Her clinical doctor has been following the cysts in her breast for 7 years. One got to be the size of an egg; it was drained. Two years ago she had a bad PAP. 1½ years ago a lesion was found in the breast. She has done nothing. She now aches over the ovary regions. She has lower back pain. She has had double periods all this year. She is so fatigued that she has to lie down after 3 hours of work. She aches all over the chest area. Her neck aches and the back of her head feels very strange. The back of her head is numb. The soles of her feet hurt. Her clinical doctor removed certain "spots" recently from her cervix.

☒ **Ortho-phospho-tyrosine (Cancer) YES at cervix and breast**

☒ **Fasciolopsis (Parasite) YES at liver and colon**

☒ **Fasciolopsis eggs (Parasite) YES at cervix, blood, breast, bladder, liver, colon**

> With such a wide distribution of fluke eggs, she must be full of solvent. She will go off her favorite beverages (colas). She had noticed that drinking Nutrasweet™ caused her cysts to enlarge immediately. She will make her own vegetable juice out of 50% carrots, 50% greens. She has not been eating red meat. Start on parasite program.

One week later

☐ **Ortho-phospho-tyrosine (Cancer) NO**

☐ **Fasciolopsis and all stages (Parasite) NO**

☒ **Mercury (Toxic Element) YES high**

> Has numerous tooth fillings.

☒ **Zirconium (Toxic Element) YES**

☐ **Toxic Elements (Remainder) NO**

> She will go off toothpaste, deodorant, shampoo, salves and lotions and substitute homemade varieties to get rid of zirconium. She is to see dentist immediately to have metal tooth fillings replaced. She had a urinalysis test with her. It showed crystals of various kinds in the urine. She is to start on kidney herb recipe. Continue parasite program.

> *Summary: I wonder if I did the right thing in telling her the cancer was already gone at her second visit. She did not return and possibly has done nothing about her mercury problem. Mercury may be the cause of the strange symptoms. At age 47, she should be trying to undo the bad health practices of her youth, not sweeping them aside. Perhaps she will surprise us and one day walk in, in radiant health.*

| 52 | **Robert Ohr** | **Prostate Cancer** |

This is a sturdy, confident looking man, age 55. He is here for prostate problems. It began 3 decades ago with blockage and acute prostatitis. Two years ago it was blocked again. The clinical doctors tried an experimental drug on him. It didn't work. He has cramping in the lower abdomen. A year ago he had prostatectomy and a cyst re-moved. A few months ago another cyst was removed from the right testicle. Nothing has helped the pain. At surgery, the doctor told him he had early cancer. But PSA was not high (1.1), as expected for pros-tate cancer. He picked up Candida after the surgery. He also has pain over the rib cage, in both elbows, and at his right knee. He is fatigued but forces himself to exercise. His urination is with extreme urgency, causing him to panic if not near a toilet.

☒ **Ortho-phospho-tyrosine (Cancer) YES at prostate**

☒ **Fasciolopsis (Parasite) YES at colon and liver**

☒ **Fasciolopsis cercaria (Parasite) YES at prostate and liver**

☐ **Fasciolopsis remaining stages (Parasite) NO**
    Start parasite program.

BLOOD TEST	Result	Comment
1. RBC	low (4.72)	parasites
2. Creatinine	high (1.2)	kidney problem
3. FBS	low (79)	unusually low - will check for pancre-atic fluke
4. Potassium	very low (3.7)	adrenals
5. Chloride	very low	adrenals
6. CO2	very high	lung problem, probable cause of panic attacks, look for air pollutant

☒ **Pancreatic fluke (Parasite) YES at pancreas**
    Probable cause of low blood sugar.

Ten days later

☐ **Ortho-phospho-tyrosine (Cancer) NO**

☐ **Protein 24 (HIV) NO**

☐ **Fasciolopsis adults (Parasite) NO**

☒ **Fasciolopsis redia (Parasite) YES at prostate**

☐ **Fasciolopsis remaining stages (Parasite) NO**

☒ **Pancreatic fluke (Parasite) YES**

☒ **Wood Alcohol (Solvent) YES**

☒ **Isopropyl Alcohol (Solvent) YES**
    Stop shampoo, shaving chemicals, mouthwash, cold cereal.

☒ **Mineral oil (Toxic Element) YES**

Stop using lotions. Continue parasite program. Note: He is full of wood alcohol, which has a tendency to accumulate in the pancreas. This allows the fluke family to develop and multiply in the pancreas. He is to stop eating undercooked chicken, turkey, beef. He will stop drinking commercial beverages.

☒ **Cadmium (Toxic Element) YES**

Plumbing or old tooth fillings.

☒ **Copper (Toxic Element) YES**

Has copper water pipes.

☒ **Iridium (Toxic Element) YES**

Needs to change metal frame glasses to plastic.

☒ **Hafnium (Toxic Element) YES**

Stop hair spray or see *Recipes*.

☒ **Thallium, Germanium (Toxic Element) YES**

Thallium and germanium together point at metal tooth fillings. Thallium is a deadly toxin, polluting the mercury alloy. He is to see dentist immediately to remove all metal. Toxic element test is not yet completed. Note: cancer is gone but Robert is still at high risk for it.

Eight weeks later

All dental work is complete. He still has abdominal cramping.

☒ **Beryllium (Toxic Element) YES**

There is a door between garage and kitchen - will cover with plastic or park vehicles outside.

☒ **Cobalt (Toxic Element) YES**

Off detergent.

☒ **Asbestos (Toxic Element) YES**

Needs to change clothes dryer belt.

☒ **Copper (Toxic Element) YES**

☒ **Chromate (Toxic Element) YES**

Needs to change metal glasses to plastic.

☒ **Cesium (Toxic Element) YES**

No source found.

⊠ **PCB (Toxic Element) YES**

Off detergents, use borax.

⊠ **Scandium, Tantalum, Rhodium, Nickel (Toxic Element) YES**

The metals are coming out of him rather slowly considering all his metal tooth fillings are gone. Start thioctic acid, 100 mg, 2/day. Note: His cadmium is gone - it must have been in his tooth fillings.

⊠ **Hexane (Solvent) YES**

Off commercial beverages.

⊠ **Petroleum ether (Solvent) YES**

Will be more careful with gasoline.

One month later

He still has a lot of pain with sitting. Still some lower abdominal pain.

☐ **Beryllium (Toxic Element) NO**

Is parking vehicles outside.

☐ **Cobalt (Toxic Element) NO**

Switched to borax.

⊠ **Asbestos (Toxic Element) YES**

Hasn't changed the dryer belt yet.

☐ **Copper, Chromate, Cesium (Toxic Elements) NO**

☐ **PCB (Toxic Element) NO**

Is off detergent.

☐ **Scandium, Tantalum, Rhodium (Toxic Elements) NO**

⊠ **Nickel (Toxic Element) YES**

Glasses frames not yet changed.

☐ **Ortho-phospho-tyrosine (Cancer) NO**

☐ **Protein 24 (HIV) NO**

⊠ **Methylene chloride (Solvent) YES**

Go off commercial beverages. The kidney tests were not done, but he will start on kidney herbs anyway.

Summary: The metal from glasses frames is usually the second highest source of body metal, coming right after metal tooth fillings, from my observation. Nickel is quite soluble in fat, so skin oils could dissolve a lot of it out of the glasses frames and absorb it. Notice that Robert has made a lot of changes already in his lifestyle and yet his pains remain. But he has two potent causes of prostate trouble still left to conquer: asbestos and nickel. The list of metals absorbed into his body was exceptionally long - probably due to many kidney stones blocking their excretion. Although the kidney stone test was not done, I am curious to see how his pains are after several weeks of stone removal. Usually we cleanse kidneys early on to give clients pain relief. Our preoccupation with toxic elements slowed down the whole program. But he is free of cancer and soon will be free of pain.

One month later (4 months and 2 weeks after the first visit)

He has no pain with sitting but pain in front lower abdomen persists as well as in testicles. (This is probably the bladder.) I suspect a missed parasite, even though he has been on maintenance parasite program.

☒ Hymenolepis dim (Parasite) YES

A small tapeworm!

☒ Schistosoma haem (Parasite) YES at bladder

Could this be causing his abdominal pain? He will take 20 wormwoods for a few days in a row and note if pain stops. This is in addition to high dose black walnut tincture and cloves. This often comes from a pet. Must ask if he owns one.

Erik Gerger	Cancer and HIV

Erik is 26 years old and has only minor problems. He is here for his underweight condition; he is 25 lbs. underweight. There is a cat in his house. He needs ten hours of sleep at night but still has low energy.

☒ Ortho-phospho-tyrosine (Cancer) YES

He has cancer, but he is incredulous and anxious to leave. There isn't time to search for its location.

☒ Protein 24 (HIV) YES high

He has a very high level of HIV virus. This seems even less likely to him. But I prevailed upon him to stay long enough to get his instructions.

☒ Fasciolopsis adults and redia (Parasite) YES at thymus

☐ Sheep liver fluke (Parasite) NO

321

☐ **Pancreatic fluke (Parasite) NO**
Others not tested. He will start on parasite killing program.

☒ **Benzene (Solvent) YES at thymus**
Uses Tom's™ toothpaste.

☒ **Hexane (Solvent) YES**

☐ **Solvents (Remainder) NO**
He is instructed to go off commercial beverages and avoid the benzene list.

Summary: Erik has not returned. I hope he at least stopped using benzene-polluted products, and is staying on a parasite maintenance program. But it's too much to hope for. Note that propanol was not listed as YES and yet ortho-phospho-tyrosine is present. Nor is Fasciolopsis listed as present in the liver. Were these tests missed? If not, this would be a unique case of cancer without both of its two chief causes. I will search for more such exceptions.

---

53   Rojer Costa   Brain Cancer

This is a young (age 29), sturdy man with one leg amputated, sitting in a wheel chair. He has had several operations for cancer, it runs in his family. His brother has brought him from his home in the northwest.

His leg was amputated for osteogenicsarcoma two decades ago. He received 19 months of chemo. Earlier, he had a brain tumor, astrocytoma. It was removed by surgery. Three years ago, he got radiation for a subsequent brain tumor. He also had surgery and chemotherapy at the time. As a result of his last surgery, he has mild seizures in his left hand and left arm.

He is on Dilantin 400™ in 2 doses plus Valium™ for muscle relaxant as necessary. He also has left side weakness in his hand, arm, and leg. He has been in a wheelchair for 2 years, since his brain surgery, due to residual weakness from surgery.

☐ **Protein 24 (HIV) NO**

☒ **Ortho-phospho-tyrosine (Cancer) YES at bone, brain, cerebellum**

☒ **Fasciolopsis (Parasite) YES at liver only**

☒ **Fasciolopsis miracidia (Parasite) YES at brain and blood**

☒ **Sheep liver fluke (Parasite) YES at liver**

☒ **Sheep liver fluke cercaria (Parasite) YES at brain and blood**

Note: We have not accounted for cancer at bone and cerebellum since the above fluke stages were not present there. Is there another fluke involved?

☐ **Pancreatic fluke (Parasite) NO**

☒ **Human liver fluke (Parasite) YES at liver, brain, bone and cerebellum**

☒ **Human liver fluke metacercaria (Parasite) YES at brain, bone, and cerebellum**

☐ **Human liver fluke eggs (Parasite) NO**

☒ **Isopropyl Alcohol (Solvent) YES at liver, brain, bone and cerebellum**

Start on parasite program. Go off all propanol containing products.

One week later

BLOOD TEST	Result	Comment
1. Seg/Lymph	low	chronic virus
2. Eos	slightly high (3%)	parasites
3. Platelet count	slightly low (170)	bone marrow toxin
4. Total protein and albumin	low	liver problem
5. SGPT, SGOT	high	liver problem

☐ **Protein 24 (HIV) NO**

☐ **Ortho-phospho-tyrosine (Cancer) NO**

☐ **Fasciolopsis and all stages (Parasite) NO**

☐ **Sheep liver fluke and all stages (Parasite) NO**

☐ **Human liver fluke and all stages (Parasite) NO**

Continue parasite program.

☐ **Isopropyl Alcohol (Solvent) NO**

He could not find "prop" on any of his body products so he did not change anything. But he has not shampooed or shaved since last visit, and he has stopped using rubbing alcohol.

☒ **Antimony (Toxic Element) YES at brain**
Go off colognes.

☒ **Cadmium (Toxic Element) YES high at brain**
Will test water sources, then dental sources.

☒ **Thallium, Germanium (Toxic Element) YES at prostate and lung**

☐ **Toxic Elements (Remainder) NO**
Thallium/germanium in his dental materials is the probable cause of his weakness, not the after-effects of surgery. He must immediately have this removed. He stands a good chance of getting out of his wheelchair again. His cancer is gone and tumors can be shrunk.
Summary: Rojer was from 2000 miles away and had only one week to spend with us, yet he accomplished his purpose. This was a most fascinating case: another parasite of the fluke family, the Human liver fluke, has joined the intestinal and other liver flukes to invade tissues like bone and brain. This is no doubt due to the presence of solvent in these tissues. Perhaps his whole family was in the habit of using a lot of rubbing alcohol. Both the cancer and the propanol were eliminated in a week's time. But will he pursue the dental problem?

Jan Whitacker	Cervical and Uterine Cancer

Jan, age 41, came with friends who had an appointment in the hope that I could work her into the schedule for a very short visit. She had cancer of the cervix and uterus twelve years ago. They both were removed by a complete hysterectomy. She got no radiation or chemo. She was told by her clinical doctors that they "got it all." But she is not in good health. She has a stomach problem, insomnia, weakness in her arms, pain in her lower back, and other problems, including mood.

☒ **Ortho-phospho-tyrosine (Cancer) YES at cervix and uterus**
This surprised and disappointed her.

☐ **Fasciolopsis adults (Parasite) NO**

☒ **Fasciolopsis miracidia (Parasite) YES at liver, cervix, uterus, and colon**

☐ **Fasciolopsis remaining stages (Parasite) NO**
She is to avoid undercooked meats and avoid propanol in her body products. Start on parasite program.

Summary: Jan did not come back. She is dependent on friends for transportation. Notice that there are fluke miracidia present without any adults! Sexual transmission seems likely. She was to bring her husband along at her next visit. There are other explanations but not enough evidence. Note that the test showed fluke stages at the cervix and uterus when these had been removed! I suppose this means there is a remnant of such tissue still present.

54	Kathryn Poore	Breast Cancer

Kathryn Poore (age 56) came to the office because of long-standing problems with shingles that were spreading into the right eye. She had a mastectomy 11 years ago but now the cancer is back, under the same breast and armpit. Her clinical doctor wants to start her on chemotherapy. She started herself on a new essential oil product as well as some other herbs. She has both upper back and lower back pain. She had a hysterectomy in the past for growths on one ovary and the uterus.

☒ **Ortho-phospho-tyrosine (Cancer) YES at breast**

☒ **Fasciolopsis (Parasite) YES at colon, liver and blood**

This is very unusual. The parasite is large. How could it be in blood vessels? Does this represent a hemorrhage?

☒ **Fasciolopsis redia (Parasite) YES at breast, pancreas and blood**

☒ **Fasciolopsis cercaria (Parasite) YES at breast and blood**

She has been running a fever and has lost weight. Start on parasite program. Note: cancer is trying to spread to pancreas. She will stop essential oil products immediately since I know they have benzene pollution in them.

Five days later

She is feeling better. The shingles in her eye seem to be gone for now. She put herself on 3 goldenseal a day.

☐ **Ortho-phospho-tyrosine (Cancer) NO**

☐ **Fasciolopsis (Parasite) NO**

☒ **Fasciolopsis eggs (Parasite) YES at colon, breast, liver, blood**

Continue parasite program. Note that the malignancy is gone.

One month later

She complains about dizziness. Shingles in eye still noticeable.

☐ **Protein 24 (HIV) NO**

☐ **Ortho-phospho-tyrosine (Cancer) NO**

☒ **Wood Alcohol (Solvent) YES**

☐ **Solvents (Remainder) NO**

She will stop drinking carbonated beverages and drink milk and water instead.

☒ **Herpes zoster (Pathogen) YES**

(Shingles virus.)

One month later

☒ **Wood Alcohol (Solvent) YES**

Off beverages and cold cereals.

☒ **Herpes zoster (Pathogen) YES**

☒ **PCB (Toxic Element) YES**

Off detergent.

One month later

She is feeling better.

☐ **Wood alcohol (Toxic Element) NO**

☐ **PCB (Toxic Element) NO**

Switched off detergents.

☐ **Herpes zoster (Pathogen) NO**

BLOOD TEST	Result	Comment
1. RBC	low	anemic, probably parasites
2. MCV	high	In need of B12. This always implicates common roundworm *Ascaris*. These worms are often pink from absorbing our B12!
3. Phosphates	high (over 4)	dissolving bones - reduce phosphate in diet, increase milk, fruit, and vegetables)
4. Cholesterol	low (123)	liver problem - use butter, not margarine; low cholesterol is also a cancer risk factor

☒ **Ascaris (Parasite) YES**

It is easy to pick this up from somebody else's dog or cat. She will start on a 5 day high dose parasite program and then continue on maintenance as before.

☒ **Barium (Toxic Element) YES at thyroid**

The usual sources are lipstick and bus exhaust, and she does not use lipstick. Also, her recent plastic fillings can not be ruled out (remember all dental composites contain barium to enable them to show up on X-ray).

☒ **Fluoride (Toxic Element) YES**

Will stop using toothpaste.

☒ **Vanadium(Toxic Element) YES very high**

Will check for a gas leak - says can smell stove.

Summary: Kathryn is happy to have the shingles under control at last. I believe they were started when she began to get benzene in the new essential oil product. The cancer was cured in 5 days but the shingles were more of a challenge. They will probably recur each time she is indiscreet and allows herself commercial beverages or goes off the parasite maintenance program. In this way, the shingles will serve as a watch dog for her and remind her to clean-up before a cancer would return.

Seven weeks later

She feels quite a bit better, more like her former self. She has brought air samples for testing.

☐ **Barium, Fluoride (Toxic Element) NO**

Evidently the barium was not from her plastic fillings.

☒ **Vanadium(Toxic Element) YES**

Have not found their gas leak and are still suffering.

☐ **Protein 24 (HIV) NO**

☐ **Ortho-phospho-tyrosine (Cancer) NO**

☐ **Herpes zoster (Pathogen) NO**

☐ **Ascaris (Parasite) NO**

5-day high dose parasite program got rid of roundworms.

☒ **Ascaris eggs, Schistosoma jap eggs, Hymenolepis dim eggs, Schistosoma haem eggs (Parasite) YES**

Notice: These eggs have survived the 5 day high dose program. She will take 1 tsp. cloves twice a day for several days.

☒ **Ascaris eggs, Schistosoma jap eggs, Hymenolepis dim eggs, Schistosoma haem eggs (Parasite) YES**
> Notice: These eggs have survived the 5 day high dose program. She will take 1 tsp. cloves twice a day for several days.

Six weeks later
> Kathryn had another dizzy spell since last seen.

☐ **Protein 24 (HIV) NO**

☐ **Ortho-phospho-tyrosine, hCG (Cancer) NO**

☒ **Fasciolopsis eggs (Parasite) YES at kidneys only**
> She has eaten no meat or any dairy products. (Possibly from her husband; he will do a 3 day high-dose parasite program.)

☒ **Vanadium(Toxic Element) YES**
> Six out of eight rooms tested had vanadium in the air; they were advised to hurriedly call the Health Department or Gas Company to fix the gas leaks. This could be the cause of her dizzy spells.

55	Beth Morato	Breast and Lung Cancer

Beth is a middle aged, pleasant woman, who had severe lower back pain before her clinical doctor found she had cancer of the lower spine. Since bone cancer is seldom the primary cancer, they searched for the primary source and found it in the lung. She was treated with chemotherapy and radiation to her lung and back. The spot on her lung has only shrunk 30%. She had to quit her job at that time, over a year ago.

☒ **Ortho-phospho-tyrosine (Cancer) YES at liver and pancreas (not lung!)**

☒ **Fasciolopsis (Parasite) YES at liver and pancreas**

☒ **Fasciolopsis eggs (Parasite) YES at breast, pancreas, intestine, lungs and bone**

☐ **Fasciolopsis remaining stages (Parasite) NO**
> Other parasites not tested. Start on parasite program. Go off all commercial cosmetics and shampoo and the whole isopropyl alcohol pollution list.

Seven days later

☐ **Ortho-phospho-tyrosine (Cancer) NO**

☐ **Fasciolopsis and all stages (Parasite) NO**

Had forgotten to pick up cloves from us so she used grocery store WHOLE cloves, and they worked.

☒ **Radon (Toxic Element) YES at kidney, breast, bone (other organs not tested)**

☐ **Toxic Elements (Remainder) NO**

Note: cancer is already gone. Only one toxic element was present: radon. There is a crawl space under their house. They will open vents and then bring in air sample to test.

Nine days later

Her fatigue is worsening. But her low back pain is gone.

☐ **Radon (Toxic Element) NO**

Opened vents.

☐ **Kidney Stones (ALL) NO**

Drinks a lot of water, eats a lot of vegetables and fruit, empties her bladder about 10 times in 24 hours. Continue parasite program.

☒ **Benzene (Solvent) YES**

☐ **Solvents (Remainder) NO**

She will go off toothpaste, chapstick, ice cream, and frozen yogurt.

BLOOD TEST	Result	Comment
1. WBC	very low (3.2)	bone marrow toxin
2. RBC	very low (3.48)	bone marrow, parasites
3. Platelet count	slightly low	bone marrow probably has benzene
4. Eos	slightly high (3%)	parasites
5. BUN	slightly high	kidney
6. Phosphate	high	dissolving bone. She will drink 2% milk, 3 glasses/day and reduce phosphate sources. She will start to make vegetable juice.
7. Cholesterol	low (169)	cancer risk

She will start on supplements, from Bronson's only, B6 (250) 1/day, magnesium oxide (300) 1/day, vitamin C (500) 1 to 6/day, vitamin E (400), 1/day, beta carotene (25,000) 1/day.

Summary: Beth planned to do everything perfectly; her lower back pain was gone, and she did not need to return. Her cancer was ready to burst out at her breast and pancreas, but she got it all stopped and was enjoying planning her future again. She appreciated all the helpful advice and her husband was supportive. She should follow up in 3 months.

56	Susan Arthur	Intestinal Cancer

This is a young 41 year old woman who is a cat lover. She has had as many as 40 cats at one time, all of them house cats. She only has 10 now. She has a constant migraine for which she is on 3 medications, including codeine. Nothing else helps. She also has total insomnia without her medications. Her entire colon has been removed surgically for colitis; there is no rectum or anus. Her clinical doctor said it was all precancerous. She also has a history of stomach ulcers and numerous smaller health problems. But her eyes light up at the mention of cats, as if they had nothing to do with her condition. She has extreme allergies - to almost everything; I would suspect Sheep liver flukes as well as Strongyloides.

☐ **Protein 24 (HIV) NO**

☒ **Ortho-phospho-tyrosine (Cancer) YES at intestine**
This comes as a surprise to her. She felt that all that surgery was protecting her.

☒ **Fasciolopsis (Parasite) YES at liver and intestine**

☒ **Fasciolopsis cercaria (Parasite) YES at kidney, bladder and intestine**

☒ **Sheep liver fluke (Parasite) YES at liver and intestine**

☒ **Sheep liver fluke miracidia and redia (Parasite) YES at kidney, bladder**

☒ **Pancreatic fluke (Parasite) YES at kidney, bladder and pancreas**
We will search urine for these stages since they are present in the bladder.

☒ **Isopropyl Alcohol (Solvent) YES at liver, kidney, intestine and bladder**

☒ **Toluene, Xylene Hexane, methyl ethyl ketone, methylene chloride (Solvents) YES**

⊠ **Wood Alcohol (Solvent) YES at uterus, stomach, pancreas**
She is to go off all commercial beverages, except fresh squeezed (in her grocery store) orange juice if she can find it. If not, she is to make all her own beverages from fruits and vegetables. She can drink 2% or more milk, if tolerated, and single-herb teas. She will be off cold cereals. She will start on parasite program for herself and cats.

Summary: Susan came to the office for migraines, never suspecting that this could be due to a tiny parasite, threadworm, that cats could bring her. Her chances of recovering from migraines are zero, but maybe she can reduce them a lot by treating her pets daily with a parasite program designed for them. Indeed, she did have the Sheep liver fluke; this causes terrible obstruction in the liver bile ducts; how can the liver detoxify food chemicals with such a severe handicap? Besides this, some intestinal flukes are nesting there. We don't often see them together in the liver. Together, these two flukes are probably keeping the pancreatic fluke out of the liver, relegating it to bladder and kidney, besides pancreas. These were the only parasites tested; she scored three out of three. And in quite untraditional organs for these parasites. One look at the solvent test gives the clue. Wood alcohol accumulates in the pancreas and induces hatching of flukes there. Propanol induces hatching in the liver. The other solvents may have their favorite target organs, too, causing parasitism there. This has not been studied yet. Happily, she was eager to correct her problems.

Eight days later
Susan came back for a follow-up.

☐ **Ortho-phospho-tyrosine (Cancer) NO**

☐ **Solvents (ALL) NO**
She feels quite different (better). The Toxic Element tests showed asbestos very high, antimony YES, arsenic very high, and PCB YES. Others were not tested since this is enough for her to cope with. She doesn't use a hair blower so the asbestos must be coming from the clothes dryer. She will persuade her husband to change the belt to a USA made belt. The antimony may be in her hand cream, she will switch to our skin softener and apricot kernel oil. She will go off detergents to get rid of PCB. But the arsenic is a real problem because she needs to treat the house and cats with pesticide frequently. I could not give her a good solution, but she will start by putting a lot of boric acid behind the stove, refrigera-

tor and in the carpet. She is enjoying her new lifestyle and wants to make changes.

Four weeks later (5 weeks after first visit)

She is still complaining about memory lapses. Her husband insisted on a CAT scan and other clinical tests which she has done; nothing showed up. She has periods of completely irrational behavior. This suggests intermittent interference with brain function. I will search for tapeworm heads (scolices).

☒ Moniezia (Parasite) YES

She will kill this extremely harmful tapeworm stage with an herbal product called Rascal (which we used before we developed the Mop Up program). After 3 weeks she will be on the usual maintenance program of twice a week treatment, including Rascal. This tapeworm head may be emerging due to solvent exposure in the past.

☒ Hexane, Methyl Butyl Ketone, Styrene (Solvents) YES

She will stay off processed food.

Carol Masters	Intestinal Cancer

Carol was accompanying another client of ours and after seeing what our diagnostic system could do, she wanted to be tested for cancer before leaving. We did not get her history or list of symptoms. Her mother had died of breastbone and pancreatic cancer. We gave her 15 minutes of office time.

☐ Protein 24 (HIV) NO

☒ Ortho-phospho-tyrosine (Cancer) YES at intestine

☒ Fasciolopsis (Parasite) YES at intestine and liver

☒ Fasciolopsis miracidia (Parasite) YES at liver, thymus, intestine

☐ Sheep liver fluke and stages (Parasite) NO

☒ Isopropyl Alcohol (Solvent) YES at liver, thymus, pancreas

☒ TCE (Solvent) YES

She will remove all propanol containing products. She will go off cold cereals and commercial beverages and drink milk, water and home made juices or simple herb tea. She will not eat beef, turkey, or chicken in restaurants, and will cook them as if they were pork at home. Start on parasite program.

| Dan Hudgins | Prostate Cancer |

Dan is a youngish man brought in by his sister in great secrecy. He did not wish to give his address, age, or fill out any paper work. His sister said he was diagnosed with prostate cancer a few weeks ago, although he was given a clean bill of health at a different clinic. His clinical doctor put him on antibiotics. His PSA is 12 (too high, indicative of prostate cancer).

☐ **Protein 24 (HIV) NO**

☒ **Ortho-phospho-tyrosine (Cancer) YES at prostate**

☒ **Fasciolopsis (Parasite) YES at liver**

☒ **Fasciolopsis eggs (Parasite) YES at liver and prostate**

☒ **Sheep liver fluke (Parasite) YES at prostate**

☐ **Pancreatic fluke (Parasite) NO**

☒ **Isopropyl Alcohol (Solvent) YES at liver and prostate**

☐ **Solvents (Remainder) NO**

He will remove all products with "PROP" on the label from his house. He will start on parasite program. His sister discreetly pointed out, here, that Dan is not likely to come in for a follow up; the implication was that we must do all we can in one visit.

☒ **Oxalate (Kidney Stones) YES**

☒ **di Calcium Phosphate (Kidney Stones) YES**

Start on kidney herbs after 3 weeks. He will avoid rare meat.

Summary: What a blessing it is for some of us to have a sister or brother, so truly interested in our welfare that idiosyncrasies are overlooked. Perhaps she will help him recover if she can't persuade him to come back. Notice that the two big flukes were thriving in his body, but the pancreatic fluke which he must be picking up frequently, too, had not gotten established. This is probably due to the absence of wood alcohol in his body. Wood alcohol accumulates in the pancreas allowing the pancreatic fluke to multiply there.

| 57 | **Greg Byrem** | **Colon Cancer** |

Greg Byrem was seen by us 1½ years ago for gout. At that time he could barely hobble about in spite of being on two medicines for it. He said that 3 days after beginning our kidney herb recipe, he was able to walk again. He got well enough to resume his job as a traveling salesperson. He is in this area now and wants to be given the same kidney program as before in order to gain energy and lose weight. He has put himself on a high protein diet and is eating a lot of rare meat. He brought a blood test with him.

BLOOD TEST	Result	Comment
1. Phosphates	very low (2.8)	He will go on Vitamin D, Rx from the dentist, 2/week.
2. Uric acid	high (7.6)	kidney problem
3. SGOT, SGPT	high (32, 42)	needs to cleanse liver
4. LDH	high (210)	cancer, heart disease, recent exercise?
5. Ferritin	high (260)	cancer?

☐ **Protein 24 (HIV) NO**

☒ **Ortho-phospho-tyrosine (Cancer) YES at intestine**

☒ **Fasciolopsis (Parasite) YES at liver and intestine**

☒ **Fasciolopsis eggs (Parasite) YES at liver, intestine, bladder, and semen**

☐ **Sheep liver fluke (Parasite) NO**

☒ **Pancreatic fluke and all stages (Parasite) YES at pancreas**

☒ **Isopropyl Alcohol (Solvent) YES at liver and intestine**

☒ **Wood Alcohol (Solvent) YES at pancreas**

He is using a lot of EQUAL™ artificial sweetener; he will switch to honey. Start on parasite program. Get off all propanol products. Go off cold cereals and commercial beverages and switch to milk, freshly made fruit and vegetable juice and simple herb teas (not blends).

Summary: This was certainly not what Mr. Byrem had expected. He felt healthy and simply wanted a weight loss diet. Fortunately, we discovered this early cancer. He is eager to eliminate it. Notice that there were fluke eggs in his bladder (urine) and semen; meaning he could sexually transmit it. Notice also that wood alcohol accumulates in the pancreas causing the pancreatic fluke, which is also abundant in our meat supply, to increase its population in the pancreas. This would soon give him diabetes. What an irony that diabetics use artificial sweeteners (which contain wood alcohol) to HELP their diabetes, thereby putting wood alcohol into the pancreas to make the diabetes WORSE.

Twelve days later

☐ **Ortho-phospho-tyrosine, hCG (Cancer) NO**

☐ **Fasciolopsis and all stages (Parasite) NO**

☐ **Sheep liver fluke (Parasite) NO**

☒ **Pancreatic fluke (Parasite) YES at pancreas**

☐ **Human liver fluke (Parasite) NO**
He will not eat undercooked meats and only eat fish in restaurants.

☒ **Styrene (Solvent) YES at prostate, intestine, pancreas**
He will stop using styrofoam.

☒ **Hexane, Kerosene (Solvent) YES**
He will be more careful at gas stations and not get any drops of gasoline on himself.

☒ **Mineral oil (Toxic Element) YES**
Stop hand lotions, use ours.

☒ **Isophorone (Solvent) YES**
He will definitely go off commercial beverages. With the cancer gone, Greg can follow his original plan which was to go on a weight loss program. To begin this, he will go on the kidney herb recipe. He will continue the parasite program. He is anxious to clean the liver to realize his weight loss.

☒ **Mercury (Toxic Element) YES**
He has a root canal, also. He is advised to remove all metal from his mouth.

Two months later
He has done 2 liver cleanses and got out about 2000 countable stones. He also lost 10 pounds at that time.

☐ **Ortho-phospho-tyrosine (Cancer) NO**

□ **hCG (Pre-Cancer) NO**
Has not gotten cancer back. He still needs to do dental work.

| 58 | Pete Mathes | Intestinal Cancer |

Pete Mathes, age 71, has had heart by-passes and several small strokes for which he is on medication. He feels fine but would like to improve his failing memory. He lives in a large city.

□ **Protein 24 (HIV) NO**

☒ **Ortho-phospho-tyrosine (Cancer) YES at intestine**
His bowel habits have changed recently.

☒ **Fasciolopsis eggs (Parasite) YES at intestine**
Note: No adults in the liver!

☒ **Fasciolopsis miracidia (Parasite) YES at intestine**

☒ **Sheep liver fluke adults, redia, cercaria, miracidia (Parasite) YES**
He is heavily parasitized with Sheep liver fluke, which is a probable explanation for his severe allergies in the past.

□ **Pancreatic fluke and stages (Parasite) NO**

☒ **Isopropyl Alcohol (Solvent) YES**
He uses no body products except Dr. Bronner's baby soap, which he has used for years. He also uses shaving cream. He will go off these and other propanol polluted products.

☒ **Acetone, Methyl butyl ketone (Solvents) YES**
He will go off all commercial beverages. He will start parasite program. After this he will start on half a dose of kidney herb recipe. He agrees to come back in a month.

One month later

□ **Ortho-phospho-tyrosine (Cancer) NO**
Bowel is normal again.

□ **Isopropyl Alcohol (Solvent) NO**
Stopped using shaving cream and uses an electric razor.

☒ **Wood Alcohol (Solvent) YES**
Artificial sweetener.

⊠ **Styrene (Solvent) YES**
Drank from a styrofoam cup yesterday - will stop.

⊠ **Europium and europium oxide (Toxic Elements) YES**
Dentures.

⊠ **Aluminum Silicate (Toxic Element) YES**
Salt. Switch to Hain's Sea Salt.™

⊠ **Scandium, Silver (Toxic Element) YES**
Teeth? He has complete dentures; yet these are metals used in tooth fillings. He will ask dentist to do a whole mouth X-ray to search for bits of left over amalgam in his jaw bone.

⊠ **PVC (Toxic Element) YES**
Hobby supplies?

⊠ **Tungsten (Toxic Element) YES**
Will test toaster and hot water system.
Summary: Pete eliminated his intestinal cancer and propanol by his second visit. His heavy burden of Sheep liver flukes may have been with him for many decades since he has been extremely allergic most of his life. They came a very long distance and would like very much to have a healthy old age. Notice that there were no adult intestinal flukes in his liver. Did the Sheep liver flukes keep them out? He, nevertheless, developed cancer!

| 59 | Rosie Veach | Bladder and Colon Cancer |

Rosie Veach is 86 years old and still sturdy looking. She had some surgery 5 years ago and ever since then she doesn't feel right. She is sore over the lower abdomen. The surgery was for cancer of the colon; a piece of the colon was removed along with the uterus (her daughter-in-law related this). She thinks her problem is the bladder.

☐ **Protein 24 (HIV) NO**

⊠ **Ortho-phospho-tyrosine (Cancer) YES at bladder; NO elsewhere**

⊠ **Fasciolopsis (Parasite) YES at liver and bladder**

☐ **Fasciolopsis other stages (Parasite) NO**

☐ **Sheep liver fluke (Parasite) NO**

☐ **Pancreatic fluke (Parasite) NO**

Start on parasite killing program. She is concerned that the herbs will bother her super- sensitive stomach. She probably has *Ascaris* (roundworm of cats and dogs) in her stomach.

☒ **Ascaris, Ascaris megalo. (Parasites) YES**

(*Ascaris* megalo is roundworm of horses.) These will certainly give her a sensitive stomach. She is to go slowly with the parasite program after day 5, increasing the dose only when she feels ready. She is to cook all meat as if it were pork.

☒ **Isopropyl Alcohol (Solvent) YES**

Probably in shampoo - will switch to borax.

☒ **Toluene (Solvent) YES**

She has been drinking 7Up™ to settle her stomach. She will switch to Bronson's digestive enzymes: 2 for breakfast, 4 for supper.

☒ **Pentane (Solvent) YES**

Will switch from Sanka™ to hot water with cream and honey.

☒ **Carbon Tetrachloride (Solvent) YES**

Will go off cold cereal.

Two weeks later

☐ **Ortho-phospho-tyrosine (Cancer) NO**

Cancer is gone. She said she had quite a difficult time with her stomach but is very pleased. Her front lower abdomen is still painful. She has to get up six times in the night to empty her bladder. This leaves her exhausted the next day. But she is afraid of taking any more herbs on account of her stomach.

☐ **Solvents (ALL) NO**

☒ **Oxalate, Cysteine, Cystine (Kidney Stones) YES**

Start on kidney herbs: only a half dose for first five days; then full dose for 2 weeks; then half a dose for 3 months.

Summary: Very elderly clients immediately strike a chord in me. Do they try harder? Do they complain less? Are they more successful, giving me pride? Is their personality sweeter? Rosie is a perfect example of all these virtues. I believe she will do everything right and earn a pain-free, pill-free old age.

| Nancy Hamper | Intestinal Cancer |

Nancy's main problem was Crohn's disease, diagnosed in 1973. The colon became cancerous in 1974 and a portion was removed that year. Additional surgery was done the next year for adhesions. She has a list of impressive illnesses: 1) Sores on her face that won't heal. 2) Fibrositis/fibromyalgia all over her body at times (probably due to Trichinella). 3) Mitral valve prolapse (probably due to tooth bacteria). 4) Stomach ulcers. 5) Low back pain.

She has dentures. She is 49.

☐ **Protein 24 (HIV) NO**

☒ **Ortho-phospho-tyrosine (Cancer) YES at intestine**

☐ **Fasciolopsis adults (Parasite) NO**
Very unusual!

☒ **Fasciolopsis miracidia (Parasite) YES**

☒ **Sheep liver fluke adult and its stages (Parasite) YES at liver**
Note: There is no intestinal fluke adult in the liver! Yet she is forming ortho-phospho-tyrosine.

☒ **Isopropyl Alcohol (Solvent) YES**
Will remove it from her dwelling and products.

☒ **Benzene (Solvent) YES at liver, thymus and intestine**
She will go off everything on the benzene list I gave her.

☒ **Toluene, Hexane (Solvents) YES at intestine**
She will go off commercial beverages and cold cereal and make her own juices and drinks and cereal. She doesn't tolerate milk, so she will make vegetable juice: 50% carrot, 50% remaining vegetables until she is well enough to try milk. She will start parasite program.

Summary: A month has passed and Nancy has not returned. Notice how the Sheep liver fluke is in the liver instead of the intestinal fluke adults. The cancer is present. Does this mean that the Sheep liver fluke can initiate a cancer as well as the intestinal fluke? Or did Nancy actually have intestinal flukes in the liver until very recently? What killed them? Nancy has both propanol and benzene accumulated in her body. Very soon some flukes would mature in the thymus, and she would get the HIV virus. Hopefully, she will prevent all this.

60	Lois Browne	Liver Cancer

Lois is 72, and looks sturdy and healthy. She embroiders for extra income; she wishes to pay us in embroidery! We agreed. She had colon cancer four years ago and part of the colon was removed. Her clinical doctor has been keeping track of the cancer marker CEA since then. This spring the cancer returned. There are 3 lesions in the liver. She had chemotherapy last month. There is also a tumor on the wall of her uterus. It is inoperable.

☐ **Fasciolopsis adults (Parasite) NO**
Very unusual.

☒ **Fasciolopsis redia (Parasite) YES at liver and colon**

☒ **Sheep liver fluke adults and eggs (Parasite) YES at liver and colon**

☒ **Sheep liver fluke (Parasite) YES**

☒ **Pancreatic fluke and stages (Parasite) YES**

☒ **Dog heartworm (Parasite) YES**
Used to have a dog.

☒ **Echinococcus granulosus cysts (Parasite) YES**

☒ **Eimeria (Parasite) YES at liver**
End Box 1.

☒ **Toluene (Solvent) YES**

☒ **Xylene (Solvent) YES**
Drinks one glass of 7Up™ a day - will stop.

☒ **Methyl ethyl ketone (Solvent) YES**

☒ **Isopropyl Alcohol (Solvent) YES**
Uses hair spray and a salve - will go off.

☒ **Mineral oil (Toxic Element) YES**
Probably in salve.

☒ **TCE, Hexane (Solvents) YES**
Note: She is very full of solvents. She will go off all commercial beverages, cold cereals and body products. She will start parasite killing program.

☒ **Ortho-phospho-tyrosine (Cancer) YES at liver and uterus**

One week later

☐ **Protein 24 (HIV) NO**

☐ **Ortho-phospho-tyrosine (Cancer) NO**
Eliminated cancer.

☒ **Styrene (Solvent) YES**
She ate fast food from a styrofoam plate earlier today. She will stop using it.

☒ **Hexane, Benzene (Solvents) YES**
She ate ice cream yesterday. She will avoid everything on the benzene list.

☒ **Barium (Toxic Element) YES**

☒ **Copper (Toxic Element) YES**
Has metal tooth fillings.

☒ **Fiberglass (Toxic Element) YES**
Source unknown.

☒ **Mercury (Toxic Element) YES**
Tooth metal.

☒ **Yttrium (Toxic Element) YES**
Probably a pill; will not use any.

☒ **Radon (Toxic Element) YES**
Will get her son to seal cracks for her.

☒ **Tantalum, Tellurium, Rhodium (Toxic Element) YES**
Tooth metals. She is to see dentist to remove all metal from her mouth. Until then, she should get a new soft toothbrush, and use only water, no toothpaste nor soda nor salt since the metal would corrode faster.

Ten days later
A telephone call from her family canceled the next appointment and reported that Lois is in the hospital for bleeding.
Summary: Lois was heavily parasitized, no doubt due to the accumulation of solvent in her tissues. Her body could no longer detoxify solvents. But by getting rid of propanol and killing the intestinal fluke, she got rid of her cancer in a week, even though it was in her liver. Notice that there were no adults of the intestinal fluke in her liver! But there were redia. Can redia by themselves make ortho-phospho-

341

tyrosine? Or had there been an adult lately which had gotten killed by her chemo treatments? Obviously, she has a terrible mouth, maybe it is all the mercury and other metals finding their way to the liver that lets it become cancerous. I do hope she makes the dental work her top priority. While we wait for her, there is some lovely embroidery here for sale!

Irene Williams   Cancer

Irene is a youngish woman, age 53, brought in by her brother, for a diagnosis of non-Hodgkin's Lymphoma given to her five years ago. It is not operable, but she has been on every kind of chemo. She has had extensive radiation, too. Her entire body is involved in the cancer. Her body is not making any antibodies, according to her clinical doctor, so she is getting shots of Gammamune™ monthly. She is not able to work and does appear very ill. She smokes. She has been drinking bottled water. I started with a discussion of smoking, she needs to stop. She will check into a nicotine patch. She will use ginseng - 2, three times a day - to give her some relaxation.

☐ **Protein 24 (HIV) NO**

☒ **Ortho-phospho-tyrosine (Cancer) YES**
  Did not search for the location.

☒ **Fasciolopsis (Parasite) YES at liver, NO at colon**

☐ **Fasciolopsis other stages (Parasite) NO**

☐ **Sheep liver fluke (Parasite) NO**

☐ **Pancreatic fluke (Parasite) NO**
  She said her WBC was very, very low (about 900). She probably has the parasite in her thymus or bone marrow, but I didn't check.

☒ **Benzene, Isopropyl Alcohol, Methyl butyl ketone (Solvents) YES all very high**

☒ **Methyl ethyl ketone (Solvent) YES**

☐ **Solvents (Remainder) NO**
  She was instructed to make all her own beverages, cereal, ice cream and frozen yogurt, to purchase only fresh squeezed orange juice made in her grocery store. She will go off Chapstick™ and all Vaseline™ products and toothpaste. (We gave her the benzene list.) She must not use Celestial Seasonings™ teas or other mixed-

herb teas. She will remove all propanol-containing items from her bathroom and kitchen. She will start on parasite program.

Two weeks later

A telephone call from her was received telling us she couldn't stop smoking and wanted to cancel her appointment.

Summary: I believe Irene was overburdened. If I had postponed the subject of smoking I probably would have kept this client and prolonged her life.

61	Barbara Kiley	Colon Cancer

Barbara came in to the office for what she believed was arthritis: she had pain in her shoulder and upper arm and upper back, which is actually due to clogging of the biliary tubing. She needs to clean this tubing with our liver cleanse, which gives immediate pain relief the next day. She also had lower back pain for which cleaning the kidney tubules of sediment is the answer. She is on pain killer each day.

☐ **Protein 24 (HIV) NO**

☒ **Ortho-phospho-tyrosine (Cancer) YES at intestine only**

Our routine start up tests showed she had a cancer growing in her intestine somewhere. She had a hysterectomy 10 years ago and a benign lump was also removed from her left breast. But she was quite shocked at the news. She is 55 years old.

☒ **Fasciolopsis (Parasite) YES at liver**

☐ **Sheep liver fluke (Parasite) NO**

☒ **Isopropyl Alcohol (Solvent) YES**

She will remove all propanol from her dwelling so nobody could ever accidentally use it again. She will start on a parasite killing program.

☒ **Oxalate (Kidney Stones) YES**

☐ **Kidney Stones (Remainder) NO**

She also had gallstones. She will start on parasite program, followed by kidney herbs in about 3 weeks. Then she may clean the liver.

Summary: colon or intestinal cancer came as a surprise to Barbara as it did to me. She had no bowel problems.

Seven weeks later

She has not yet followed-up, but if she complies with all my instructions she will never get cancer again. She took the kidney herb pack with her, so she may be in the process of taking that; this should bring her relief from lower back pain. The gallstone test is for cholesterol crystals. Since we nearly all have them in our bile ducts, I seldom test for them. I tested her for gallstones for the persuasion value and motivation to clean her liver. Barbara had a shortened appointment to spare her financially, since she did not expect to have to purchase something like the parasite killing ingredients.

Two weeks later

We are happy to see Barbara. She has been traveling a lot, explaining her long lapse. She has had an X-ray of her shoulder but can't take the pain killers which were prescribed because they bother her a lot.

☐ **Protein 24 (HIV) NO**

☐ **Ortho-phospho-tyrosine, hCG (Cancer) NO**

☒ **Acetone, Wood alcohol (Solvent) YES**

☐ **Solvents (Remainder) NO**

Off commercial beverages. Start on kidney program.

62	Judy Olesen	Cancer, Unknown Location

Judy, age 31, from a neighboring state, brought in a long list of symptoms. The most serious were: psoriasis in 4 locations, thyroid disease, migraine headaches, irritable bowel syndrome, stomach trouble with lactose intolerance, and a severe upper and lower back pain which keeps her from sleeping at night. She had a long list of medicines to take. She is drinking water that has come from the refrigerator. Because of severe allergies she eats a lot of tofu cheese. I explained to her that in order to get well, she would need to : 1) Cleanse her kidneys for 3 weeks; 2) Kill all her parasites; 3) Eliminate toxic elements from her body; and 4) Cleanse her liver. All this could take several months so she should be patient. At least it wouldn't be expensive.

☐ **Protein 24 (HIV) NO**

344

⊠ **Ortho-phospho-tyrosine (Cancer) YES**

This positive cancer result was so shocking to her that I did not search for a location, but simply reassured her that she could completely cure it quite quickly.

⊠ **Fasciolopsis miracidia (Parasite) YES**

There were no adults in the liver! Does it mean that the miracidia by themselves can start ortho-phospho-tyrosine forming? Or had there been an adult in the liver recently to start it all, but then got killed somehow?

⊠ **Sheep liver fluke adult (Parasite) YES at liver**

⊠ **Sheep liver fluke cercaria, redia, eggs, and miracidia (Parasite) YES**

⊠ **Pancreatic fluke and stages (Parasite) YES**

⊠ **Isopropyl Alcohol (Solvent) YES very high everywhere**

She will go off commercial body products and use our replacements.

⊠ **Methylene chloride, methyl ethyl ketone (Solvents) YES**

She will go off commercial beverages and cold cereals. Start parasite killing program.

Summary: What an unusual case. Judy was smothered in Sheep liver flukes and all their stages. Could the Sheep liver fluke also induce a cancer by starting ortho-phospho-tyrosine formation? It is an intriguing question. It is 6 weeks already, and she has not returned. We wonder what happened.

Three months later

Judy has appeared. We are happy to see her. She stated she did not believe a thing we told her at her earlier visit. But she was too afraid not to take our herbs and follow the rules about products. Suddenly she began to feel amazingly well and wondered if it was all in her head. Although she was done with the recipe she was too afraid to stop. She was also afraid to continue and this indecision brought her back.

☐ **Protein 24 (HIV) NO**

☐ **Ortho-phospho-tyrosine, hCG (Cancer) NO**

⊠ **TCEthylene (Solvent) YES**

☒ **Mercury, Silver (Toxic Elements) YES**

> Others not tested. She is advised to replace all tooth metal with metal-free plastic.

> *Summary: This was certainly a happy ending for us since we had waited anxiously to hear what might have happened to her. We were not at all sure she was complying with instructions after the first visit. But her intelligence (and perhaps a little fear) saw her safely through this ordeal.*

Juanita Holden	Colon Cancer, Metastasized

Ms. Holden is only 57 but her clinical doctor has given her 2 months to live and doesn't mind if she goes to see alternative therapists. She had surgery for colon cancer five years ago, and now it is in her liver. She has been getting chemo once a month, but it is getting worse. Her doctor is using the CEA test as a cancer marker. She will bring in future results of CEA tests, although she hadn't expected to do any more since she was so terminal.

☐ **Protein 24 (HIV) NO**

☒ **Ortho-phospho-tyrosine (Cancer) YES at liver, brain, pancreas and vagina**

☒ **Fasciolopsis (Parasite) YES at liver, thymus, brain and colon**

☐ **Fasciolopsis other stages (Parasite) NO**

☒ **Sheep liver fluke (Parasite) YES at thymus and colon, NO at liver**

☒ **Pancreatic fluke (Parasite) YES**

> Note: All three large flukes are present. The sheep liver fluke is not in the liver, but in the thymus! She probably has benzene in her body.

☒ **Isopropyl Alcohol (Solvent) YES**

☒ **Hexanedione (Solvent) YES**

> Drinks a variety of teas.

☒ **Benzene (Solvent) YES**

> Uses toothpaste - will go off.

☒ Methyl ethyl ketone (Solvent) YES

Start on parasite program. Off all commercial beverages except herb teas (not Celestial Seasonings™, not mixtures) and off cold cereals. She will avoid Vaseline™ products like Chapstick™ and ice cream and frozen yogurt as well as all toothpastes. She will remove all body products that say "PROP" on the label. She will eat no meat that isn't cooked in the oven until the meat falls off the bone. And order only fish and seafood in restaurants.

Summary: Six weeks have passed, and we haven't seen Ms. Holden for follow-up. She had the deadly benzene solvent in her, and it was difficult for her to believe it was in her toothpaste. But she had a chance to save herself and recover. Did she take it?

| Alan Anderson | Multiple Cancer Sites |

Alan has a son who is an oncologist and recommended a PSA test for him a few years ago. This is a marker for prostate cancer. It was over 100! It should be less than 4. Doctors found cancer metastases into lymph nodes and bone. Chemo brought his PSA down to one. Recently it began to rise again. He was switched from Lupron™ (antitestosterone drug) to Cytradin™ plus cortisone to replace his own. He had a hip replacement several years before the prostate problem. He also now has arthritis in his knees. They have a water softener.

☐ Protein 24 (HIV) NO

☒ Ortho-phospho-tyrosine (Cancer) YES at adrenals, kidneys, bone, testicles and intestine

Beginning a massive invasion of cancer.

☒ Fasciolopsis (Parasite) YES at liver, intestine

☒ Fasciolopsis eggs (Parasite) YES at adrenals, kidneys, bone, testicles, blood

☐ Sheep liver fluke (Parasite) NO

☐ Pancreatic fluke (Parasite) NO

☒ Isopropyl Alcohol (Solvent) YES at liver, adrenals, kidneys

Off propanol sources.

☒ Methyl ethyl ketone (Solvent) YES

- ☒ **TCEthylene (Solvent) YES**

  Make own fruit and vegetable juices.

- ☒ **Uric Acid (Kidney Stone) YES**

- ☒ **di Calcium Phosphate (Kidney Stones) YES**

  Start on kidney herb recipe 2 weeks after starting parasite killing recipe. We will follow up in a month.

  Summary: We will also use the PSA test to follow up on his prostate cancer. He was very eager to solve his prostate problem. He seemed to have enough determination for us to let him start his second program, the kidney herbs, on his own without visiting the office in between. This is not generally good policy since it tends to become overwhelming. But he begged for progress with his pain when sitting and lives two states away, too far away for frequent visits.

Two months and two weeks after the first visit

His PSA has gone up. He will need urethral cleaning.

- ☐ **Protein 24 (HIV) NO**

- ☐ **hCG (Pre-Cancer) NO**

- ☒ **Ortho-phospho-tyrosine (Cancer) YES very high**

  Worse than before; still using hair spray and has not searched for propanol.

- ☒ **Nickel, Chromium, Gadolinium, Rubidium (Toxic Elements) YES**

  Tooth fillings.

- ☒ **Molybdenum (Toxic Element) YES**

  Automotive?

- ☒ **Lead (Toxic Element) YES**

  Root canal, water?

- ☒ **PVC (Toxic Element) YES**

  Source unknown.

- ☒ **Tungsten (Toxic Element) YES**

  Comes from an electrical heating element. There is no electric water heater. He does not use a wok or electric frying pan. We will test his toasters. He will not eat toast till then.

⊠ **Radon, Uranium (Toxic Elements) YES**

They are living on the 2nd floor. He will read a pamphlet on clearing up radon.

Summary: We are anxiously waiting to hear about him. Hopefully he carried out our instructions and got himself well this time. It was a mistake to let him start out with more than one program in spite of his eagerness.

| 63 | **Lynette Sarda** | **Breast and Liver Cancer** |

Lynette is a 51 year old woman from three states away who came for a number of problems she thought were stemming from her taking Tamoxifen™ for several years. So she took herself off recently but the problems are getting worse. The Tamoxifen™ was given to her to block estrogen uptake after she had a mastectomy on the right side. She had breast cancer in 1986. She now has severe migraines, insomnia and sees her moles are growing. She has had a hysterectomy. They have a water softener.

☐ **Protein 24 (HIV) NO**

⊠ **Ortho-phospho-tyrosine (Cancer) YES at liver and breast**

Cancer spread to the liver.

⊠ **Fasciolopsis (Parasite) YES at liver and colon**

⊠ **Fasciolopsis eggs (Parasite) YES at liver, colon and blood**

⊠ **Isopropyl Alcohol (Solvent) YES at liver and breast**

She has a pet (no doubt the source of Strongyloides, causing her migraines). She will start her pet on pet parasite program and herself on the human parasite program. She will remove all propanol from use *without using up any first.*

Two weeks later

☐ **Ortho-phospho-tyrosine (Cancer) NO**

⊠ **Fasciolopsis miracidia (Parasite) YES**

Note: She took the parasite treatment carefully, she got to 12 wormwood capsules, but one stage is still present. She has had a frozen turkey breast to eat recently. She will give herself a 3 day high dose program and then maintenance parasite treatment. She will stop eating meats. We have recent blood test results:

BLOOD TEST	Result	Comment
1. Calcium	very low (8.7)	She has been drinking lots of milk, but always skim. She will switch to 2%. Also take magnesium oxide (300mg), one/day.
2. LDH	slightly high (175)	recent cancer
3. SGOT, SGPT	low	Take B6 (250 mg) one/day, forever.
4. Cholesterol	low (172)	cancer risk. Eat butter and olive oil, not margarine.
5. Estrogen	very low	clean adrenals with kidney herb recipe
6. WBC	very low (3.65)	toxin in bone marrow
7. Eos	high (4%)	parasites
8. Atyp lymphs	high (4.7%)	cancer risk

☒ **Aluminum Silicate (Toxic Element) YES at breast**
Change salt to Hain, bypass water softener.

☒ **Aluminum (Toxic Element) YES high at breast**
Deodorant, cookware.

☒ **Iridium, Mercury (Toxic Elements) YES at breast**
Tooth fillings. Obviously, this is quite a burden to her breasts. She needs all amalgam fillings out of her mouth, all aluminum out of her kitchen, and the water softener taken out.

☒ **Platinum, Gallium (Toxic Elements) YES**
Tooth fillings.

☒ **Gold (Toxic Element) YES at breast and ovaries**

☒ **Tellurium (Toxic Element) YES at breast**

☒ **Zirconium (Toxic Element) YES**
Off deodorant and toothpaste.

☒ **Terbium (Toxic Element) YES**
Off foil packed foods, off all lozenges and pills except from Bronson's Pharm.

☒ **Wood Alcohol (Solvent) YES**
Drinks Coke™ products.

☒ **Ethyl denatured alcohol (Solvent) YES**
Uses this to clean bathroom. She will go back to simple chlorine bleach for cleaning the bathroom.

⊠ **TCEthylene, Methylene chloride (Solvents) YES**

She will stop drinking commercial beverages and eating cold cereals.

Summary: What a toxic build-up there is in Lynette's body! She is dissolving her tooth fillings but instead of passing the metals through the kidney and bowel they are staying stuck in her breast. She probably has numerous kidney stones from all this which, in turn, then slow down excretion. She is full of solvents; no doubt her detoxifying mechanisms are so overtaxed that no solvent can be oxidized any more. The aluminum silicate is probably coming from the water softener. She has not returned. Perhaps her husband did not like to hear all this. We hope he will come along if she comes back.

64	Sarah Hor	Kidney and Colon Cancer

Sarah is 47 years old, and came for her kidney disease. She was given interleukin 1 and interleukin 2 plus Interferon shots for her multiple kidney tumors. That was 9 months ago. She was scanned recently, and the tumors are growing again. She has only one kidney left. The other kidney was removed, full of tumors, 2 years ago, and at the same time half of her thyroid was removed for renal cell carcinoma. She listed ringing in her ears and stomach problems as her other problems. She has had a complete hysterectomy and wears an estrogen patch. She is presently on chemo-drip (a catheter implanted in her chest).

☐ **Protein 24 (HIV) NO**

⊠ **Ortho-phospho-tyrosine (Cancer) YES at kidney (very high) and colon only**

⊠ **Fasciolopsis (Parasite) YES at liver, kidney and colon**

⊠ **Fasciolopsis cercaria (Parasite) YES at kidney and in blood**

⊠ **Sheep liver fluke (Parasite) YES at liver, kidney and colon**

⊠ **Sheep liver fluke cercaria Parasite) YES at kidney, liver, colon, and in blood**

Start on parasite program.

⊠ **Isopropyl Alcohol (Solvent) YES high**

Other solvents not tested. She cleanses her catheter with rubbing alcohol. She will switch to grain alcohol or food grade hydrogen

351

peroxide. We will give her some 17½% "peroxy" to get started. She usually orders medium-cooked beef in restaurants, will stop.

Nine days later

☐ **Ortho-phospho-tyrosine (Cancer) NO**

☒ **Fasciolopsis miracidia(Parasite) YES at kidney, blood only**

☒ **Sheep liver fluke redia (Parasite) YES at kidney, blood only**
Other stages and adults are gone.

☒ **Pentane (Solvent) YES**

☐ **Solvents (Remainder) NO**
The propanol is gone. She drinks coffee and Pepsi™. She will switch to home made beverages.

☒ **Gallium (Toxic Element) YES**

☐ **Toxic Elements (Remainder) NO**
She wears rings. They were YES (positive) for gallium. She will stop wearing them. She will start on thioctic acid (100 mg), 4 per day. She has dentures. We hope they do not contain gallium. Continue parasite program.
Summary: Sarah did not return after hearing her cancer was gone. This is probably for financial reasons. She was very pleased with how she felt and could not believe these simple herbs succeeded where interleukin and interferon had failed. Hopefully, she is staying on our meat rule (beef, turkey, and chicken must be cooked at home, as well done as if it were pork, never grilled. And only fish or seafood in restaurants). The thioctic acid will speed up removal of gallium from her body.

65	Bryan Myers	Colon Cancer

Bryan, age 57, came for his painful feet, which began after an aortic bypass was done in 1990. At first the leg from which the blood vessel was taken was painful, too. His clinical doctor told him there was no connection. He smokes. My first thoughts were thallium or cadmium toxicity.

☐ **Protein 24 (HIV) NO**

☒ **Ortho-phospho-tyrosine (Cancer) YES at intestine**

This was a surprise. His wife had had cancer and had a breast removed. She also smokes. They have a water softener.

☒ **Fasciolopsis (Parasite) YES at liver only; NO at intestine**

☒ **Fasciolopsis eggs (Parasite) YES at lung and blood only; NO at intestine**

Obviously, he picked up the infective stages from somewhere other than if he had adults in his own intestine. This could be from eating raw meat or by sex or kissing. Smoking probably drew it to his lung. Another possibility is that his intestinal flukes were somehow killed while the stages survived in the blood. He will start on parasite program. He will use ginseng capsules and Chinese herbs to help him stop smoking. His wife will smoke outdoors only. He will switch his shampoo and shaving supplies to our varieties.

☒ **Oxalate, Phosphates (Kidney Stones) YES**

Sixteen days later

He has done parasite program. He will start kidney program.

☐ **Ortho-phospho-tyrosine (Cancer) NO**

☐ **Protein 24 (HIV) NO**

His cancer is gone. He says his bowel movement is normal again. He has not stopped smoking but likes the ginseng. His wife stopped smoking for his sake. He would like to do his share.

☒ **Cadmium, Europium oxide (Toxic Element) YES**

He has dentures. He will stop abrasive brushing and will use strong salt water and food grade hydrogen peroxide for brushing instead. We will see if this clears it up.

☒ **Ruthenium (Toxic Element) YES**

Dentures?

☐ **Toxic Elements (Remainder) NO**

His glasses frames are YES (positive). They may contain cadmium, adding to cadmium from cigarettes. Cadmium is the usual cause of leg pain (smoker's leg). It could, of course, be in his water supply if there is galvanized piping, but we will try to emphasize the smoking first, for his sake. He will get plastic framed glasses. He had a blood test done and will bring a copy next time.

Summary: Although Bryan's cancer cleared up within 16 days without stopping smoking, we emphasize stopping a lot. His lung lesions will probably continue to enlarge, and he may not get his foot pain relieved without stopping. We may not see him again, though, since heavy emphasis on stopping addictions loses us nearly every client.

66	Leo Stafford	Liver and Intestinal Cancer

This young man in his early thirties came to the office for a skin rash in the groin area. Although it is no doubt Candida, I suspect PCBs are weakening his immunity. He has tried every medication given by clinical doctors, as well as over-the-counter products. Nothing works. Also, any little sore he gets from his work (he works with lumber) does not heal for a long time. I suggested stopping using detergents, where PCBs are found, and using simple borax for all purposes: dish washing, laundry, shampoo, bathing, and citric acid to rinse his hair and body (¼ tsp. to a pint of water).

⊠ **Aluminum Silicate (Toxic Element) YES**
In salt, switch to Hain's.

⊠ **Bromine (Toxic Element) YES**
Rare, could it be in lumber treatment? Stop eating bread made with brominated (bleached) flour.

⊠ **Europium (Toxic Element) YES**
Tooth metal?

⊠ **Platinum (Toxic Element) YES**
Tooth filling or metal watch or glasses rims.

☐ **Solvents (ALL) NO**

⊠ **Candida (Pathogen) YES**
He will use only our home made skin lotions or apricot kernel oil, or 50% glycerin.

⊠ **Cholesterol crystals (Gallstones in liver) YES**
Crystals deposited somewhere. Clean liver.

One month later
He says there is some improvement but some lesions, especially on legs, are two years old!

BLOOD TEST	Result	Comment
1. WBC	high (8.2)	infection somewhere
2. RBC	low (4.7)	there is a blood loss somewhere. Parasites?
3. Eos	very high (12%)	parasites at high level
4. Urinalysis	shows urinary tract infection	
5. Cholesterol	very low	cancer risk - will test; eat butter and olive oil)
6. Ferritin	high (137)	cancer risk

☐ **Protein 24 (HIV) NO**

☒ **Ortho-phospho-tyrosine (Cancer) YES at liver and intestine**

☒ **Fasciolopsis (Parasite) YES at liver and intestine**

☒ **Fasciolopsis miracidia (Parasite) YES at blood only**

☒ **Sheep liver fluke redia, miracidia, and eggs (Parasite) YES at intestine**

☒ **Ancylostoma (hookworm) duod. (Parasite) YES at skin**

☐ **Pancreatic fluke, Ascaris, Trichinella, Strongyloides, Necator (Parasites) NO**
He will start on parasite killing program.

☒ **PCB (Toxic Element) YES**
Off detergent.

One month later
He is healing better. Leg lesions are better. Scrotum is still raw and flaking. He has chest pain today, over breast bone.

☐ **Protein 24 (HIV) NO**

☐ **Ortho-phospho-tyrosine (Cancer) NO**

☒ **Fasciolopsis (Parasite) YES at thymus; NO at liver**
Suspect benzene.

☒ **Sheep liver fluke (Parasite) YES at thymus; NO at liver**
No stages found for either fluke. Repeat 5-day high dose parasite program, then maintenance.

☒ **Benzene (Solvent) YES at thymus; NO at liver**
He will go off all toothpaste and Vaseline products, ice cream, and frozen yogurt.

☐ **Aluminum Silicate, Europium. Bromine (Toxic Elements) NO**
Now wears gloves to handle lumber.

☒ **Platinum (Toxic Element) YES**
Must be tooth fillings since he has changed glasses and wrist watch to plastic - replace tooth fillings with composite.

☒ **Candida (Pathogen) YES**
PCBs probably still in clothing.

☒ **tri Calcium Phosphate, Oxalate, Uric Acid (Kidney Stones) YES**
Summary: What a tragedy it is to fill up a young person, the same age as my children, with PCBs. My generation did not have this handicap. Body yeast in the genital area must be a difficult problem. If all the people with this problem were to join hands, could they persuade authorities to protect them? Could the responsibility be placed on the suppliers to analyze their products for a list of harmful substances (like PCBs or solvents) rather than having the responsibility be with the individual person to prove that the ailment was caused by a particular product? We shall soon all be in this young man's situation! Notice that in the first solvent test there was no benzene, and in the second test it was YES. He had picked it up between tests. He was still healthy enough to detoxify and clear it from his body. But he is very near to getting the HIV virus from the fluke in his thymus.

Five weeks later
He feels better and has more energy. Skin purple spots (reddish, but not open lesions) are still on both legs. He has had 2 bouts of the flu. Groin itch is better. He has not yet done dental work.

67	Sue Weeks	Cancer at Multiple Sites

This 52 year old woman gave a hair-raising account of brushes with death. In the early 80s, she was diagnosed as having Chronic Fatigue Syndrome. Her clinical doctors found she had 80% blockage of carotid arteries and leg arteries. She chose chelation instead of standard clinical treatment but stopped after 60 treatments without responding. She was on 90 supplements a day but was still bedridden. She picked up active mononucleosis and went down to 84 pounds in weight. She got all amalgams out but it made no difference. She tried acupuncture for pain. She was in pain all over and had terrible fatigue. She tried the macrobiotic diet for 2 years; this made her feel better, but she didn't gain weight or energy. She went to an Oklahoma clinic and a Reno clinic for homeopathy. No improvement. Near death, she went to an alternative hospital in Mexico. She was on Gerson therapy for 2 years but couldn't get well. Suddenly she improved without explanation for 3 months. Then she worsened and was hospitalized. Her relationship broke, and she had to return to her mother's home. At the same time she was pursuing clinical routes with CAT scans, hematologists, neurologists, and other specialists too numerous to mention. Her mother died of cancer.

☒ Ortho-phospho-tyrosine (Cancer) YES at liver, kidney, bladder, intestine, stomach

Cancer everywhere! How has she survived?

☐ Protein 24 (HIV) NO

☒ Fasciolopsis (Parasite) YES at liver, kidney, bladder, intestine, stomach

☒ Fasciolopsis miracidia (Parasite) YES at liver, kidney, bladder, stomach

She used to eat rare meat. She craved meat. Start on parasite program.

Two weeks later

☐ Ortho-phospho-tyrosine (Cancer) NO

Client says she is cured, feels fine. She can't believe it was simply a parasite and that she probably ate it many times. She wonders why nobody is looking for such things.

☐ Fasciolopsis and all stages (Parasite) NO

☒ Ancylostoma can. (Parasite) YES

Has a dog and will treat it

☒ Human liver fluke (Parasite) YES

☒ Ancylostoma br. (Parasite) YES

☒ Dog heartworm (Parasite) YES

Raised horses, had dogs, was a nail biter.

☒ **Eimeria (Parasite) YES**
Used to have ducks.

☐ **Parasites (Remainder) NO**

☒ **Isopropyl Alcohol (Solvent) YES**

☒ **Benzene (Solvent) YES**
Uses Tom's Toothpaste™, will stop. She will use Milk Thistle, 2 a day. She will get all solvents out of her house, except grain alcohol. She will avoid the benzene list I gave her and the propanol list.

Summary: A ten year torment was ended in 2 weeks by killing this large parasite that had invaded so much of her body; it is a wonder she was alive to tell the story. Possibly all her alternative therapies helped her to survive, each in its own way. She was undoubtedly reinfecting herself many times and letting parasites proliferate due to having the two worst solvents accumulated in her. Her intelligence and courage saw her through. Hopefully she will follow-up in the near future.

Esther Santos   **Breast Cancer**

This 49 year old woman came to the office for a list of peculiar symptoms: numbness of lips, arms and tip of tongue occasionally. Tingling sensation in her back. Leg veins turn blue and painful, also the wrist veins. Her clinical doctor diagnosed pulmonary angina and put her on 2 aspirins a day for the last 4 months. The symptoms haven't changed. She had a polyp in a milk duct in her right breast removed a year ago and another one in the left cheek sinus, not removed. She recently discovered a lump in her breast and is scheduled for a biopsy in 10 days. They have a water softener. There is pain in her left collar bone.

☐ **Protein 24 (HIV) NO**

☒ **Ortho-phospho-tyrosine (Cancer) YES**

☒ **Fasciolopsis (Parasite) YES at liver, side of breast and intestine**

☒ **Fasciolopsis redia (Parasite) YES at liver, side of breast, blood**

☐ **Fasciolopsis other stages (Parasite) NO**

☒ **Isopropyl Alcohol (Solvent) YES**

☐ **Solvents (Remainder) NO**
Start on parasite program.
Summary: Esther only made this one visit to our office. She feared her insurance company would not pay for anything. Perhaps the breast lump biopsy showed a malignancy, and she pursued the clinical route of removing the breast. Perhaps it did not show a malignancy (the parasite program could have turned it around in 5 days), and she lost confidence in our testing. Whatever happened, we will never know. Hopefully she began to avoid propanol containing cosmetics as we suggested.

68	**Rosa Lee Kestler**	**Pancreatic Cancer**

Rosa Lee, age 63, came in because her clinical doctor found gall-stones in her gallbladder. She had a serious attack where she passed out and was hospitalized. They did a blood test then, which showed that the pancreas had some blockage, too, because the pancreatic enzyme, lipase, was very high in the blood. The doctor wanted to do surgery to investigate the problem and possibly remove stones from the pancreas, too. But she declined the offer and doesn't know what to do next. She brought in a recent blood test when all this happened.

BLOOD TEST	Result	Comment
1. FBS	slightly high (135)	clean the liver
2. BUN and Creatinine	slightly high	clean the kidneys
3. Calcium	very low (8.7)	Drink 2% milk, 3 glasses a day (cow or goat); take Vitamin D (50,000 iu, from doctor or dentist), 3 a week; take magnesium oxide (300 mg), one a day.
4. Chloride and potassium	very low (95, 3.8)	adrenal problem; clean kidneys
5. Albumin and Total protein	slightly low	clean liver
6. GGT, SGOT, SGPT	all very high (74, 130, 140)	liver disease
7. LDH	very high (359)	heart stress or cancer
8. WBC	very high (20.8)	gallbladder disease
9. RBC	high (5.25)	check for cobalt toxicity
10. Lymphs	very low (5%)	toxin in bone marrow
11. Platelet count	very high (383)	parasites
12. Amylase	very high (548)	pancreas problem

☐ **Protein 24 (HIV) NO**

☒ **Ortho-phospho-tyrosine (Cancer) YES at liver, pancreas**
Her doctor may have suspected cancer when he wanted to look inside her body.

☒ **Fasciolopsis (Parasite) YES at liver, intestine, pancreas**

☐ **Sheep liver fluke and its stages (Parasite) NO**

☒ **Pancreatic fluke and stages (Parasite) YES**
Start on parasite program. Remove all propanol from her house.

Eight days later
She has a lot more energy. In fact she looks happy.

☐ **Ortho-phospho-tyrosine (Cancer) NO**
She got up and hugged me. She brought in a jar with dead flukes in it. She passed them in her stool, they came to the top. They appeared to have black hairy legs. I recognized them as either intestinal or Sheep liver flukes; the "black hairy legs" are strings of eggs.

☐ **Fasciolopsis and all stages (Parasite) NO**

☐ **Sheep liver fluke and all stages (Parasite) NO**

☐ **Pancreatic fluke and stages (Parasite) NO**

☐ **Human liver fluke and stages (Parasite) NO**
She'll continue parasite program and go off all commercial beverages and cold cereals.
Summary: Rosa Lee was a model client, a joy to work with. In eight days she had eliminated cancer and begun to regain her health. I hope she carries out her whole program and learns to live into her 90's in a healthy state.

69	Kathy Doyle	Breast Cancer

Kathy is 29 years old and has been watching a breast lump for 3 years. Mammograms were "sometimes positive, sometimes negative." She also has low back pain and very crampy menstrual periods. She drinks coffee, tea and cola to control her weight but feels she is still overweight. She seems of normal weight to me.

☐ **Protein 24 (HIV) NO**

☒ **Ortho-phospho-tyrosine (Cancer) YES at breast**

☒ **Fasciolopsis (Parasite) YES at liver, uterus, intestine, breast**

☒ **Fasciolopsis cercaria (Parasite) YES at breast, blood, uterus**

☐ **Sheep liver fluke (Parasite) NO**

☒ **Isopropyl Alcohol (Solvent) YES at liver**
Since she came late to her appointment, it had to be cut short. Only these essentials were tested. She will start a parasite killing program and go off all propanol containing products.

One month later

☐ **Protein 24 (HIV) NO**

☐ **Ortho-phospho-tyrosine (Cancer) NO**

☐ **Fasciolopsis and all stages (Parasite) NO**
She was late for her appointment, and I will need to cut her time short again.

☒ **Chromium (Toxic Element) YES**
The source of chromium is not clear since she does not use eye make-up, and they do not have a water softener. She'll go off her supplements and use only Bronson's Pharm brand.

☒ **Gallium, Gadolinium (high), Platinum, Silver (Toxic Elements) YES**
Tooth metal.

☒ **Strontium (Toxic Element) YES**
Off toothpaste.

☒ **Zirconium (Toxic Element) YES**
Go off deodorant.

☒ **Benzene (Solvent) YES**
Was just one step away from getting the HIV virus.

☒ **Pentane, Methyl ethyl ketone, Toluene, Methyl butyl ketone (Solvents) YES**
She will remove all solvent type cleaners from the house and stop drinking pop. She will go off toothpaste, chapstick, ice cream, and frozen yogurt to get rid of benzene.

Summary: Kathy was very lucky to be told about her benzene problem and how to stop getting it into herself; otherwise she would have soon had the HIV virus. Notice how her metal tooth fillings are dissolving. The toxic metals are probably attaching themselves to her breast tissue; there wasn't time to check this. She is to get dental work done before returning.

Three months after first visit

She is on the birth control pill for excessive bleeding. She has not done dental work yet.

☐ Ortho-phospho-tyrosine (Cancer) NO

☐ hCG (Pre-Cancer) NO

Her breast lump is still there.

☒ Wood Alcohol, TCE (Solvents) YES

She will go off commercial beverages, definitely, this time. She will start drinking 2% milk, 3 glasses a day and take magnesium, 300 mg, one a day. She had a blood test done.

BLOOD TEST	Result	Comment
1. SGOT, SGPT	slightly low (16, 18)	take B6 500 mg/day
2. Triglycerides	slightly high (157)	kidney problems
3. Iron	low	parasites and excessive bleeding
4. Urinalysis	shows urinary tract infection	kidney

She will go back on the kidney herbs for 2 weeks. She will also repeat a 3 day high dose parasite program.

70	Elizabeth Iler	Cancer Of Pancreas

This 54 year old woman looks like 74. Her sister-in-law and daughter-in-law brought her from the West for treatment of cancer of the pancreas. It is inoperable, and she is losing weight fast. She has a tube implanted in her stomach to give herself extra feedings. She is on Percocet™ and morphine for pain. Her complexion is yellow, and she knows she is being treated like a terminal patient. She smokes. She does not want to stop.

☒ Ortho-phospho-tyrosine (Cancer) YES at liver, pancreas

☒ Fasciolopsis (Parasite) YES at liver and intestine, NO at pancreas

☒ **Fasciolopsis eggs (Parasite) YES at pancreas**

☒ **Fasciolopsis cercaria (Parasite) YES at pancreas**

☒ **Sheep liver fluke redia (Parasite) YES at pancreas**

☐ **Pancreatic fluke and stages (Parasite) NO**

☒ **Human liver fluke metacercaria (Parasite) YES at pancreas, NO at liver**

☒ **Isopropyl Alcohol (Solvent) YES at liver and pancreas**

☒ **Wood Alcohol, Methyl butyl ketone (Solvent) YES**
She will start parasite program. She will go off all "prop"-containing products, meaning isopropanol. She will go off commercial beverages and make herself fruit and vegetable juices and cereals. She will be totally vegetarian for 3 months. She will use Bronson's Digestive Enzymes to assist the pancreas temporarily; 6 with larger meals, 4 with breakfast.

Two days later

☐ **Ortho-phospho-tyrosine (Cancer) NO**
She was incredulous that her cancer could be gone in 2 days. She is off propanol (it was in her face cream and hair spray). She is off meat. She is off commercial beverages; she has found fresh squeezed juice in the grocery store. She is using Bronson's Digestive Enzymes and is feeling better.

☒ **Barium (Toxic Element) YES at pancreas**
Check lipstick.

☒ **Cesium (Toxic Element) YES**
She has been drinking distilled water from plastic bottles; will switch to cold faucet water.

☒ **Palladium, Mercury (high), Gold (high), Samarium (Toxic Elements) YES at pancreas**
Tooth fillings.

☒ **Tin (Toxic Element) YES high at pancreas**
Will go off toothpaste.

☒ **Uranium (Toxic Element) YES at pancreas**
Seal cracks.

☒ Radon (Toxic Element) YES

Summary: Elizabeth had perked up at her second visit when I told her her cancer was already gone. She reeked strongly of tobacco smoke. When I brought this up to her, she replied that since she was dying there was no need to quit. The women with her disagreed and tried to support my view. Then I pointed out to her that she was one of the fortunate ones who have only 2 problems of any difficulty: She merely needed her teeth replaced by plastic and to seal cracks in her basement. Checking in her mouth, there were only 4 on each side that needed replacement, but she began to sob about the cost. She whined and groaned about having to borrow money from her family, and said she couldn't do it. I personally believe she was looking for any excuse to die rather than survive, so that she would not have to quit smoking. What devilish games our addictions play with us. And to think that wonderful, moral-minded people allow themselves to grow tobacco for money, knowing that the addiction spells death for other humans, perhaps their own grandchildren! I hope her wonderful family will persuade her to choose life for herself and transport her to the dentist.

71	Betty Naylor	Cervical Cancer and HIV

Betty is 24 years old, arriving from a neighboring state for Chronic Fatigue Syndrome. However, she had an impressive list of additional symptoms involving her lower back, stomach, chest (tightness and the need for long breaths of air), throat, skin, ears, neck, and PMS. They have a water softener. The chest problem suggested the possibility of HIV-illness. She sleeps all day and has burning over the chest. She has been sick all winter.

☒ Protein 24 (HIV) YES at thymus, vagina

There are no known risk factors.

☒ Ortho-phospho-tyrosine (Cancer) YES at cervix only

☒ hCG (Pre-Cancer) YES at thymus, cervix, NO at vagina

This was quite a surprise. Betty volunteered that she had never had sex in her life and had never been in a hospital except at birth. I assured her that this virus, HIV, did not originate with sex and blood and could be quickly cleared up, provided she followed instructions meticulously. She was very eager to do so.

☐ Fasciolopsis adults (Parasite) NO

☒ Fasciolopsis miracidia (Parasite) YES at cervix and vagina

☒ Fasciolopsis cercaria (Parasite) YES at cervix

☒ Fasciolopsis eggs (Parasite) YES at vagina

☒ Sheep liver fluke adults (Parasite) YES high at liver (one side) and intestine

☒ Sheep liver fluke eggs (Parasite) YES at liver (one side) and cervix and vagina

☒ Human liver fluke adults and eggs (Parasite) YES at liver (same side as above)

These findings suggest both benzene and isopropanol have accumulated in Betty's body. There isn't enough time to test for all solvents.

☒ Benzene (Solvent) YES at thymus and vagina

☒ Isopropyl Alcohol (Solvent) YES at liver (same side as above) and thymus, NO at vagina

Remainder of solvents not tested. She is to go off all toothpaste, Vaseline™ products, ice cream and frozen yogurt, cold cereals and cooking oils, except olive oil. This is to avoid benzene. She is to go off all body products that have "PROP" on the label to avoid propanol. She will go off her shampoo, mouthwash, hair mousse and hair spray because they contain it without labeling. She is to go off all commercial beverages to avoid other solvents, not yet tested. We will follow-up very soon. She is very anxious. She will start on parasite killing program. She will be strictly vegetarian for 3 months. She will use our replacement shampoo, etc.

Five days later

She has a lot more energy and went off her antibiotics. She is very apprehensive, though.

☐ Protein 24 (HIV) NO

☐ Ortho-phospho-tyrosine, hCG (Cancer) NO

☐ Solvents (ALL) NO

☐ Fasciolopsis and all stages (Parasite) NO

☐ Pancreatic fluke and all stages (Parasite) NO

☐ Sheep liver fluke and all stages (Parasite) NO

☐ **Human liver fluke and all stages (Parasite) NO**

She is elated. She will continue the parasite killing program and other lifestyle changes.

☒ **PCB (Toxic Element) YES**

Go off detergent; use borax, washing soda and homemade or Amish soap.

☒ **Gadolinium, Tantalum (Toxic Elements) YES**

Tooth fillings.

☒ **Holmium (Toxic Element) YES**

Probably with the PCBs.

☐ **Toxic Elements (Remainder) NO**

She needs metal tooth fillings replaced. After 3 months of vegetarian diet she will eat only fish and seafood in restaurants and super-well done meats at home.

Summary: This young woman fairly bounced out of the office at the good news of her second visit. The entire story of how she could have gotten the HIV virus and developed cancer of the cervix was like a revelation to her - almost unbelievable. Yet her mother, she said, was witness to her health improvement in just 5 days, and so she is forced to believe it. At any rate, she is much too scared not to believe that she had HIV virus.

Notice a peculiarity: There is no adult intestinal fluke in the liver. Not even a stage of it is in the liver! Yet there is ortho-phospho-tyrosine being produced. It is being produced at the cervix where the miracidia and cercaria are and where the Sheep liver fluke eggs are. Now, the Sheep liver fluke adults are found in the liver. Could they orchestrate the production of ortho-phospho-tyrosine for the intestinal fluke? Or was there an adult intestinal fluke at some earlier time which died? One very seldom sees both adult flukes together. Do they kill each other somehow? Notice, too, that the cancer marker, hCG, was present along with the cancer marker, ortho-phospho-tyrosine, at the cervix. But only hCG was being produced at the thymus. Is a particular parasite stage responsible for producing hCG? I explained to Betty that she must take great care to protect her thymus for two years so that it will completely regain its health. It would be tempting to neglect the dental work but this would be a tragic mistake. Benzene leaves the thymus in a weakened condition so that other solvents and toxic substances continue to get accumulate there. This would, surely, give her lowered immunity, perhaps even AIDS.

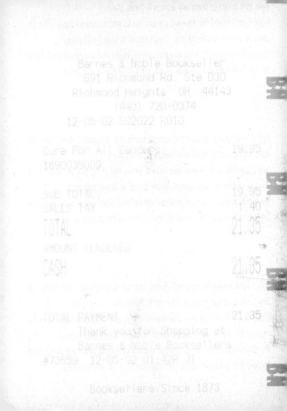

days with a receipt from any Barnes & Noble store.

Store Credit issued for new and unread books and unopened music after 30 days or without a sales receipt. Credit issued at <u>lowest sale price</u>.

We gladly accept returns of new and unread books and unopened music from bn.com with a bn.com receipt for store credit at the bn.com price.

Full refund issued for new and unread books and unopened music within 30 days with a receipt from any Barnes & Noble store.

Store Credit issued for new and unread books and unopened music after 30 days or without a sales receipt. Credit issued at <u>lowest sale price</u>.

We gladly accept returns of new and unread books and unopened music from bn.com with a bn.com receipt for store credit at the bn.com price.

Full refund issued for new and unread books and unopened music within 30 days with a receipt from any Barnes & Noble store.

Store Credit issued for new and unread books and unopened music after 30 days or without a sales receipt. Credit issued at <u>lowest sale price</u>.

We gladly accept returns of new and unread books and unopened music from bn.com with a bn.com receipt for store credit at the bn.com price.

| 72 | Ken Kitsinger | Brain Cancer |

Ken is a quiet but highly attentive young man of 19. He said his parents had brought him to our office for depression but he disagreed with this opinion. Both parents were respectfully quiet while he spoke. He is currently getting psychiatric counseling. I explained the cause of serious depression to be brain parasites and toxic elements accumulated in the brain. It was therefore quite shocking to see the initial test results.

☐ **Protein 24 (HIV) NO**

☒ **Ortho-phospho-tyrosine (Cancer) YES at brain**
He has brain cancer!

☒ **hCG (Pre-Cancer) YES at brain, blood**

☒ **Fasciolopsis (Parasite) YES at liver, intestine; NO at brain**

☒ **Fasciolopsis redia, cercaria, eggs, miracidia (Parasites) YES at brain**
Note: Every stage of the fluke is present, suggesting a high level of solvents. Note that the cancer marker hCG is present in the blood; it could have been found clinically by a blood test. Finding this brain cancer was rather shocking. But his mother stated that Ken's first cousin, a boy, had died of brain cancer at the age of 18. So the news of Ken's brain cancer was not totally unbelievable. I could assure them of a complete recovery.

☒ **Sheep liver fluke redia (Parasite) YES at brain**
Here the presence of a developmental stage of Sheep liver fluke without an adult present to produce it, suggests another source, most likely raw meats. They will stop eating rarely cooked meats (they do a lot of grilling).

☒ **Pancreatic fluke stages (Parasite) YES at brain**
Again no adults.

☒ **Human liver fluke (Parasite) YES at brain and thymus**
Apparently the thymus is involved, too, suggesting benzene accumulation there. He will start on parasite killing program.

☒ **Benzalkonium (Solvent) YES at brain**
Go off toothpaste.

⊠ **Asbestos (Toxic Element) YES high at brain**

Change dryer belt to USA made; bring in old belt for testing; test hair blower. He will make his own hair spray, switch shampoos and go off the benzene-containing items on the benzene list. He will stop eating out of styrofoam.

⊠ **Mercury (Toxic Element) YES at brain**

Remove amalgam tooth fillings.

Summary: brain cancer is fairly rare; yet two persons, both very young, had this disease in his family. Could it all be inherited through the placenta from the mother or through sex during pregnancy? Had his body defended him all these 19 years, only now to be losing the battle? Surely, he had not been using propanol all this time, nor benzene. My guess is that the fluke resided quietly in the intestine for all family members. Then, as usage of propanol and benzene began in early adulthood, they colonized the brain and thymus. This still does not answer why the brain was selected by the parasite stages, rather than another tissue. Possibly, the brain-seeking solvents, xylene and toluene, were present, the cousins choosing the same brands of beverages.

Seventeen days after first visit

The dentist took panoramic X-rays and found no mercury fillings. He will get a tooth extracted, though. He will take vitamin D (50,000 u) 2/week to help heal the bone cavity when the tooth is extracted. He is not drinking milk but will start with 3 glasses of 2% a day. He will also take magnesium oxide, (300 mg), 1 per day.

⊠ **Asbestos, Mercury, Gadolinium, Indium, Fiberglass (Toxic Elements) YES**

They have brought air samples, but there is no time to test for them - he has just taken a job and must be on time for it!

☐ **Solvents (ALL) NO**

⊠ **Mycoplasma (Pathogen) YES at brain (cerebrum)**

⊠ **A strep, Measles (Pathogens) YES at brain**

⊠ **Shigella flex (Pathogen) YES high at brain**

Shigella produces a toxin that causes intense irritability, even anger. Could this be the major cause of his depression? We will see him after the dental work. These are very rare pathogens to be seen in the brain!

Seven weeks later

There are no changes in his condition. He has had one tooth extracted by a non-Huggins trained dentist, so the socket wasn't cleaned.

☐ **Ortho-phospho-tyrosine, hCG (Cancer) NO**

☒ **Benzene, Isopropyl alcohol (Solvents) YES**

☐ **PCB (Toxic Element) NO**

☒ **Mercury (Toxic Element) YES at teeth 10, 18, 22, and 29**

☒ **Fiberglass (Toxic Element) YES**

☒ **EBV, Bacteroides fragilis, Streptococcus pneumoniae, L strep, Haemophilus influenzae, Herpes zoster, Herpes simplex, FLU (Pathogens) YES in brain**

He will try harder to exclude benzene and propanol and other solvents from food and body products. He is showing an AIDS-like syndrome in the brain.

73	Alyce Dean	Lung Cancer and HIV

Alyce is a low key, sweet tempered person, age 48, brought in by her brother for a spreading numbness in her body. She has pain and numbness at the same time in her arms, legs and hands. Three years ago Alyce had a mastectomy on the right side for cancer. Now a lump is developing on the back of her neck. (I suspect this is a PCB cyst.) Her father died of liver cancer a few years ago.

☒ **Ortho-phospho-tyrosine (Cancer) YES at lungs only**

☒ **Fasciolopsis (Parasite) YES at liver and intestine**

☒ **Fasciolopsis redia (Parasite) YES in blood**

She will start on parasite killing program.

Four days later

☐ **Ortho-phospho-tyrosine (Cancer) NO**

☐ **Fasciolopsis and all stages (Parasite) NO**

Her cancer is gone, but her symptoms have not improved; in fact, she is worse, and walks slowly.

☒ **Terbium (Toxic Element) YES**
Probably in a pill.

☒ **Zirconium (Toxic Element) YES**
Off deodorant. These are not enough to explain her nerve-muscle deterioration.

☒ **Benzene (Solvent) YES**
There are building supplies (paint thinner) on the back porch. Also insect spray and chemicals for dairy animals. She lives alone but will have one of her children remove it all and make an air sample in her home for us to test. She is to return within the week, this is urgent.

Fifteen days later
She is much worse. It is tragic to see this young woman losing ground. If she can't find the benzene source, she may not survive. She missed 2 earlier appointments due to transportation problems.

☐ **Ortho-phospho-tyrosine (Cancer) NO**
Cancer has not returned.

☒ **Protein 24 (HIV) YES**
Now has HIV illness.

☒ **Benzene (Solvent) YES, and in bedroom air sample, bathroom air, kitchen air, porch air**
Cattle spray supplies have not yet been removed.

☐ **Fasciolopsis and all stages (Parasite) NO**

☒ **Fasciolopsis cercaria (Parasite) YES at thymus, bone marrow, and blood**
This is evidently from eating undercooked meat since they were all absent last week. Her children are cooking for her. It is impossible to say no to their cooking, Some of the chemicals have been removed from the porch. She has seen her clinical doctor who has scheduled radiation for her.

☒ **Salmonella (Pathogen) YES throughout body (is septic)**

☒ **EBV, Coxsackie B #4 (Pathogens) YES**
Others not tested. She is to clear the whole house of chemicals; her highest priority is to get the benzene out of her body. Her family is sympathetic but isn't taking seriously the need to clear the house of

chemicals. Alyce does not have enough immune power to combat the simplest infections anymore.

Summary: This is the last time we saw Alyce. She cleared her cancer in the first four days and the future looked bright. But she was not strong enough to clean up the solvent benzene, which was polluting the air in her house and let 2 weeks slip by. Her family did not come with her to learn the details of cleaning up and so the job was left undone. Without immunity, she was helpless against the most common bacteria and viruses.

74	Stan Spillman	Prostate Cancer

Stan is 76 and was brought in by his sister because he has refused to go to a clinical doctor for almost 20 years. He has difficulty urinating and is up 4-5 times a night to try to empty his bladder.

☐ **Protein 24 (HIV) NO**

☒ **Ortho-phospho-tyrosine (Cancer) YES at prostate**

☒ **hCG (Pre-Cancer) YES at prostate**

☒ **Isopropyl Alcohol (Solvent) YES at prostate, liver**
He uses a hair thickener, not a hair spray. He will go off, also off shampoo and after-shave lotion. He will use our products.

☒ **Isophorone, Pentane, Styrene, Methyl Ethyl Ketone (Solvents) YES**
Will be careful not to use styrofoam dishes. He drinks mostly root beer, thinking it is good for him to drink so much water to help his urination. He will go off all commercial beverages and stick to our list of six.

☒ **Fasciolopsis (Parasite) YES at prostate and liver**
Note: We seldom see an adult fluke in the prostate, but here is a case of it.

☒ **Fasciolopsis redia (Parasite) YES at bladder and semen**
Note: If he were sexually active, he would transmit redia to his spouse. We will search for them in his urine specimen.

☒ **Sheep liver fluke (Parasite) YES at prostate, NO at liver**
Note: quite unusual for a liver fluke that ought to be in the liver to be in the prostate. It often seems as though *Fasciolopsis* keeps the Sheep liver fluke out of the liver and vice versa.

371

☒ **Sheep liver fluke cercaria and metacercaria (Parasite) YES at prostate, bladder and semen**

☐ **Pancreatic fluke and all stages (Parasite) NO**

☐ **Human liver fluke and all stages (Parasite) NO**
He will start on parasite program.
Summary: Both cancer markers ortho-phospho-tyrosine and hCG were present in the white blood cells and prostate. It is tempting to speculate that propanol can cause the Sheep liver fluke, as well as the intestinal fluke, to produce ortho-phospho-tyrosine. This would mean the Sheep liver fluke could give us cancer, too. But if they don't let each other into the liver, whoever gets there first may stay there. Or perhaps the intestinal fluke can chase the Sheep liver fluke out of the liver. Could it be that sheep flukes can defend against invasion by intestinal fluke? The relationship between them should be a fascinating study.

Five weeks later

☐ **Ortho-phospho-tyrosine, hCG (Cancer) NO**

☐ **Isopropyl Alcohol (Solvent) NO**
He is rid of his cancer. We will now search for the heavy metals and other toxic accumulations in the prostate that enabled the cancer to develop there.

☒ **Mercury (Toxic Element) YES at prostate**
Tooth fillings.

☒ **Nickel (Toxic Element) YES at prostate**
Tooth fillings. Remainder not tested. He is advised to have all metal removed from his mouth and replaced with metal-free plastic. Note: nickel is <u>almost always</u> seen accumulated in the prostate.

75	Sharon Brownie	Liver and Lung Cancer and HIV

Sharon Brownie came to the office for pain behind her shoulder blades, behind her ears, in both legs, and on top of her head at the scalp. These are unusual symptoms to occur together.

☒ **Protein 24 (HIV) YES at thymus**
Quite a surprise.

☒ **Ortho-phospho-tyrosine (Cancer) YES at liver and lungs**
She also has liver and lung cancer, another surprise, since there is no smoker in the house.

☒ **Fasciolopsis (Parasite) YES at thymus and blood**
The meaning of this result is not clear. How could an adult fluke fit into a blood vessel? She has both cancer and HIV. Yet, the adult intestinal fluke is not in the liver, only in the thymus and, apparently, blood.

☒ **Fasciolopsis redia (Parasite) YES at blood, thymus, liver and lung**
She will start on parasite program. She will go off items on the benzene and propanol lists.

Four days later

☐ **Ortho-phospho-tyrosine (Cancer) NO**

☐ **Fasciolopsis and all stages (Parasite) NO**

☐ **Protein 24 (HIV) NO**

Fifteen days later
She feels considerably better. She still gets weak spells in her arms and legs (but not pain, now).

☐ **Protein 24 (HIV) NO**

☒ **Gallium, Gold, Ruthenium (Toxic Elements) YES**
Tooth fillings. She has no tooth fillings but wears a metal partial denture. She will get a new metal-free plastic one.

Thirteen days later

☐ **Protein 24 (HIV) NO**

☐ **Ortho-phospho-tyrosine (Cancer) NO**

☒ **Oxalate (Kidney Stones) YES**
Start on kidney herb recipe.

☒ **Isopropyl Alcohol (Solvent) YES**

☒ **Pentane (Solvent) YES**

☒ **Kerosene (Solvent) YES**
Used in cook stove.

⊠ **Denatured alcohol (Solvent) YES**
Used in lamps. She will be much more careful when pouring these fuels and will stop drinking soda pop.

⊠ **Diphyllobothrium (Parasite) YES**
Dog/fish tapeworm. She will increase parasite dosage.

Eleven days later
She still has pain at left lower abdomen, upper back and lower back. This is probably still due to parasites, plus liver gallstones.

☐ **Kidney Stones (ALL) NO**
Continue kidney herbs at half dose.

☐ **Protein 24 (HIV) NO**

☐ **Ortho-phospho-tyrosine (Cancer) NO**

☐ **Denatured alcohol (Solvent) NO**

⊠ **Pentane (Solvent) YES**
Can't give up soda pop.

⊠ **Isopropyl Alcohol (Solvent) YES**
Source unknown, since she uses no commercial body products.

⊠ **Gastrothylax, Trichomonas (Parasites) YES**
Continue parasite program.

☐ **Parasites (Remainder) NO**
She will start taking peroxy and 07 in preparation for a liver gallstone cleanse. She will do a 5 day high dose parasite treatment.

Another month later
Her left arm is numb, both feet are numb. There is shoulder and shoulder blade pain. She is still putting off the dental work.

☐ **Protein 24 (HIV) NO**

☐ **Ortho-phospho-tyrosine (Cancer) NO**

☐ **Diphyllobothrium Gastrothylax, Trichomonas (Parasites) NO**

☐ **Solvents (ALL) NO**

☒ **Diplococcus pneu, Histomonas, Salmonella typh, Haemoph inf (Pathogens) YES**
Two of these are teeth bacteria. She is getting a lot of headaches. Remainder of box 1 and 2: NO.

Five weeks later
She is still getting a lot of headaches, probably from tooth bacteria. She did a liver cleanse and got numerous tan-colored stones.

☐ **Protein 24 (HIV) NO**

☐ **Ortho-phospho-tyrosine (Cancer) NO**

☒ **Clostridium sept. (Pathogen) YES**
Probable cause of pain behind both ears. Needs to do dental work.

☒ **Wood Alcohol (Solvent) YES**
Is drinking Pepsi™ again.

☒ **Kerosene (Solvent) YES**
They are using it again; must change.
Summary: Sharon eliminated the HIV virus and her liver cancer in record time: 4 days. What was more difficult was eliminating headaches; in fact, it was not accomplished. Her isopropanol disappeared after she switched off commercial shampoo. It remains to be seen whether her arms and feet will recover. She does plan to get the dental work done.

76	Kimberly Maston	Brain Cancer

Kimberly is a middle aged person from a midwest state, seemingly quite anxious about her condition. Her whole left side feels as though electric shocks were traveling up and down it. It seems paralyzed, too. But she walks normally and can use her arm. This began after surgery 2 years ago at the base of her brain for cancer. She went through physical therapy after that and is exercising, but this new kind of paralysis set in just as she was discharged from the physical therapy program.

☐ **Protein 24 (HIV) NO**

☒ **Ortho-phospho-tyrosine (Cancer) YES at cerebellum**

☒ **hCG (Pre-Cancer) YES at cerebellum**

☒ **Fasciolopsis (Parasite) YES at liver and intestine**

⊠ **Fasciolopsis miracidia (Parasite) YES at intestine, spleen, kidney, bladder and cerebellum**

The remaining large fluke parasites were not tested because I felt she had too much anxiety already to cope with more information. I discussed avoiding rare meats with her; she is a lover of rare beef, but she agreed. I discussed avoiding propanol in her shampoo, hair spray and other products. She will switch to borax for shampoo. She will start on the parasite killing herb program.

Summary: Kimberly is having a recurrence or continuation of her brain cancer. Possibly this is the cause of her left side strange paralysis. However, it could also be bacterial in origin; the bacteria having gotten entrenched in the cerebellum during surgery, or simply coming along with the parasite stages. Bacteria such as Shigella produce powerful nerve toxins. There could be a metal involvement, too, but all this must wait till she returns.

Four weeks later

Kimberly has had a fall, due to the weak knee, she believes. She is in a wheel chair but very sprightly.

☐ **Protein 24 (HIV) NO**

☐ **Ortho-phospho-tyrosine, hCG (Cancer) NO**

⊠ **Isopropyl Alcohol (Solvent) YES throughout her body**

Didn't switch body products.

⊠ **Benzene, mothballs, kerosene, MBKetone, methyl propanol, butyl nitrite (Solvents) YES**

She was so engrossed in her fall and wheelchair adventure that she neglected the restrictions I gave her. But she took the parasite program carefully and got rid of her cancer. She will be careful about restrictions now, so she can recover.

⊠ **Arsenic (Toxic Element) YES**

There is no pesticide in her home; she will steam clean her carpets.

⊠ **Europium, Silver, Copper, Mercury (Toxic Elements) YES**

Tooth fillings. Others not tested. She is advised to replace all tooth metal with metal-free plastic.

Kitty Klipper | Intestinal Cancer

Kitty is 46 years old and has written down a long list of symptoms. One would be tempted to think of hypochondria since she looks well. Her symptoms seem minor, such as weak hands, bad digestion, weak knees, tight throat, stiff neck. But 2 dozen of these is surely not hypochondria! She stated her anxiety about cancer. Her mother, aunt and sister had breast cancer. (This could unnerve anybody.)

☐ **Protein 24 (HIV) NO**

☒ **Ortho-phospho-tyrosine (Cancer) YES at intestine**

☒ **hCG (Pre-Cancer) YES at intestine and breast**

Kitty's suspicion and anxiety proved correct; she had cancer, and it was beginning to move toward the breast in the family tradition. Note the cancer marker, hCG, was not in the blood yet, so it could not be detected this way, although it was present in the breast.

☒ **Fasciolopsis (Parasite) YES at intestine and liver**

☒ **Fasciolopsis eggs, cercaria (Parasite stages) YES at intestine, side of breast and center of breast**

She had, indeed, felt a sharp twang from under the arm into the breast occasionally for the past 2 years, but it would always go away. Due to shortness of time, we could not finish testing for the remaining flukes. She will start on parasite program.

☒ **Isopropyl Alcohol (Solvent) YES at liver, NO at breast**

She will remove all propanol containing body products from her house and use our substitutes for shampoo, soap, etc. She might try making her own hair spray.

Summary: Kitty's first visit came shortly before this book was begun so that her next visit could not be included.

Frances Ibsen | Cervical Cancer

We have seen Frances several times over the past 6 years for chemical sensitivities, depression and fatigue syndrome. She has been exceptionally well this past year, until now. Her last PAP smear showed abnormal cells on the cervix. She also has intense burning in the vagina, but her clinical doctor says it is not yeast nor a urinary tract infection. Her husband also complains of burning. She had a papilloma wart removed from the cervix 2 years ago.

377

☐ Protein 24 (HIV) NO

☒ Ortho-phospho-tyrosine (Cancer) YES at cervix

☒ hCG (Pre-Cancer) YES at cervix

☒ Fasciolopsis (Parasite) YES at liver and intestine

☒ Fasciolopsis eggs (Parasite) YES at intestine, bladder, kidney, and cervix

☒ Sheep liver fluke miracidia and redia (Parasite) YES at kidney and bladder
> She will start parasite program.

☒ Kerosene (Solvent) YES high
> Source unknown, probably in gasoline.

☒ Regular leaded gas (Solvent) YES
> Stopped for gas this morning.

☒ Wood Alcohol (Solvent) YES high

☒ Acetone (Solvent) YES

☐ Solvents (Remainder) NO
> She eats a lot of cold cereal. She will stop and also go off commercial beverages.

☒ Isopropyl Alcohol (Solvent) YES
> She will switch off hair spray, shampoo and cosmetics.

Jerry, her husband

☐ Protein 24 (HIV) NO

☐ Ortho-phospho-tyrosine (Cancer) NO

☒ Kerosene (Solvent) YES
> Will be more careful with gasoline.

☒ TCE (Solvent) YES

☒ Styrene (Solvent) YES
> Will stop using styrofoam cups. Note: he has much less solvent in his body than Frances. He does not eat cold cereal or use a lot of body products.

☒ Fasciolopsis redia (Parasite) YES at kidney, bladder, semen, penis, saliva

☒ **Fasciolopsis miracidia (Parasite) YES**

☒ **Sheep liver fluke (Parasite) YES at liver**

☒ **Sheep liver fluke eggs (Parasite) YES at kidney, bladder, semen, penis, saliva**

Summary: Their appointment came just before the cut-off point for this book was reached so a follow-up was not included.

77	Lori Ellis	Skin Cancer

Lori is 62, about the same age as myself. She came from a city a day's drive away for 2 purposes: to talk about her son's leukemia (he is presently on interferon) and to talk about her chronic yeast infection. It began 5 years ago, making blotches on her neck and face. She was advised to get the mercury fillings removed which she did, but it didn't help. She has tried other alternative therapies like a strict yeast-free diet. It helps somewhat. I suspect PCB accumulation in her skin and will test later. First, I assured her that if her son should worsen, she could bring him here and help him get cured.

☐ **Protein 24 (HIV) NO**

☒ **Ortho-phospho-tyrosine (Cancer) YES at skin**

This is a surprise to me. However, she said she has had basal cell cancers removed before. She had just been carefully checked 1 month ago (some moles were removed and biopsied) and was pronounced clear of it, so this was a disappointment.

☒ **Fasciolopsis (Parasite) YES at liver and skin**

Says she gets dark spots under skin.

☒ **Fasciolopsis eggs, cercaria (Parasite) YES at saliva and skin**

☒ **Sheep liver fluke miracidia, eggs (Parasite) YES at saliva and skin**

☐ **Pancreatic fluke (Parasite) NO**

☒ **Human liver fluke (Parasite) YES at saliva and skin**

We searched saliva for the stages under the microscope. Miracidia and eggs were immediately found. She will start on parasite program and avoid beef, chicken and turkey in restaurants.

☒ **MEKetone (Solvent) YES high in all her organs**

☒ **Xylene, Toluene, MBKetone, TCE, Pentane, Hexanedione (Solvents) YES**

☒ **Isopropyl Alcohol (Solvent) YES at liver and skin**
She will go off commercial beverages and cold cereal, hair spray and shampoo.

Sixteen days later
Lori's itchy eyes and other yeast-like symptoms are gone.

☐ **Protein 24 (HIV) NO**

☐ **Ortho-phospho-tyrosine, hCG (Cancer) NO**

☐ **Isopropyl Alcohol (Solvent) NO**
Her blood test results have arrived (it is dated one month ago, before we first saw her).

BLOOD TEST	Result	Comment
1. Cholesterol	very low (157)	cancer risk
2. Ferritin	very high (593)	cancer suspect
3. SGOT, SGPT	slightly low	take 1 B6, 250 mg, daily
4. WBC	very high (12.9)	infection?
5. Lymphs	low (18.5 %)	bone marrow toxin

☒ **Hafnium (Toxic Element) YES**
Off hair spray.

☒ **Mercury (Toxic Element) YES**
Still has a root canal.

☒ **Lead (Toxic Element) YES**
Root canal? Will test her water.

☒ **Platinum, Tellurium (Toxic Elements) YES**
Tooth fillings. Remainder not tested. She is instructed to have all metal removed from her mouth, including root canal. She feels ready to go on vacation. I have added PABA to our skin softener to give her some sun screening. She is also advised to wear a hat and not use sunscreen lotion.
Summary: Lori is free of her cancer and ready to enjoy life again.

78	Fred Ross	Intestinal and Prostate Cancer

Fred is 66 and has been getting his prostate checked regularly because of inflammation and swelling and infection. He must get up 6 times in the night to empty his bladder. During the day he panics when not near a toilet. He is not on any medication. His eyes itch a lot and are blurry. He has a hiatal hernia. He will start on Bronson's digestive enzymes for this (6 for dinner, 4 for lunch, 2 for breakfast). Our kidney herb recipe should be able to clear up his prostate problem, I assured him. He uses a water softener.

☐ **Protein 24 (HIV) NO**

☒ **Ortho-phospho-tyrosine (Cancer) YES at intestine and prostate**

>This news dismayed him, wondering why his clinical doctor had not caught it when he was so frequently checked. I assured him he would quickly correct this by himself.

☒ **Fasciolopsis (Parasite) YES at liver and intestine**

☒ **Fasciolopsis cercaria, redia (Parasite) YES at prostate**

☒ **Sheep liver fluke redia (Parasite) YES at prostate; NO at liver**

☐ **Pancreatic fluke and stages (Parasite) NO**

☐ **Human liver fluke and stages (Parasite) NO**

☒ **Isopropyl Alcohol (Solvent) YES at liver and prostate**

>Remaining solvents not tested. He will start on parasite killing program and postpone the kidney program. He will avoid all pro-panol products: it has been used on his skin for his B12 shots. He will bring his own grain alcohol or vodka for this purpose.

Seven weeks later

>Fred has not started kidney program yet. He is still as troubled with night urination.

☐ **Ortho-phospho-tyrosine, hCG (Cancer) NO**

☒ **Cesium (Toxic Element) YES, high**

>Does not drink anything out of clear plastic bottles.

☒ **Cadmium (Toxic Element) YES, high**

>Not certain what kind of plumbing is at home.

☒ **Chromium (Toxic Element) YES, high**

>Needs to take out water softener.

☒ **Scandium (Toxic Element) YES, high**

Tooth metal is dissolving.

☒ **Lead (Toxic Element) YES, high**

No obvious source; will check water supply.

☒ **Vanadium(Toxic Element) YES, high**

Gas leak - check gas lines.

☒ **Yttrium (Toxic Element) YES**

Will take vitamins from Bronson's only. He is to see dentist to get metal replaced by plastic. Continue parasite program.

Summary: Fred cured his cancer but not his prostate disease as yet. I suspect these metals are nearly all coming from his tooth fillings, including the lead. We will see if it is gone after doing dental work. Notice he had very high levels of metals in his white cells. He has not begun washing out his prostate with the kidney herbs yet. We are waiting for dental work to be done since these toxic metals are the highest priority.

| 79 | Joyce Chambers | Breast Cancer |

At age 49, Joyce came specifically for her extreme hot flushes.

☐ **Protein 24 (HIV) NO**

☒ **Ortho-phospho-tyrosine, hCG (Pre-Cancer) YES at breast and under breast**

She is quite shocked and disappointed although she had been experiencing twinges at the side of her breast under the arm.

☒ **Fasciolopsis (Parasite) YES high at liver and intestine**

☒ **Fasciolopsis miracidia (Parasite) YES high at blood, kidney, bladder only**

☒ **Sheep liver fluke (Parasite) YES at pancreas**

Note: are the intestinal flukes in the liver keeping the liver flukes out?

☒ **Sheep liver fluke redia (Parasite) YES at blood only**

☒ **Sheep liver fluke miracidia (Parasite) YES at kidney and bladder**

☒ **Pancreatic fluke (Parasite) YES high at pancreas, breast, sides of breast**

☐ **Human liver fluke (Parasite) NO**

She will start on parasite killing program, stay off rare meats and eliminate propanol from use.

Two weeks later

☐ **Protein 24 (HIV) NO**

☐ **Ortho-phospho-tyrosine, hCG (Cancer) NO**

While she was using the herbs at first, the twinges under the breast were strong. Now they are gone. She has only eaten very well cooked meat.

☐ **Fasciolopsis and all stages (Parasite) NO**

☐ **Sheep liver fluke (Parasite) NO**

☐ **Pancreatic fluke (Parasite) NO**

☐ **Human liver fluke (Parasite) NO**

She stopped using propanol, has been off commercial beverages and cold cereal.

☒ **Asbestos (Toxic Element) YES, high**

Uses no clothes dryer—test hair blower, radiator paint.

☒ **Lanthanum (Toxic Element) YES**

Has a typewriter at home - will keep it covered.

BLOOD TEST	Result	Comment
1. WBC	low	bone marrow toxin
2. RBC	very low	anemic; bone marrow toxin and parasites
3. MCV	very high (110)	B12 deficiency - will test for *Ascaris*
4. Eos	very high (6%)	parasites
5. CO2	slightly high (27)	due to B12 deficiency?
6. Creatinine	high (1.2)	kidney problem
7. Calcium	very high (10.00)	
8. Phosphates	very high	is dissolving bones. She will begin to drink milk. Will also take magnesium oxide (300 mg), 1/day.
9. LDH	low (134)	muscle fatigue

She will add Vitamin C, at least 1 gm/day, from Bronson's Pharm.

☒ **Ascaris (Parasite) YES**

Go on 3- day parasite program. She will start on kidney herb recipe as well as continue the parasite program.

Summary: Joyce was very happy to learn what those twinges under her arm and toward the breast meant. She cured her cancer quickly. Hopefully, she will return to follow up on her asbestos problem.

| Lucy Lindbeck | Intestinal Cancer |

Lucy is 42 and is concerned about her weight loss without a reason - she eats as much as ever. She has a few other minor complaints. She works for a doctor.

☐ **Protein 24 (HIV) NO**

☒ **Ortho-phospho-tyrosine (Cancer) YES at intestine**

☒ **hCG (Pre-Cancer) YES at intestine, NO in blood**
   Note: A clinical cancer test for serum hCG would not have found this early cancer.

☒ **Fasciolopsis adults and cercaria (Parasite) YES at liver and intestine**

☐ **Sheep liver fluke (Parasite) NO**

☐ **Pancreatic fluke (Parasite) NO**

☐ **Human liver fluke (Parasite) NO**

☒ **Isopropyl Alcohol (Solvent) YES at liver, thymus and throughout her body**

☒ **TCE (Solvent) YES high**

☐ **Solvents (Remainder) NO**
   She will stop eating health food brand cold cereal. She was very disappointed that health food brands are not pollution-free. She will switch off her body products to propanol-free kinds. She will start parasite killing program.
   Summary: Lucy's case came up near the end of this series so her follow-up is not available to us.

| Wes Yerkley | Breast Cancer |

This is a 52 year old man from Michigan who came with his wife and parents. He was very anxious about his condition. He had a large mass the size of my hand under his right chest wall. He was diagnosed with cancer 1 year ago in his right arm pit. Since this was not the primary location they searched very hard for it, but could not find it. So he was given extra heavy doses of chemotherapy and radiation. However, 5 weeks after ending the treatments, this very large lump appeared on his chest. He has a lot of pain on the right side and is on pain killers continually. His fingers and elbow on his right side are numb. He has no other problems. He appears well, except for cringing with pain throughout the appointment (despite the pain killers).

☐ **Protein 24 (HIV) NO**

☒ **Ortho-phospho-tyrosine (Cancer) YES at intestine, side of breast and breast**
Note: I believe this is the only breast cancer in a man that I have seen.

☒ **hCG (Pre-Cancer) YES high at all organs!**
His body electrical resistance is exceptionally high, possibly due to PCBs. Will test later.

☐ **Fasciolopsis and all stages (Parasite) NO**
Most unusual.

☒ **Pancreatic fluke (Parasite) YES**

☒ **Pancreatic fluke stages (Parasite) YES in saliva**

☐ **Human liver fluke (Parasite) NO**

☒ **Isopropyl Alcohol (Solvent) YES**
Other solvents not tested. He will go off cold cereals and body products with propanol in them. He will switch to our shampoo and shaving products.

☒ **PCB (Toxic Element) YES high**
He will go off detergents and use borax for all purposes. He will start parasite killing program.
Summary: Wes did not return, for reasons unknown. Hopefully, he carried out our instructions. Note his high level of PCBs. They reduced the body current from 55 microamps to about 40 microamps when 5 volts is applied across the hands. Perhaps they block or obliterate the conductance channels in our cells. Perhaps they raise capacitance. This would be interesting to study.

| 80 | Richard Nunley | Intestinal Cancer |

Richard, age 49, came for his tinnitus in both ears. It was preceded by dental work. He also has chronic low back pain. He is a tall intellectual person who enjoys gardening and would like to be able to do this again but can't bend down because of his ear condition.

☐ Protein 24 (HIV) NO

☒ Ortho-phospho-tyrosine (Cancer) YES at intestine and pancreas

☒ Fasciolopsis (Parasite) YES at liver and intestine

☒ Sheep liver fluke (Parasite) YES at liver
Note: These two flukes are not excluding each other, perhaps they are in different places in the liver.

☒ Pancreatic fluke (Parasite) YES at pancreas

☒ Human liver fluke (Parasite) YES at liver and pancreas

☒ Human liver fluke metacercaria (Parasite) YES at pancreas

☒ Isopropyl Alcohol (Solvent) YES at liver and pancreas

☒ Benzene (Solvent) YES

☒ Methyl Butyl Ketone, Mineral oil (Solvents) YES
Note: He has both propanol and benzene. This may explain having all 4 large flukes! He will go off rare meats; he eats very little anyway. He will go off the benzene list, commercial body products and commercial beverages.

Two weeks later

☐ Protein 24 (HIV) NO

☐ Ortho-phospho-tyrosine (Cancer) NO

☐ hCG (Pre-Cancer) NO

☒ Adenovirus, Strep pyog and Bacillus anthracus (Pathogens) YES at tooth #17
I am searching pathogens for cause of tinnitus.

☒ Sphaerotilus nat (Pathogen) YES

☒ Haemophilus infl (Pathogen) YES at teeth 15, 16, 17

☐ **Pathogens (Remainder) NO**

He needs cavitations cleaned at teeth 15, 16, 17. He will continue parasite program. Note: the usual bacterium for tinnitus, Strep pn, is not present!

Summary: Richard cleared up his cancer promptly but clearing up tinnitus is a lot harder. He will need to clean up his mouth of chronic infection and cleanse his liver of bacteria.

| 81 | Iris Kilpatrick | Bone Cancer |

Iris was diagnosed with bone cancer a week ago, involving hip, shoulder, and knee. It was first found as a tumor on the kidney. It began with bleeding from the bowel. She had 2 colonoscopies, but nothing was found.

☐ **Protein 24 (HIV) NO**

☒ **Ortho-phospho-tyrosine (Cancer) YES at intestine, kidney, bone**

☒ **hCG (Pre-Cancer) YES throughout her body**

☒ **Fasciolopsis (Parasite) YES at liver and intestines**

☒ **Fasciolopsis miracidia (Parasite) YES at bone**

☐ **Sheep liver fluke (Parasite) NO**

☐ **Pancreatic fluke (Parasite) NO**

☒ **Human liver fluke (Parasite) YES at liver and bone**

Note bone invasion.

☒ **Isopropyl Alcohol, TCEthylene, Hexane, Xylene (Solvents) YES**

She will go off commercial beverages, cold cereal, shampoo, hair spray and mouthwash. She will start on parasite killing program.

Twelve days later

☐ **Protein 24 (HIV) NO**

☐ **Ortho-phospho-tyrosine, hCG (Cancer) NO**

Various cancers are gone.

☒ **PCB (Toxic Element) YES**

Will go off detergents.

☒ **Gold, Mercury (Toxic Element) YES**
Tooth metals. Other tooth metals not tested.

☒ **Arsenic (Toxic Element) YES**
She is careful to avoid indoor pesticide treatment, has no wallpaper - only other source is stain-proofed carpets - will steam clean.

☒ **Aluminum (Toxic Element) YES**
Will switch to Hain's salt.

☐ **Toxic Elements (Remainder) NO**
She needs to replace tooth metal with metal-free plastic.
Summary: Iris is planning to bring in her recent test results from her clinical doctor's office. She will stay on the parasite program, avoid meat and get all the metal removed from her mouth and replaced with plastic. Her cancer is gone but I hope she finishes this health program.

| 82 | Nancy Hampson | Cancer Of The Pancreas and Intestine |

Nancy came with her brother for her general poor health. She had learned from a friend how to do a liver cleanse and has already gotten out a lot of stones.

☐ **Protein 24 (HIV) NO**

☒ **Ortho-phospho-tyrosine (Cancer) YES at intestine and pancreas**
Cancer of the pancreas and intestine came as quite a shock to her. She is only 36 years old and has never drunk alcohol. In fact, she has a strange sugar problem; when she eats sugar she gets panic attacks and weird symptoms like partial blindness, dizziness, mood change. (I suspect numerous parasites in the pancreas.) Yet, if she does not eat she gets very shaky and nervous.

☒ **hCG (Pre-Cancer) YES at many body tissues**

☐ **Fasciolopsis adults (Parasite) NO**

☒ **Fasciolopsis eggs (Parasite) YES high at pancreas**
With such numerous eggs, she must have had an adult to release them; perhaps the adult was killed.

☒ **Sheep liver fluke cercaria (Parasite) YES at pancreas**

☒ **Sheep liver fluke metacercaria (Parasite) YES**

☒ **Pancreatic fluke adults, stages (Parasite) YES at liver and pancreas**

☐ **Human liver fluke (Parasite) NO**

I suspect she is full of wood alcohol which targets the pancreas. Also, note the absence of both large flukes in the liver. How is ortho-phospho-tyrosine being produced? By the stages themselves?

☒ **Wood Alcohol (Solvent) YES at pancreas and liver**

Needs to go off carbonated beverages and sugar substitutes.

☒ **Isopropyl Alcohol, Acetone, Isophorone (Solvent) YES at pancreas and liver**

She drinks Folger's™ decaf and TofuMu™. She will stop all commercial beverages and drink only milk, water and single-herb teas (she doesn't tolerate fruit juice due to sugar in it). She will also start taking Bronson's Digestive Enzymes (6 with lunch and supper, 2 with breakfast) to assist her pancreas. She will start a parasite killing program.

Three weeks later

She has complied with all instructions except that she is still eating cold cereals occasionally. She misses her TofuMu™ and has brought it with her for testing.

☐ **Protein 24 (HIV) NO**

☐ **Ortho-phospho-tyrosine, hCG (Cancer) NO**

She expressed joy at this news.

☒ **Xylene, Decane (Solvent) YES**

☐ **Solvents (Remainder) NO**

She has gotten rid of the wood alcohol, propanol, acetone, and isophorone in her system, but now has xylene and decane, undoubtedly from eating cold cereal. She will take the whole family off it.

☒ **Aluminum (Toxic Element) YES**

☒ **Chromate (Toxic Element) YES**

She will stop using aluminum cookware and foil, aluminized salt, deodorant, and regular soap. She will make borax soap concentrate. The chromium source is mysterious since she uses no make-up and there is no water softener.

⊠ **Gadolinium (Toxic Element) YES**
Tooth fillings.

⊠ **Fluoride (Toxic Element) YES**
Off toothpaste. Sodium fluoride is a well known metabolic poison, in fact it was widely used in my graduate lessons in understanding metabolism. It inhibits the anaerobic part of general animal metabolisms. Traces of fluoride in organic form are beneficial, and the body may convert some of the inorganic type, but it is inadvisable to expose yourself to the amounts of inorganic fluoride found in toothpaste, even though it is present as a "non-toxic" compound such as stannous fluoride.[61] Fluoride in toothpaste greatly overshadows the fluoride consumed in city water, because I do not see toxicity after stopping toothpaste even when still drinking city water.

⊠ **Strontium (Toxic Element) YES**
Off toothpaste.

⊠ **Zirconium (Toxic Element) YES**
Off toothpaste and deodorant.

⊠ **Thulium (Toxic Element) YES**
Off multi-vitamins. She will get her metal tooth fillings replaced with metal-free plastic.
Summary: All these metals, as well as the solvents, were accumulated in her pancreas. There is a possibility that the chromate will also disappear after she stops the supplements. So we will wait until this is done before searching harder for its source.

83	Lenore Dale	Intestinal Cancer and HIV

This is a 34 year old person who works for a clinical doctor and has already tried a number of alternative health procedures. She has a long list of bizarre symptoms, such as swollen and itching lips, gagging when eating (suggesting AIDS), and chest heaviness (making it even more probable).

⊠ **Protein 24 (HIV) YES at thymus, vagina and ovaries**

---

[61] The Merck Index (10th Ed.) states the solubility of stannous fluoride is about 30%. Thus there is a high probability of forming sodium fluoride, the metabolic poison.

☒ **Ortho-phospho-tyrosine (Cancer) YES at intestine**

☒ **hCG (Pre-Cancer) YES everywhere**

What a shocking realization this brought to her, both HIV and cancer in a single diagnosis. She could hardly bear the news in spite of my assurance that she could eliminate them both within 10 days. Perhaps she was also angry or disbelieving.

☒ **Fasciolopsis (Parasite) YES at liver and intestine**

☒ **Fasciolopsis eggs (Parasite) YES at intestine, adrenals, saliva**

☐ **Sheep liver fluke (Parasite) NO**

☐ **Pancreatic fluke (Parasite) NO**

☐ **Human liver fluke (Parasite) NO**

☒ **Benzene (Solvent) YES at thymus**

Will go off items on benzene list.

☒ **Isopropyl Alcohol (Solvent) YES at liver**

Will eliminate propanol. Others not tested. She will start parasite program.

Ten days later

☐ **Protein 24 (HIV) NO**

☐ **Ortho-phospho-tyrosine, hCG (Cancer) NO**

Both HIV and cancer are gone; she did everything correctly.

☒ **Aluminum Silicate (Toxic Element) YES**

Will disconnect water softener.

☒ **Bismuth (Toxic Element) YES**

Will get rid of fragranced items.

☒ **Radon (Toxic Element) YES**

She will open the vents to the crawl space.

☒ **Thallium, Germanium (Toxic Elements) YES**

Tooth metal pollutant. This coincidence of thallium and germanium is only found when the tooth filling metal has these pollutants. She is very upset about this since she states that she has had weak hands (very weak) for many years already (caused by thallium). She had all her mercury fillings taken out by Dr. S. who is a

Huggins Institute trained dentist. Five gold crowns were put back in her mouth and she spent $3,000 on this last fall.

☒ Gold (Toxic Element) YES

☒ Mercury (Toxic Element) YES at tooth #29 and #15

Tooth #29 has a gold crown. She says this tooth has been bothering her. I then searched for the location of the thallium and found it at tooth #29, 10, and 18. She will ask the dentist to do a fresh panoramic x-ray to search for tattoos. I shone a flashlight in her mouth and could see 2 tattoos. However, these metal pinpoint leftovers might be left from the braces she used to wear. She states she remembers seeing them after the braces were removed.

☒ PCB (Toxic Element) YES

Uses Dr. Bronner's Peppermint™ soap - will go off.

Summary: Lenore's case is especially tragic and an early warning sign for all people. She was given 16 mercury fillings starting in early childhood, some of which were polluted with thallium. This was the probable cause of having a child with microcephaly. In an effort to improve her health, she turned to health brand soap, only to be poisoned with PCBs. Only her strong intelligence and survival instinct kept her from self-destructive anger. Instead, she will probably set herself and her family on the road to good health.

84	Phylis Zink	Liver and Breast Cancer and HIV

Phylis is a 46 year old woman who drove by herself 150 miles for reasons of her history of breast cancer. It was discovered by mammogram. She had a mastectomy and they took out 3 lymph nodes two years ago and has been followed since then by annual mammograms. She has a heart murmur, occasional pain in knees and wrists, and a long history of period-related problems. They have a water softener and use reverse osmosis (R.O.) water for drinking.

☒ Ortho-phospho-tyrosine (Cancer) YES

☒ Protein 24 (HIV) YES

Since these results seemed impossible to her and I was afraid she might leave, do nothing about her status, and never return, I suggested she get a clinical test (p24 antigen test) for HIV.

Six weeks later

She waited two weeks before doing the test and it came back NO (negative) for the HIV virus. This was most unfortunate since she waited another month before returning.

☒ **Ortho-phospho-tyrosine (Cancer) YES at liver and breast**
The cancer has spread to the liver.

☒ **hCG (Pre-Cancer) YES at liver, breast and blood**

☒ **Protein 24 (HIV) YES at thymus only**
Perhaps the clinical test didn't find the virus because the lab examines blood serum, not the white blood cells or their contents. A case must be further advanced for the virus to be so prevalent that the virus is in the blood serum.

☒ **Fasciolopsis (Parasite) YES at intestine, liver, thymus**
Adults in the liver are giving her cancer; adults in the thymus are giving her HIV. However, she has no sensations over the breastbone nor chest tightness.

☒ **Fasciolopsis redia (Parasite) YES at liver and thymus**

☐ **Sheep liver fluke and all stages (Parasite) NO**

☐ **Pancreatic fluke and all stages (Parasite) NO**

☒ **Human liver fluke (Parasite) YES high at liver, thymus, bladder, kidney, breast**

☒ **Human liver fluke metacercaria (Parasite) YES high at liver, thymus, kidney, bladder, saliva**
Notice: she could transmit these very tiny infective stages by kissing! She will start on parasite killing program.

☒ **Benzene (Solvent) YES at liver, thymus, breast, etc.**
Brushes teeth twice a day with Colgate™, Crest™, and Tom's™ toothpastes–eats cold cereal daily–go off the entire benzene polluted list.

☒ **Isopropyl Alcohol (Solvent) YES at liver, thymus, breast, etc.**
Remainder not tested. She will check her cosmetics for propanol and make her own hair spray. She will switch shampoo to borax.

Seven days later

She is having some loose bowels, probably due to parasite killing herbs.

☐ **Protein 24 (HIV) NO**

☐ **hCG (Pre-Cancer) NO**

☐ **Ortho-phospho-tyrosine (Cancer) NO**

☒ **Regular leaded gasoline, Petroleum ether (Solvent) YES**

Put gas in her car yesterday. She will be much more careful.

☒ **Methyl Ethyl Ketone (Solvent) YES**

Instead of stopping cold cereal, switched to a health brand, will stop.

☒ **Titanium, Thallium/Germanium (Toxic Elements) YES**

Tooth fillings.

☐ **Toxic Elements (Remainder) NO**

See dentist immediately to remove all metals; save grindings for me to add to my thallium collection.

Summary: Phylis cleared up her HIV and cancer in 7 days. But will she complete her program of getting well again? Thallium is to the body what termites are to a wood frame house—just a question of time before health collapses.

85	Joe Osborn	Skin, Prostate, Intestinal Cancer

Joe is 45 and came in for seemingly minor problems like bursitis, low back pain, and hip pain. But I found cancer present.

☐ **Protein 24 (HIV) NO**

☒ **Ortho-phospho-tyrosine (Cancer) YES at intestine, skin, and prostate**

He showed me a lump under his left armpit the size of a golf ball. He stated he had first noticed it one year ago and had seen his doctor. His doctor had said it was not malignant.

☒ **hCG (Pre-Cancer) YES high throughout his body**

☒ **Fasciolopsis (Parasite) YES at liver and intestine**

☒ **Fasciolopsis eggs (Parasite) YES in blood, saliva, etc.**

Remainder not tested.

☒ **Isopropyl Alcohol (Solvent) YES at liver and prostate**

☒ **Benzene (Solvent) YES**

☒ **Carbon Tetrachloride (Solvent) YES**

☐ **Solvents (Remainder) NO**
The news of his cancer came as a shock since his clinical doctor had cleared him of suspicion. He will go off commercial beverages, cold cereal and body products. He will go off the benzene list. He will start parasite program. Note: he has benzene and the intestinal fluke but he does not have HIV virus yet. It is not far away, though.

One week later
Joe still has no appetite. His pains continue. The cyst under his arm is bothering him. He is instructed to put a hot, wet towel under his armpit daily to draw it to the surface.

☐ **Ortho-phospho-tyrosine, hCG (Cancer) NO**

☐ **Benzene (Solvent) NO**

☐ **Isopropyl Alcohol (Solvent) NO**

☒ **Carbon Tetrachloride (Solvent) YES**
Probably from store-bought drinking water.

☒ **Mercury, Platinum (Toxic Elements) YES**
He is instructed to remove all metal from his mouth. He may begin readiness program (07, peroxy) for liver cleanse to clear his bursitis.
Summary: Joe and his wife made the changes in their family's habits that were necessary to get rid of his cancer and protect the whole family from getting cancer or HIV illness in the future.

86	Ray Broyles	Cancer and HIV

We first saw Ray two years ago. He was age 40 at that time and had just had an unusual experience. He had always been healthy and energetic. Then for no reason he passed out. He began vomiting, felt extremely weak and had other strange symptoms. His regular doctor prescribed a tranquilizer, Oxazepam™, after ruling out numerous possibilities. However, these attacks recurred, and he lost about 10 pounds in a few months. I did not suspect nor test for cancer. I found the parasite, Trichuris, and heavy metals from tooth fillings as well as tungsten from his electric hot water heater. He was put on a parasite program. He became well but did not clear up the metal problems. He did not stay on a maintenance program for killing parasites. We did not see him till recently. He had no further episodes of passing out but was unable to recover from a recent flu.

This time the parasite test revealed *Fasciolopsis* in the liver. He was put back on the parasite killing recipe. The cancer test, ortho-phospho-tyrosine, was positive, and tungsten was showing its presence in all his body tissues. He soon got rid of his cancer and by changing his water sources and doing dental work he got rid of the tungsten problem. (He stopped all use of electrical frying pans and toasters.) He felt fine, his former self, and was released with food and body product restrictions.

We saw him again a half year later for frequent burping and difficulty swallowing. There was some similarity to his original attacks. There was pain over his chest and heart area, but I did not suspect HIV at that time. The parasite test showed heartworm and dog tapeworm eggs. The cancer test was negative.

He was put on a high dose parasite killing program and dental repair was recommended. This cleared up his health problems, again, temporarily. He was not given food or product restrictions. A half year later he became ill again with prolonged flu and pressure on his chest.

☐ **Ortho-phospho-tyrosine (Cancer) NO**

☒ **Protein 24 (HIV) YES**

☐ **Fasciolopsis and all stages (Parasite) NO**
I did not search his tissues, only the white blood cells. Could I have missed a few?

☒ **Sheep liver fluke redia (Parasite) YES at thymus, penis**

☒ **Sheep liver fluke metacercaria (Parasite) YES at pancreas only**

☒ **Pancreatic fluke (Parasite) YES at thymus, pancreas**

☐ **Human liver fluke (Parasite) NO**

☒ **Benzene (Solvent) YES at thymus**
Uses Nivea™ brand cream after shaving - will go off entire list of benzene containing products.

☒ **Wood Alcohol (Solvent) YES high at thymus and pancreas**

Others not tested at this time. He was to switch off commercial beverages and will take Milk Thistle capsules temporarily, to assist the liver. And he will return to a high dose parasite killing program followed by a maintenance program. He must avoid eating meats in restaurants.

Three days later

☐ **Protein 24 (HIV) NO**

Virus is gone but he is still very ill.

☒ **Benzene (Solvent) YES**

Has not stopped eating cold cereals.

Ten days later

His pains are gone. His digestion continues to be a problem. I suspect tapeworm heads have been released in his liver by the solvents; they are shedding eggs. He feels well enough to return to work. He will add Rascal to his daily routine for 2 weeks to kill tapeworms.

☒ **Decane, Methyl Butyl Ketone (Solvent) YES**

Hasn't stopped eating processed foods.

☒ **Toluene (Solvent) YES**

Summary: Ray's patience has paid off, in spite of imperfect compliance. If he had accepted the tranquilizer a few years ago, without pursuing the true cause of his illness, namely parasites and solvents, he would be a permanent invalid today.

---

87 Gorge Matte	Mesothelioma

This is a heavy-set tall man, only 59, but appearing so much older and fatigued. He smokes. He must burp constantly and pass gas for the little comfort he feels. About 3 months ago he suddenly couldn't breathe. There was fluid accumulated in his right lung. He was put in the hospital where he had fluid drained, but it returned. Because of his past work in an asbestos factory, mesothelioma was suspected. When it was found, he was told it was inoperable and untreatable so he is not on chemotherapy or radiation. But one year ago, he had radiation therapy for prostate cancer. That was considered to be corrected. He started smoking again after that because it didn't seem to make any dif-

397

ference to his health - he got cancer anyway. He had quit for 6 years. He feels this is the end for him, but I assured him he had a lot of life left, so he had better quit smoking again.

☐ **Protein 24 (HIV) NO**

☒ **Ortho-phospho-tyrosine (Cancer) YES at intestine, prostate and lung**

☒ **hCG (Pre-Cancer) YES throughout his body**

☒ **Fasciolopsis (Parasite) YES at liver, prostate, and lung!**
One seldom sees adults in the lung, only the developmental stages.

☒ **Isopropyl Alcohol (Solvent) YES at liver, prostate and lung**
He doesn't eat cold cereal. It is probably in his shaving products. He will switch to homemade soap. No other parasites or solvents were tested for at this time since his appointment time was extra short. He will start on a parasite killing program and avoid picking up new parasites in undercooked meats. He travels 4 hours to reach our office.

Seven days later
His right side is still sore from recent drainage of fluid. He must burp constantly. He hasn't slept decently for 2 years, being awake 4 hours in the night. For 5 years he cleaned his hands daily in mineral spirits. He will increase the digestive enzymes we started him on to double the amount and see if he gets some relief from abdominal pains.

☐ **Ortho-phospho-tyrosine (Cancer) NO**

☒ **hCG (Pre-Cancer) YES throughout his body**

☐ **Isopropyl Alcohol (Solvent) NO**
The cancer is gone, but the cancer marker hCG is still present. He only began the parasite killing program two days ago.

☒ **Lead (Toxic Element) YES**
Test water - has no root canals but some tooth fillings.

☒ **Mercury, Platinum (Toxic Elements) YES**
Tooth fillings.

☒ **Fiberglass (Toxic Element) YES**
Will test home air.

☒ **Thulium (Toxic Element) YES**
Off supplements.

☒ **Asbestos (Toxic Element) YES**
Will test hair blowers and the clothes dryer.

☒ **Barium (Toxic Element) YES**
Teeth? Bus exhaust inhaled during trip to office?

☒ **Zirconium (Toxic Element) YES**
Off deodorant.

☒ **Aluminum Silicate (Toxic Element) YES**
Off regular table salt, onto Hain's sea salt.

☒ **Formaldehyde (Toxic Element) YES**
Has a new large foam mattress. He is instructed to get rid of his foam mattress. Remainder of elements were not tested, since this is as much as he can cope with in the next week. He is instructed to get all dental metal removed.

Two weeks later
He missed an appointment due to transportation problems; this is very unfortunate.

☐ **Ortho-phospho-tyrosine (Cancer) NO**

☐ **hCG (Pre-Cancer) NO**
He still has a lot of pain over stomach area at surgery site (over the spleen); the digestive enzymes don't help.

☒ **Mineral oil (Toxic Element) YES**

☒ **2 Methyl propanol, Xylene (Solvents) YES**

☐ **Solvents (Remainder) NO**

☒ **Lead (Toxic Element) YES and in hot and cold water**
He must search his cold water line for lead solder joints.

☒ **Fiberglass (Toxic Element) YES**
His daughter works near rolls of it and brings it home on her clothing. She should shed work clothes in the garage before coming into the house.

☒ **Formaldehyde (Toxic Element) YES**
Has a new carpet; test house air.

☒ **Asbestos (Toxic Element) YES**
Changed the dryer belt and discarded hair blower only 2 days ago.

☐ **Zirconium (Toxic Element) NO**
Is off deodorant.

☐ **Aluminum Silicate (Toxic Element) NO**
Now using Hain's Sea Salt.

☒ **PCB (Toxic Element) YES high**
Go off detergent.

☒ **PVC (Toxic Element) YES**
New carpet? He will get started on dental work and continue parasite program.
Summary: Gorge has an unusually long list of toxic elements stuck in his tissues. But he is making progress. Hopefully, he can clean them up before his lungs are completely out of commission.

88	Mick Gammon	Myelo Monocytic Leukemia

This is an elderly man with some slowness of movement and thought. His wife was very helpful in telling us about the situation. Four months ago, his CBC showed an abnormality: an extremely low lymphocyte count (8%). They have arrived from Iowa on a snowy day and will be here for 6 days. As I began testing, it was extremely difficult to get a current flow, suggesting PCB toxicity.

☐ **Protein 24 (HIV) NO**

☒ **Ortho-phospho-tyrosine (Cancer) YES**

☒ **hCG (Pre-Cancer) YES**
It was too difficult to determine the location of his cancer, due to low current levels.

☒ **Fasciolopsis (Parasite) YES at liver**
Other parasites not tested. He will start on a parasite program.

☒ **PCB (Toxic Element) YES**
Will go off detergents and soap and use borax and homemade soap for all purposes.

☒ **Acetone, Methyl Butyl Ketone, Methylene Chloride, Ethyl (grain) Alcohol (Solvents) YES**
Off alcoholic beverages until recovered.

⊠ **Xylene, TCE, Decane, TCEthylene, MEKetone, Isopropyl Alcohol (Solvents) YES**

☐ **Solvents (Remainder) NO**

He will go off commercial beverages, the benzene list and cold cereals. (Note: although he does not have benzene build-up I gave him the benzene list to avoid because the same foods and products have many of the same solvents he tested YES for.) We got a saliva sample to search for parasite stages.

Two days later

⊠ **Arsenic (Toxic Element) YES**

Will search out and remove pesticide; will avoid lawn treatments at home.

⊠ **Bismuth (Toxic Element) YES**

Off colognes and antacids.

⊠ **Aluminum (Toxic Element) YES**

Off deodorant, detergents, aluminum cookware, and regular table salt.

⊠ **Beryllium (Toxic Element) YES**

Has an upper denture; we will test it.

⊠ **Strontium (Toxic Element) YES**

Off toothpaste.

⊠ **Gallium, Nickel, Silver, Samarium, Tantalum, Gold, Mercury, Thallium (Toxic Elements) YES**

Tooth metals. I am astounded to find this much thallium.

⊠ **Aluminum Silicate (Toxic Element) YES**

Off regular table salt.

⊠ **Europium (Toxic Element) YES**

⊠ **Niobium (Toxic Element) YES**

Uses vitamin pills and Chinese herbs.

⊠ **Niobium (Toxic Element) YES in vitamin pills**

Will switch to Bronson's Pharm brand.

☐ **Niobium (Toxic Element) NO in Chinese herbs**

May continue using them.

☒ **Thulium (Toxic Element) YES**

In his vitamin pills. At this point, I omitted testing other metals often found in tooth metal to save time.

☒ **PCB (Toxic Element) YES**

Off detergents.

☒ **Rubidium (Toxic Element) YES**

☐ **Toxic Elements (Remainder) NO**

Note: This is an exceptionally long list of toxic metals burdening his body and immune system. He is to see the dentist tomorrow if they can take him. Also, he is discouraged over what he can eat. I did not have time to discourse over it.

Two days later

Mr. Gammon appeared healthier today, in better command of his communication; he spoke for himself instead of letting his wife do it for him. The dentist removed all metal yesterday. He will get new plastic dentures at home in Nebraska after calling the Huggins Institute for the name of a dentist. He will start on thioctic acid, 100 mg, taken twice daily for 6 months to remove metal from his tissues.

☒ **PCB (Toxic Element) YES**

Has not lessened during his stay, probably in clothing.

☐ **Thallium (Toxic Element) NO**

Was in tooth fillings.

☐ **Protein 24 (HIV) NO**

☐ **Ortho-phospho-tyrosine, hCG (Cancer) NO**

☐ **Isopropyl Alcohol (Solvent) NO**

☐ **Fasciolopsis and all stages (Parasite) NO**

He will continue his parasite program, unless he is ill, and return to it after any illness.

☒ **Uric Acid, Oxalate (Kidney Stones) YES**

Remainder NO. Start on kidney herb recipe.

Summary: Like so many other cancer clients, Mr. Gammon experienced a quantum leap of improved health after the metal was removed from his mouth. After laundering out the PCBs at home with borax, he may decide to continue on his job instead of retiring.

| Jonathon Kohl | Liver Cancer and HIV |

This very young man is here with his family mainly for low energy, but nothing more specific than that. He does not feel well, especially after eating. He is attentive and interested in his health. He has no addictions and no risky behaviors. He has chronic Herpes simplex 1 (cold sores). He sleeps eight hours at night but still can't get up in the morning.

☒ **Protein 24 (HIV) YES at thymus and penis**

This is certainly a shock for all of us; I explained the basis for it as "parasites plus benzene pollution". He took the news in a calm manner.

☒ **Ortho-phospho-tyrosine (Cancer) YES at liver**

He has cancer, too, of the liver! His parents are distraught.

☐ **hCG (Pre-Cancer) NO**

☒ **Fasciolopsis (Parasite) YES at liver and thymus**

☒ **Sheep liver fluke redia (Parasite) YES at liver and thymus; NO in saliva**

☒ **Sheep liver fluke miracidia (Parasite) YES at liver, thymus, saliva and semen**

☐ **Pancreatic fluke and all stages (Parasite) NO**

☒ **Human liver fluke (Parasite) YES at liver and thymus**

He will start on parasite killing program.

☒ **Benzene (Solvent) YES at thymus**

☒ **Isopropyl Alcohol (Solvent) YES everywhere**

☒ **Kerosene (Solvent) YES**

He uses kerosene to heat his work area. I suggested electric heat.

☒ **Carbon Tetrachloride, Methyl Ethyl Ketone, TCE, Acetone, TCEthylene (Solvents) YES**

☐ **Solvents (Remainder) NO**

He will be off commercial beverages and the benzene list as well as body products with propanol in them.

Summary: Unfortunately, Jonathon did not return. Perhaps his parents were angry with him. His mother tested NO for HIV, ortho-phospho-tyrosine and hCG; his father complained of chest pains but declined to be tested. No doubt, Jonathon still has several years of moderately good health left. Hopefully, he has made some changes in his product usage.

Steven Aust	Synovial Cell Sarcoma

Steve is 24 years old and is here from Detroit for a sarcoma (Synovial Cell Sarcoma) on the outer thigh of his left leg. It is about the size of a grapefruit. A left groin lymph node has been surgically removed. He has a catheter in place in preparation for further therapy. He is on pain medicine, blood thinner and tranquilizers.

☐ **Protein 24 (HIV) NO**

☒ **Ortho-phospho-tyrosine (Cancer) YES at intestine, muscle**
Very unusual location.

☒ **hCG (Pre-Cancer) YES everywhere**

☒ **Fasciolopsis (Parasite) YES at liver**

☒ **Fasciolopsis eggs (Parasite) YES at liver, muscle, saliva**

☐ **Sheep liver fluke (Parasite) NO**

☐ **Pancreatic fluke (Parasite) NO**

☒ **Human liver fluke (Parasite) YES at muscle**

☒ **Isopropyl Alcohol (Solvent) YES everywhere**

☒ **Benzene (Solvent) YES**
Remainder not tested We are short on time; it is 4 PM; I must check dental metal so he can make a dental appointment, if needed, before returning home.

☒ **Arsenic (Toxic Element) YES high everywhere**
They are living in a trailer and have not put pesticide anywhere. I suggested opening the trailer skirting and searching under the trailer. Also steam clean carpets. There is no wallpaper (one small panel in bathroom).

☒ **Bismuth (Toxic Element) YES**
Off aftershave, colognes, all fragrances.

☒ **Cobalt (Toxic Element) YES**
Off detergent.

☒ PCB (Toxic Element) YES

Will test well water; off detergent.

☒ Mercury (Toxic Element) YES

Tooth fillings. Remainder not tested. He needs all metal removed from his mouth and replaced with metal-free plastic.

Summary: Steve has not returned. Hopefully, he has carried out his instructions and will surprise us with a visit soon.

---

89 Jason Willy	Lung Cancer and HIV

Jason is a 43 year old man whose medical record, which he brought with him, gave his diagnosis as "undifferentiated large cell carcinoma of the lung with metastases to the left neck and brain area." More recently, the cancer has spread to the liver. His sister-in-law drove him to our office. Jason smokes, and I reminded him that smoking is incompatible with lung health. He is on Dilantin™ and Decatron™ to prevent brain swelling.

☐ Protein 24 (HIV) NO

☒ Ortho-phospho-tyrosine (Cancer) YES at liver, thymus, lung, brain

Note that cancer in the thymus is quite rare.

☒ Fasciolopsis (Parasite) YES at liver, intestine, lung

☒ Fasciolopsis cercaria (Parasite) YES at lung, etc.

☒ Sheep liver fluke (Parasite) YES at thymus; NO at liver

Note: the normal habitat for the Sheep liver fluke is the liver. Is the intestinal fluke keeping it out somehow?

☐ Pancreatic fluke and all stages (Parasite) NO

☒ Isopropyl Alcohol, Benzene (Solvent) YES at liver, thymus, kidney, etc.

With this critically ill person here from so far away, I made a second office visit possible for him 7 hours later in the same day. He went off all benzene products and propanol products and took a shower in the meanwhile. He also took a massive amount of parasite killing herbs instead of starting at "day one."

Seven hours later

☐ **Ortho-phospho-tyrosine (Cancer) NO**

His cancer is already stopped. He doesn't believe what I am telling him, but his sister-in-law is ecstatic. He will stay off rare meats.

☒ **Cryptocotyl, Hypodereum con (Parasites) YES**

End box 1.

☒ **Asbestos (Toxic Element) YES high**

☐ **Toxic Elements (Remainder) NO**

He had only one toxic element out of the entire set. They agree to change his clothes dryer belt to a USA model as soon as they get home.

☒ **Candida, CMV, Herpes simplex, Flu (Pathogens) YES**

☐ **Mycoplasma (Pathogen) NO**

Only 5 tests done. Since Jason had 4 out of 5 pathogens as I began to test him, I realized he had extremely low immunity due to having benzene and propanol in his thymus. We will wait until his next visit to test the rest of the pathogens. I did not use the word AIDS when talking to him but this is what he has. And the HIV virus is not far away.

Seventeen days later

He did not keep the appointment which was scheduled for 10 days earlier. Perhaps he is not committed to surviving. He appears very ill today.

☒ **Protein 24 (HIV) YES**

☒ **Ortho-phospho-tyrosine (Cancer) YES**

He now has his cancer back and HIV in addition. What went wrong? He has been eating meats as usual. He has not checked out his body products for propanol, simply used all of them, nor stayed off benzene polluted products.

☒ **Fasciolopsis (Parasite) YES at thymus**

☒ **Isopropyl Alcohol (Solvent) YES**

Rubbing alcohol used on his arm at hospital to draw blood yesterday - he is advised to bring own alcohol, Vodka.

☒ **Benzene (Solvent) YES**

Hasn't stopped using toothpaste or Vaseline.

☐ **Asbestos (Toxic Element) NO**

Changed the dryer belt.

☒ **Trich vag, Bacteroides fr, Chlamyd trach, Campyl pyl, Bacillus cereus, Strep pneu, Proteus mir, Herpes simplex 1, Gardnerella vag, B strep, Adenovirus (Pathogens) YES**

Because he had Bacteroides fr, he must have *Ascaris*, since they are always found together. He is still smoking. I emphasized the importance of stopping. At his first visit, Jason had AIDS but without the HIV virus; the picture of AIDS is seen in the 4 out of 5 YES (positive) tests. At his second visit, the parasites had reached adulthood in his thymus and the virus is present; his AIDS is worsened.

Summary: Maybe I was too harsh with Jason about his smoking, so that he won't come back. But if he doesn't stop he can't survive. It is weeks past his appointment time. I am afraid it is only his sister-in-law who wants Jason to survive, not Jason himself.

Ralph Smith	Multiple Cancer and HIV

Ralph, age 43, came to our office because of his sarcoidosis which was diagnosed six years ago, although he had had it earlier than that. At that time, he had pain on the center front chest so that he couldn't breathe deeply. He was put on cortisone for it and the pain was reduced, but it is still minimally present. This location suggests the thymus. He is still on prednisone.

☒ **Protein 24 (HIV) YES at thymus and penis; NO in semen and saliva**

☒ **Ortho-phospho-tyrosine (Cancer) YES at thymus, intestine, lung, bronchii**

He has both cancer and HIV! He stated that he had been tested for HIV antibody twice already, both times with negative results.

☒ **hCG (Pre-Cancer) YES in all tissues**

He is pre-cancerous throughout his body! This was a shock.

☒ **Fasciolopsis (Parasite) YES at thymus and liver**

☒ **Fasciolopsis cercaria (Parasite) YES at thymus, liver, semen, penis**

Other flukes not tested. Start on parasite program.

☒ **Isopropyl Alcohol (Solvent) YES high at liver**

Since he does not eat cold cereal nor use body products, his only source is shampoo. Considering his high levels, there must be an unknown source of propanol. He will be watchful. He will switch off commercial shampoo.

☒ **Benzene (Solvent) YES high throughout his body**

Go off the benzene list. This youngish man had tried many things to improve his health. His medical file is ½ inch thick. It seems incredible that so massive a cancerous state could be missed by clinical routines.

Five weeks later

☐ **Protein 24 (HIV) NO**

Very good news.

☒ **Ortho-phospho-tyrosine (Cancer) YES at intestine only**

☒ **hCG (Pre-Cancer) YES at intestine, lung, bronchii**

☒ **Fasciolopsis (Parasite) YES at intestine and liver; NO at thymus**

☒ **Fasciolopsis cercaria (Parasite) YES at intestine and liver; NO at thymus**

☐ **Benzene (Solvent) NO**

☒ **Isopropyl Alcohol (Solvent) YES**

He is still using his favorite shampoo but will switch.

Summary: Ralph has solved part of his problem, the HIV virus and benzene pollution. But the propanol level was still high and the flukes were still thriving (due to eating hamburgers) so the cancer continued. He is determined, though, to cure it all.

| 90 | Jack Lindsey | Colon and Lung Cancer |

This 56 year old man came for his asthma. His breathing is labored and he is on asthma medicine. They have a water softener. He has had colon surgery for cancer and 15 inches were removed. He is also very allergic and is getting allergy shots every week. (He probably has Sheep liver fluke which causes severe allergies.)

☐ **Protein 24 (HIV) NO**

☒ **Ortho-phospho-tyrosine (Cancer) YES at intestine and lung**
Surgery had not cured cancer; now in lungs.

☒ **hCG (Pre-Cancer) YES at intestine and blood**

☒ **Fasciolopsis (Parasite) YES at liver and intestine**
Other flukes not tested.

☒ **Ascaris (Parasite) YES at lungs**
Cause of asthma. He will start on parasite killing program.

☒ **Isopropyl Alcohol (Solvent) YES high everywhere**
Other solvents not tested. He will go off commercial body products, rare meats, and cold cereal.

One week later
He has complied with our restrictions perfectly.

☐ **Protein 24 (HIV) NO**

☐ **Ortho-phospho-tyrosine (Cancer) NO**

☒ **hCG (Pre-Cancer) YES at intestine only; NO at blood, etc.**

☐ **Isopropyl Alcohol (Solvent) NO**

☒ **Benzene (Solvent) YES at kidney, bladder, thymus**

☐ **Solvents (Remainder) NO**
He is using a Vaseline™ chapstick and several cooking oils. He will go off the benzene list of products.

☒ **Arsenic (Toxic Element) YES at lungs**
Remove pesticide from house.

☒ **Cadmium (Toxic Element) YES at lungs**
Plumbing?

☒ **Silver, Mercury, Gallium (Toxic Elements) YES at lungs**
Tooth fillings. Remainder not tested. It is obvious that Jack's corroded tooth metal has accumulated in his lungs, inviting the cancer parasites to reproduce there. He is advised to remove all metal from his mouth and replace it with metal-free plastic.

Summary: Jack, with his wife's help, got rid of his cancer in 1 week. However, Jack still has a precancerous condition at the intestine. We will follow up on him after his dental work.

91   Elsie Avalos   Breast, Bronchial and Bone Cancer

This 30 year old woman came in complaining of the following symptoms: 1) Occasional pain in her left wrist and right leg. 2) She experiences nausea and has a stomach ulcer. 3) Her energy level is moderate to low. 4) She has occasional migraines, usually before her menstrual period. 5) She has cancer in her right breast and is currently being treated with radiation and chemotherapy. She had a mastectomy. 6) Her clinical doctor suspects pneumonia in her left lower lung, and there is something on her x-ray there. The doctor also found some cancer attached to the breast bone.

She is on the following medications: Advil™, Zantac™, Ceclor™, Pepto Bismol™, Zanax™, and Zofran™. She has a water softener at home. She is a tea drinker.

⊠ **Ortho-phospho-tyrosine (Cancer) YES at bronchii and bone; NO at breast**

Note: the clinical treatment has eliminated the cancer from her breast.

⊠ **hCG (Pre-Cancer) YES high everywhere**

☐ **Protein 24 (HIV) NO**

⊠ **Isopropyl Alcohol (Solvent) YES high everywhere**

☐ **Solvents (Remainder) NO**

⊠ **Fasciolopsis (Parasite) YES at liver, bronchii, part of the thymus (is set to get HIV); NO at other part of thymus**

One seldom sees an adult developed in the lungs!

⊠ **Fasciolopsis miracidia (Parasite) YES at liver, thymus, bone**

Remainder not tested. She will start a parasite killing program. She will go off rare meat, commercial beverages, and cold cereal. She will search out propanol in her body products and throw them out. She will use borax for shampoo.

Note: The cancer has indeed spread to the bronchii of her lungs and the breast bone. The cancer marker, hCG, is throughout her body, in every tissue tested. The solvent propanol is everywhere in her tissues also. Surprisingly, there was NO build-up of other solvents. I'm sure she takes in some benzene with her foods as well, and yet there is no buildup, although benzene is thought of as being more difficult to oxidize. Apparently, her body can detoxify everything except propanol. Certainly, being drenched in propanol as her tissues are, did not inhibit them from oxidizing the other solvents. This is probably the action of aflatoxin, a byproduct of common mold, in her diet.

Twenty days later

She only got to day 6 with the parasite program because her stomach was too upset with the chemotherapy she has been on.

☐ **Protein 24 (HIV) NO**

☐ **Ortho-phospho-tyrosine, hCG (Cancer) NO**
Cancer is gone.

☒ **Isopropyl Alcohol (Solvent) YES**
She is still using cosmetics that may contain it. She will check.

☒ **Terbium (Toxic Element) YES**
Takes several kinds of pills.

☒ **Neodymium (Toxic Element) YES**
Pills. She will rotate brands of pills as long as she stays on them.

☒ **Tungsten (Toxic Element) YES**
She is drinking tea with the hot water from coffee maker, will stop. Remainder not tested.

☒ **mono-, di-, tri-Calcium Phosphate (Kidney Stone) YES high**
She will start to drink milk, 3 glasses a day, at least 2% cream. And take magnesium oxide (300 mg), one a day.

☒ **Cysteine, Cystine, Uric acid (Kidney Stones) YES**
She will start on kidney herbs.
Summary: Elsie is luckier than most! She still has the propanol but because the intestinal fluke is gone, all her cancer is gone. Having such good luck could put her off her guard. Hopefully, she will not try to live dangerously.

92	Bill Hutcheson	Malignant Adenoma

Bill is in his mid-fifties and is here for his bursitis and unexplained fatigue. He also had a "polyneuropathy" diagnosed a year ago and a list of minor problems. He came with his wife from three states away. Two years ago a tumor was seen on his adrenal gland. It was called "adenoma" but it did not continue to grow so nothing is being done clinically. He has a chronic cough.

☐ **Protein 24 (HIV) NO**

☒ **Ortho-phospho-tyrosine (Cancer) YES at adrenal glands**

☒ **hCG (Pre-Cancer) YES at adrenals and blood**

☒ **Fasciolopsis (Parasite) YES at pancreas and adrenals**
Not in the liver? Note: adults are seldom seen in the adrenals!

☒ **Fasciolopsis redia (Parasite) YES at adrenals**

☒ **Sheep liver fluke (Parasite) YES at one layer of adrenals**

☒ **Pancreatic fluke (Parasite) YES at pancreas**

☒ **Human liver fluke (Parasite) YES at adrenals; NO at liver**
He will start on a parasite killing program.

☒ **Kerosene (Solvent) YES at kidney, spleen, adrenals**

☒ **Isopropyl Alcohol (Solvent) YES at adrenals**

☒ **Methylene chloride (Solvent) YES**

☒ **Carbon Tetrachloride (Solvent) YES at adrenals**

☐ **Solvents (Remainder) NO**
He will go off commercial beverages and cold cereals and rarely cooked meats.

Three weeks later
He is still fatigued and has a chronic cough.

☐ **Ortho-phospho-tyrosine, hCG (Cancer) NO**

☒ **Formaldehyde (Toxic Element) YES at lungs**
They have recently acquired 2 new sofas and 2 new easy chairs. He is instructed to move them all into a single room and keep it locked until he is well. (Hopefully, when he is well, he will not be so foolish as to try to live with new furniture.)

☒ **Fiberglass (Toxic Element) YES at lungs**

☐ **Toxic Elements (Remainder) NO**
He is to search for a hole in ceiling or wall where bits of fiberglass could blow into the living space. He will bring air samples for testing next time.

Note: He had no other toxic element problem, although he has metal tooth fillings and assorted environmental hazards. He may prepare to cleanse his liver by starting on 07 and peroxy, beginning with 1 drop each in a beverage at mealtime (3 times daily) and increasing gradually to 10 drops each.

Summary: Bill conquered his adrenal cancer easily but getting rid of his fatigue, bursitis, cough and neuropathy will require that he clean up his environment of lung-related pollutants. I believe he is motivated, since he has traveled very far.

93	Shawn Halverson	Colon, Liver and Skin Cancer

Shawn is a very fair-skinned person, with a reddish hue to her face and neck. She is 69 years old and was brought in by her daughter-in-law for liver cancer. She was told about this office by a cured cancer client. A year ago she had pain over the stomach; ultrasound showed cancer of the liver. A scan then found it in the colon. Surgery removed 1½ feet of colon. Three weeks later the bowel had kinked and was corrected with another surgery. But she refused to take chemo and radiation since she was only given six months to live anyway.

☐ **Protein 24 (HIV) NO**

☒ **Ortho-phospho-tyrosine (Cancer) YES at liver and skin; NO at colon, etc.**

☒ **hCG (Pre-Cancer) YES in liver; NO in WBCs**

☒ **Isopropyl Alcohol, Wood Alcohol, Carbon tetrachloride, Benzene (Solvents) YES**

Remainder not tested. She will go off cold cereal, other flavored foods, and commercial beverages, as well as all body products. She will use our list of safe items.

☒ **Fasciolopsis (Parasite) YES at liver and colon**

Others not tested. She will be off meats, and she will start on parasite program.

Note: Finding the cancer in the skin instead of the colon shows that her earlier surgery removed all of the cancerous part.

One week later

- ☐ **Ortho-phospho-tyrosine, hCG (Cancer) NO**
  She is rid of her cancer at all locations. She is incredulous. She reminded me that four locations of cancer in the liver had been seen. They did an ultrasound, CAT-scan, etc. She is delighted.

- ☐ **Isopropyl Alcohol (Solvent) NO**
  We will now search for the metals and other toxins that facilitated her cancer.

- ☒ **Asbestos (Toxic Element) YES at liver, skin**
  Change dryer belt to USA-made brand.

- ☒ **Arsenic (Toxic Element) YES at liver, skin**
  Remove ant poison from house.

- ☒ **Cobalt (Toxic Element) YES at liver, skin**
  Switch off detergents and use borax.

- ☒ **Copper (Toxic Element) YES at liver, skin**
  A look inside her mouth revealed very discolored and corroded metal. She is advised to replace all metal with metal-free plastic.

- ☒ **Rhenium (Toxic Element) YES**
  Tooth fillings.

- ☒ **Mercury (Toxic Element) YES everywhere**
  Tooth fillings.

- ☒ **Vanadium (Toxic Element) YES high**
  Gas leak in the house. They had a gas leak last year and will get this one taken care of immediately, too. She will continue the parasite program.
  Summary: Shawn was a model client - she complied in everything. She made no complaints. She expressed joy at having her life preserved and, moreover, may be healthy again. She is enjoying her new lifestyle. Perhaps she has a lot to live for and appreciated being alive. She is also interested in how all of these pieces fit together to cause cancer. We will see her again after her dental work.

Carmen Miller	Liver Cancer

Ms. Miller has been diagnosed with fibromyalgia (I suspect it will be a Trichinella infection). It began with numbness of her feet about 1½ years ago. Ten years ago she had Hepatitis A for 5 months. She has pain everywhere. Now her legs, especially shins, are numb, too (I will test for thallium toxicity). She has a sleep problem and heart problems also. In fact, there is a long list of health problems.

☐ **Protein 24 (HIV) NO**

☐ **hCG (Pre-Cancer) NO in WBCs**

☒ **Ortho-phospho-tyrosine (Cancer) YES at one part of liver**
This beginning cancer in her liver came as a shock.

☒ **Fasciolopsis (Parasite) YES at liver and muscle**
Note: It is most unusual for an adult to be present in muscle tissue! This could cause a fibromyalgia no doubt!

☒ **Fasciolopsis eggs (Parasite) YES at liver and throughout muscles**

☒ **Fasciolopsis redia (Parasite) YES at liver and muscle**

☒ **Pancreatic fluke (Parasite) YES at pancreas**
Other flukes not tested.

☐ **Hookworm, 4 kinds, Ascaris, 2 kinds (Parasites) NO**

☒ **Trichinella (Parasite) YES high at muscles**

☐ **Strongyloides (Parasite) NO**
Other parasites not tested.

☒ **Isopropyl Alcohol (Solvent) YES high throughout her body**

☒ **Benzene (Solvent) YES**
Others not tested. She will switch her body products to our safe kinds. She will go off cold cereals and the whole benzene list and commercial beverages. She has a cat and a dog that are house pets (probably the source of Trichinella). They use well water and a water softener. She is only 27 years old and solvent pollution of the environment has already ruined her health. What will become of the next generations' health? She will start on our parasite killing program and include pets.

Summary: Ms. Miller has not returned. We are waiting to hear from her.

| 94 | Ray Broz | Follicular Lymphoma small cleaved cell type |

This is a short, 22 year old man, rather emaciated, appearing quite ill. He is fatigued and barely able to get up from a chair and move about. Breathing is difficult, he is grunting at each breath. He is from several states South and came with his wife. His body current is low (I suspect PCBs). He was recently diagnosed with follicular lymphoma small cleaved cell type.

☐ **Protein 24 (HIV) NO**

☒ **Ortho-phospho-tyrosine (Cancer) YES at genital tract, cerebellum and high at pancreas**

☒ **hCG (Pre-Cancer) YES throughout his body**

☒ **Fasciolopsis (Parasite) YES at pancreas, genital tract and cerebellum**

Note: These are unusual locations for the adults.

☒ **Fasciolopsis cercaria, redia (Parasite) YES in saliva, etc.**

☒ **Pancreatic fluke (Parasite) YES high at pancreas**

Other parasites not tested.

☒ **Isopropyl Alcohol (Solvent) YES throughout his body**

☒ **Wood Alcohol (Solvent) YES at pancreas**

Remainder not tested. He will start on Bronson's digestive enzymes, 6 with each meal. He will go off commercial beverages, cold cereals and body products. He will start on parasite killing program.

Two days later

He says he is feeling a lot better. He got a little sleep last night, after taking 12 ornithines. He is still grunting with breathing but only half as much. His body current is very low, suggesting PCBs.

☒ **PCB (Toxic Element) YES**

Go off detergents.

☒ **Benzalkonium (Toxic Element) YES**

Is already off toothpaste.

☒ **Aluminum (Toxic Element) YES**

Will go off table salt, deodorant

☒ **Silver, Gallium, Gadolinium, Tellurium (Toxic Element) YES**

Tooth metals.

☒ **Arsenic (Toxic Element) YES**

Search for pesticide and steam clean the carpets without using stain-proofing.

☒ **Bromine (Toxic Element) YES high**

Has worked with siding and lumber a lot. Go off brominated bread.

☒ **Yttrium (Toxic Element) YES**

Vitamin pills? Will go off vitamins.

☒ **Thallium and Germanium (Toxic Elements) YES**

Polluted tooth mercury. This is an exceptionally long list of metals in his WBCs. He is to see dentist immediately to remove all metal from his mouth. We will now finish the solvent tests.

☐ **Isopropyl Alcohol (Solvent) NO**

Already eliminated it.

☒ **Wood Alcohol (Solvent) YES**

Had orange juice yesterday.

☒ **Petroleum ether, Regular gasoline (Solvents) YES**

In gasoline. Will stop gassing up car.

☒ **Denatured ethyl alcohol (Solvent) YES**

Source unknown.

☒ **Methyl Butyl Ketone, TCEthylene (Solvents) YES**

Processed food.

☒ **Decane, Paint thinner, Acetone (Solvents) YES**

☐ **Solvents (Remainder) NO**

Presumably, some of these solvents date back to the time prior to his restricted diet. He will accelerate their removal with charcoal tablets (take 2, three times a day). Also thioctic acid (100 mg) to remove metals (take 2, three times a day).

☐ **Protein 24 (HIV) NO**

☐ **hCG (Pre-Cancer) NO in WBCs**

417

⊠ **Ortho-phospho-tyrosine (Cancer) YES**
Still has cancer but the precancerous substance, hCG, is apparently eliminated. He is on day 3 of the parasite killing program.

The next day
He appears about the same as yesterday, panting and grunting for breath.

☐ **Protein 24 (HIV) NO**

☐ **hCG (Pre-Cancer) NO**

☐ **Ortho-phospho-tyrosine (Cancer) NO**
Cancer is gone.

⊠ **Acetone, Hexane dione (Solvent) YES**
He has been eating desserts in restaurants, will stop.

⊠ **Petroleum ether (Solvent) YES**

⊠ **Isopropyl Alcohol (Solvent) YES**
Used regular shampoo. He will get dental work done today. He will take vitamin C (2 tsp. throughout the day), Bronson's digestive enzymes (6 with each meal).

Next day
He has had one half of his dental work done on one side. He could feel an improvement in breathing and less pressure over the stomach as soon as a particular tooth was pulled.

☐ **hCG (Pre-Cancer) NO**

☐ **Ortho-phospho-tyrosine (Cancer) NO**

☐ **PCB (Toxic Element) NO**

⊠ **Thallium (Toxic Element) YES**
Tooth filling.

⊠ **Aluminum (Toxic Element) YES**

☐ **Bromine (Toxic Element) NO**

☐ **Benzalkonium (Solvent) NO**

⊠ **Arsenic (Toxic Element) YES borderline**

☒ **Yttrium (Toxic Element) YES**

He will take a Selenium supplement from Bronson's Pharm to recover from arsenic damage.

☒ **Cysteine, Cystine, Oxalate (Kidney Stones) YES**

☐ **Kidney Stones (Remainder) NO**

Start on kidney herbs to dissolve these crystals.

☒ **Moniezia scolex (Tapeworm) YES in muscles and spleen**

☒ **Taenia scolex and eggs (Parasite) YES in muscles and spleen**

He will complete dental work tomorrow and leave for home.

Summary: Ray was a model client with a model family to support him. He will probably survive to return and kill his tapeworms stages.

Brandi Rosette	Cancer and HIV

This 3 month old baby is ill. She is filled with mucous. She has already had pneumonia once. She frequently does not want to feed - she is on Enfamil™ with iron. She saw her clinical doctor yesterday, he is giving her antibiotic shots twice a week and told her parents he is at a loss to understand her illness. She has very little leg motion. She does not sleep much.

☒ **Protein 24 (HIV) YES**

☒ **Ortho-phospho-tyrosine (Cancer) YES**

The baby has cancer and HIV, how tragic.

☒ **Isopropyl Alcohol (Solvent) YES at liver and thymus**

☒ **Benzene (Solvent) YES**

The baby has been on a lotion, Forever Living Aloe Heat Lotion™ since shortly after birth. This lotion tested YES (positive) to both benzene and propanol when rubbed into my arm!

☒ **Fasciolopsis (Parasite) YES at liver and thymus**

☒ **Fasciolopsis eggs (Parasite) YES at saliva**

☒ **Strep pneu, EBV, Influenza, B strep, Proteus, Gardnerella vag, Chlamydia tr, Candida, CMV, Resp Sync v (Pathogens) YES**

One half of box 1 tested. Note: She is YES (positive) to 10 out of 15 pathogens tested, this qualifies as AIDS. She will start on parasite killing program for babies.

Mother, Argella

☐ **Protein 24 (HIV) NO**

☒ **Ortho-phospho-tyrosine (Cancer) YES at liver**

Cancer of the liver is in the mother.

☒ **hCG (Pre-Cancer) YES at one part of liver only; NO in WBCs**

☒ **Isopropyl Alcohol (Solvent) YES**

Will go off body products. Other solvents not tested

☐ **Fasciolopsis adults (Parasite) NO**

☒ **Sheep liver fluke adults (Parasite) YES**

Others not tested. Note: this is unusual, not to have the adults in the liver. But it is nearly always liver cancer where this unusual situation is seen.

Father, Fred

☐ **Ortho-phospho-tyrosine (Cancer) NO**

☐ **hCG (Pre-Cancer) NO**

☒ **Protein 24 (HIV) YES**

☒ **Benzene (Solvent) YES throughout his body**

☐ **Isopropyl Alcohol (Solvent) NO**

Other solvents not tested. They will keep her off all body products except olive oil. She will get only fruits and vegetables and milk, no crackers and other processed foods. The whole family will go off propanol and benzene polluted foods.

Summary: This case nearly brought tears to the eyes of all of us. They have not returned. Parasites and pollution are claiming the life of this beautiful child.

Later: This story has a happy ending. The baby recovered her health; the family was perfectly observant of the rules to keep her healthy. She is now a happy, growing infant.

---

95   Roberta Vanwart   Kidney, Spleen and Intestinal Cancer

Roberta has been our client for 10 years. She is one of our most notable failures, since she has never become well. For this reason, I suspect tapeworm disease. It has been only recently that I learned how to detect the encysted heads (scolices) of tapeworms buried in some tissue, since it is not present in the white blood cells where I make my initial searches. For this reason, we invited her into our office, specifically, to test.

⊠ **Taenia solium scolex (Tapeworm) YES at muscle and spleen**

⊠ **Moniezia scolex (Tapeworm) YES at muscle, intestine and spleen**

I suspect these "bladder cysts" have become eroded by solvent, releasing eggs and some segments into the tissue. I will search for solvents.

⊠ **Toluene (Solvent) YES**

⊠ **Isopropyl Alcohol and Benzene (Solvents) YES**

This is unexplained since she has always lived a very careful natural lifestyle. She says she is using commercial shampoo and will switch. The presence of propanol raises the possibility of cancer, and the presence of benzene raises a similar possibility of HIV.

☐ **Protein 24 (HIV) NO**

⊠ **Ortho-phospho-tyrosine (Cancer) YES at intestine, spleen and kidney**

⊠ **hCG (Pre-Cancer) YES at blood only, not at WBCs**

⊠ **Fasciolopsis (Parasite) YES high at liver and intestine**

⊠ **Fasciolopsis redia (Parasite) YES**

Other flukes not tested. She will start on parasite program and avoid meats at restaurants except for fish and seafood. In other respects, her lifestyle appears impeccable. Her parasite program will include *Rascal*, an herbal combination, for 2 weeks. We are out of it, though, and will send it to her.

Two weeks later

☐ **Protein 24 (HIV) NO**

☐ **Ortho-phospho-tyrosine, hCG (Cancer) NO**

☐ **Isopropyl Alcohol (Solvent) NO**

☐ **Benzene (Solvent) NO**

☒ **Kerosene, Gasoline, Ether (Solvents) YES**

☐ **Solvents (Remainder) NO**

She probably got all these together while having gas put in her car this morning. She will be careful to keep car windows closed.

Summary: Roberta did an exemplary job of ridding herself of all solvents and parasites, thereby curing her cancer. She will probably be able to prevent it in the future due to her intelligent approach and determination to be well. She will include Rascal once a week with her parasite maintenance program. We are looking forward to losing Roberta as a client after her tape infestation is gone.

| 96 | Michelle Murdock | Stomach and Intestinal Cancer |

Michelle is a middle aged, cheerful person quite concerned about her inability to swallow food. The food just won't go down. Her clinical doctor has looked in her stomach more than once and attributes it to a hiatal hernia. She has pain from her throat down to her stomach. Her doctor put her on a medicine, Prilosec™, for it. He also recommended Pepto Bismol.™ She takes a lot of it, but the pain is getting worse.

☐ **Protein 24 (HIV) NO**

☒ **Ortho-phospho-tyrosine (Cancer) YES at intestine, stomach**

Has cancer of the stomach - swallowing often difficult with this condition.

☒ **hCG (Pre-Cancer) YES everywhere**

☒ **Fasciolopsis (Parasite) YES at intestine, liver and stomach**

Note: It is very unusual to see an adult in the stomach!

☒ **Fasciolopsis eggs (Parasite) YES high in stomach, saliva**

☒ **Sheep liver fluke (Parasite) YES at liver**

Had allergies her whole life.

☒ **Pancreatic fluke and stages (Parasite) YES**

☒ **Human liver fluke and metacercaria (Parasite) YES**

She will stop eating rare meat. She will start the parasite killing program.

☒ **Isopropyl Alcohol (Solvent) YES high throughout the body**

She will go off cosmetics that say "Prop" on the label, shampoo and cold cereal.

☒ **Wood Alcohol (Solvent) YES high**

☒ **Benzene (Solvent) YES high**

She will go off all items on the benzene list. Remaining solvents not tested.

Ten days later

Michelle feels much better and can swallow without pain but still has stomach distress.

☐ **Protein 24 (HIV) NO**

☐ **Ortho-phospho-tyrosine, hCG (Cancer) NO**

☒ **TCEthylene, Wood alcohol, Toluene, Isophorone, Hexane, MBKetone (Solvents) YES**

☒ **Styrene (Solvent) YES**

Will stop using styrofoam dishes.

☐ **Solvents (Remainder) NO**

Michelle still has an impressive list of solvents in her. She will stop using processed foods like fake pancakes.

☒ **Mercury, Silver (Toxic Element) YES very high at stomach**

This explains the severe indigestion. She is advised to get all metal out of mouth.

Summary: Michelle discovered the true nature of her problem just in time. We are waiting to see her after her dental work is done.

423

Deborah is 65 years old and came for her skin cancer which was diagnosed 2 weeks ago. She refused clinical treatments, although she was respectful and even fond of her clinical doctor. She has purple spots the size of quarters all over the backs of her legs. The skin is itchy and red and flakes off. She began getting these about 1 year ago and her doctor told her to use a cortisone cream. She knew that wouldn't be useful and never did it.

☒ **Ortho-phospho-tyrosine (Cancer) YES**

☒ **Fasciolopsis (Parasite) YES at liver and skin**
Cause of purple spots?

☒ **Fasciolopsis redia (Parasite) YES at skin**

☐ **Sheep liver fluke (Parasite) NO**

☐ **Pancreatic fluke (Parasite) NO**

☐ **Human liver fluke (Parasite) NO**
She will start on parasite killing program.

☒ **Hexane (Solvent) YES at spleen**

☒ **Pentane (Solvent) YES at skin**

☒ **Isopropyl Alcohol (Solvent) YES at liver**

☒ **Methylene chloride, Carbon Tetrachloride (Solvents) YES**

☐ **Solvents (Remainder) NO**
She is an avid tea drinker and has only one kidney. She is cautioned about tea drinking since it has too much oxalic acid to be a healthful beverage. She will go off tea. She will switch shampoo and cosmetics and stop eating cold cereals.

One month later

☐ **Protein 24 (HIV) NO**

☐ **Ortho-phospho-tyrosine, hCG (Cancer) NO**
Her legs feel very much better. The purple spots are smaller and dimmer. She is on the parasite maintenance program. She has been off rare meats which she always loved dearly in the past.

☐ **Isopropyl Alcohol (Solvent) NO**

☒ **ME Ketone (Solvent) YES**

☐ **Solvents (Remainder) NO**

☒ **Mercury (Toxic Element) YES**

Remainder not tested. She is advised to get metal tooth fillings replaced by metal-free plastic.

☒ **Campyl fet and Campyl pyl (Pathogens) YES**

These are bacteria living in veins causing varicosities and may be contributing to purple spots.

☒ **Oxalate, Uric acid (Kidney Stones) YES**

Remainder not tested. She may start on kidney herbs - only one half dose - and cutting back even further to begin with if pressure in bladder is noticed. She is still drinking 2 glasses of tea a day but will try to stop.

Summary: Deborah has cleared up her skin cancer and knows how to avoid it in the future. Stopping drinking tea was the most difficult of all the rules she was trying to follow. But her intelligence is strong and she will probably clear up all her problems.

| 98 David Adair | Lung Cancer and HIV |

This is a very ill-appearing tall man, with labored breathing and hot hands to the touch. He was concentrating poorly as we greeted each other. His parents drove him here from a neighboring state for his HIV positive diagnosis on the recommendation of a friend. He is extremely lethargic, but not able to sleep. Very little history was taken because he was barely able to sit in a chair.

☒ **Protein 24 (HIV) YES at thymus and penis**

☒ **Ortho-phospho-tyrosine (Cancer) YES at bronchii**

Also has lung cancer. He was diagnosed HIV positive 5 weeks ago, after several bumps appeared on his right leg. But he had not been well for two years and has moved back to his parents' home.

☒ **Benzene (Solvent) YES at thymus**

☒ **Methylene chloride (Solvent) YES at thymus**

☒ **Acetone (Solvent) YES high at thymus**

☒ **Kerosene (Solvent) YES high**

He will go off commercial beverages and drink only milk, water and homemade fruit and vegetable juices. Note: no propanol was found; yet he is producing ortho-phospho-tyrosine in his lung.

Could this be an error? Or did I fail to test for propanol? Perhaps it was only present in the liver, not the white blood cells, so I failed to catch it. He was cleaning paint brushes in kerosene recently; he will never do this again. His parents will cook for him and buy the new products he needs.

☒ **Fasciolopsis eggs (Parasite) YES at thymus and penis**

☐ **Sheep liver fluke (Parasite) NO**

☐ **Pancreatic fluke (Parasite) NO**

He will start parasite program. He will switch from soap and detergent to borax concentrate. He will use only our body products. Note: there is no adult fluke in either liver or thymus; his clinical drug for HIV may have killed it. He will be vegetarian for 3 months.

The next day

He is feeling very ill, barely able to sit for the appointment. His mother is anxious, sitting upright. His father is standing, pacing the floor with his hands together.

☐ **Protein 24 (HIV) NO**

☐ **Ortho-phospho-tyrosine (Cancer) NO**

Both the virus and cancer are gone. This quick result may be due to his having only fluke eggs in the body at the present time.

☒ **Herpes simplex 1, Trich vag, Norcardia, Borellia burg, B strep, A strep, Haemophillus inf, Coxsackie B4, Coxsackie B1, Histoplasma, Campyl pyl, Bacillus cereus, Bacteroides fr, Staph aureus, Plantar wart, Gardnerella, Propiono, Adenovirus, Strep pneu (Pathogens) YES**

☐ **EBV, CMV, Flu, Resp Sync Virus, Chlamydia, Shigella, Proteus, Salmonella (Pathogens) NO**

End box 1. Note: he has 19 out of 27 pathogens in an active stage, obviously AIDS. He will use our L-G, 1 tbs. four times a day. Also vitamin C, 3 grams a day. L-G is an immune booster we use for serious viral conditions.

They left for home, feeling that a test that shows NO (negative) for HIV without showing any improvement in symptoms must surely be worthless and they must prepare for their son's death.

Eight days later

He is less lethargic today.

☐ **Protein 24 (HIV) NO**

☐ **Ortho-phospho-tyrosine (Cancer) NO**

☒ **PCB (Toxic Element) YES high**

Off all detergents; may eat on paper plates and cups using plastic cutlery to avoid soap residue on dishes.

☐ **Solvents (ALL) NO**

Is complying very well with instructions.

☒ **CMV, Gardnerella, B strep, Bacteroides fr, Salmonella ent, Histoplasma cap (Pathogens) YES**

☐ **EBV, Flu, Resp Sync Virus, Chlamydia, Shigella, Proteus, (Pathogens) NO**

Note: he has only 6 positives out of 27 in box 1! He is improving.

☒ **Anaplasma, Strep pyog, Mycobact TB, Shigella dys, Campyl fetus, Strep G, Clostridium sept (Pathogens) YES**

☐ **Mycoplasma, Candida (Pathogens) NO**

End box 2. Note: he has only 7 positives out of 40 in box 2. He is making good progress. I suspect teeth are source of most of the bacteria.

Twelve days later

He looks better. He walks without apparent neuropathy. He is taking his own notes on this visit. He has moved back to his own apartment.

☒ **TCE (Solvent) YES**

Drinks flavored coffee - will stop.

☐ **PCB (Toxic Element) NO**

Uses borax for everything. He is on maintenance parasite program.

☐ **Protein 24 (HIV) NO**

☐ **Ortho-phospho-tyrosine, hCG (Cancer) NO**

☒ **A strep (Pathogen) YES at tooth #17**

Left lower wisdom.

427

☒ **Klebsiella (Pathogen) YES at tooth #17 and 1**
Upper right wisdom tooth.

☒ **Corynebacterium, Campyl fetus (Pathogens) YES tooth #1**

☒ **Pneumocystis carnii (Pathogen) YES at lungs**
Note: he has only 5 pathogens that are growing, out of 67 tested, and these are mainly at 2 tooth locations. He needs to see dentist for cavitations at teeth #1 and 17.

☒ **Asbestos (Toxic Element) YES**
No clothes dryer or hair blower in apartment - test house air.

☒ **Bismuth (Toxic Element) YES**
Using cologne - he will go off.

☒ **Copper, Mercury (Toxic Elements) YES high**
Tooth fillings.

☒ **Palladium (Toxic Element) YES**
Tooth fillings.

☒ **Arsenic (Toxic Element) YES high**
Remove all pesticide. Remaining toxins not tested. He is advised to remove all metal from his mouth in addition to having cavitations done.

Ten days later
He is smiling now, walking briskly, and taking charge of his own case. He says he has more energy. But his right leg is a problem. He has difficulty walking on it. It is considered to have neuropathy by his clinical doctor. A new dark spot has appeared beside the old spot on his shin. It is thought to be Kaposi's sarcoma by his clinical doctor. His doctor says he has permanent HIV neuropathy. His breathing is still labored and audible.

☐ **Protein 24 (HIV) NO**

☐ **Ortho-phospho-tyrosine, hCG (Cancer) NO**

☒ **Fasciolopsis (Parasite) YES at skin; NO in thymus, liver, intestine**
Cause of Kaposi's.

☒ **Fasciolopsis redia (Parasite) YES at skin, blood, bladder**

☒ **Sheep liver fluke cercaria (Parasite) YES at skin, bronchii**

☒ **Pancreatic Fluke adults (Parasite) YES at skin, penis and bronchii**

☒ **Human liver fluke (Parasite) YES at skin and bronchii**

He has been eating at Arby's™ but will stop. He will go on our 5 day high dose parasite program. Note: the parasites are growing in the skin, causing the purplish lumps to appear. He did not get his cancer or HIV back because he did not have propanol or benzene in him. He must have another solvent, though. Will check.

☐ **Moniezia tapeworm head (Parasite) NO**

☒ **Herpes 1 (Pathogens) YES at skin**

☒ **Resp Sync Virus, B strep, Staph aureus, Adenovirus, Norcardia, Candida (Pathogens) YES at skin and bronchii**

He needs to get his dental work done.

☒ **Wood Alcohol, Methylene chloride (Solvents) YES at skin**

He has been drinking an herb tea blend. He will stick to single herbs.

☐ **Arsenic (Toxic Element) NO**

Carpets were steam cleaned.

☒ **Asbestos (Toxic Element) YES**

He brought air samples.

☒ **Asbestos (Toxic Element) YES bedroom air, kitchen air**

☐ **Asbestos (Toxic Element) NO living room air, bathroom air**

The kitchen has a radiator, the bedroom is next to the kitchen. We will test the paint on the kitchen radiator for asbestos with a wet towel rubbing.

Nine days later

His breathing is still audible. He has made a dental appointment; is on his way there. He has done a 5 day high-dose parasite program and is on maintenance again.

☒ **Pinworm eggs, Strongyloides larvae (Parasites) YES**

☐ **Parasites (Remainder) NO**

☒ **Petroleum ether, Regular gasoline (Solvents) YES**

Gassed up car this morning. He will be more careful at gas stations.

Seven days later

He appears normal in walking and in energy but his breathing is still audible. His leg is worse, with increased purple blotches.

☐ **Protein 24 (HIV) NO**

☐ **Ortho-phospho-tyrosine, hCG (Cancer) NO**

☒ **Hexane (Solvent) YES**

He has been using artificial creamer for coffee but will stop.

☒ **Asbestos (Toxic Element) YES**

Brought paint chips from radiator in the kitchen - are YES (positive) for asbestos - remove radiator.

☒ **Campylobacter pyl and Campylobacter fet (Pathogens) YES**

Causes varicose veins. May contribute to purple blotches.

☒ **Salmonella para (Pathogen) YES**

☒ **Strep G, Diplococcus pn, and Staph mitis (Pathogens) YES**

Tooth bacteria.

☒ **Mycobacter TB (Pathogen) YES**

Lung bacteria.

☒ **Klebsiella, Corynebact diph, Blepharisma, Anaplasma (Pathogens) YES**

He is in process with dental work and appears well enough to repeat the clinical HIV test soon.

One month later

He has not been ill; he looks well. He had part of his dental work done this morning, but there is still quite a bit more to do.

☐ **Protein 24 (HIV) NO**

☐ **Ortho-phospho-tyrosine, hCG (Cancer) NO**

We will give him a requisition to do his HIV antigen test today.

☐ **Benzene (Solvent) NO**

☐ **Isopropyl Alcohol (Solvent) NO**

☒ **TCE (Solvent) YES**

Eats flavored croutons - will stop. He is on the parasite mainte-nance program, 2 times a week.

☐ **Herpes zoster, Candida, Measles (Pathogens) NO**

☒ **Herpes simplex 1, Mycoplasma (Pathogen) YES at thymus**

☒ **CMV (Pathogen) YES**

I picked some possible infections but only got 50% YES (positive), definitely not the picture of AIDS. His legs have healed; his doctors decided not to biopsy after all.

Ten days later

His clinical HIV test results arrived. They are NEGATIVE.

Five weeks later

He had remaining cavitations done yesterday and is scheduled for metal removal from dental ware in several weeks. His symptoms of "HIV neuropathy" are probably due to mercury toxicity. He is also very stiff after sitting. He also lost his peripheral vision. He has not had any illness in the past month. He has started drug testing studies at a hospital. His T count is still under 300. He has been on AZT for 6 months.

☐ **Protein 24 (HIV) NO**

☐ **Ortho-phospho-tyrosine, hCG (Cancer) NO**

☐ **Benzene (Solvent) NO**

☒ **Isopropyl Alcohol (Solvent) YES**

Is still using prescription shampoo; will use borax. He will stay on parasite maintenance program. Next time we will check for tape-worm stages and aflatoxins.

Summary: David got rid of his cancer and HIV virus in 24 hours but getting rid of his AIDS was much more difficult. With his parents' assistance and his own stick-to-it-iveness he succeeded.

| **Arlette Shapiro** | **Intestinal Cancer** |

Arlette is only 23 years old and has been diagnosed with Rheu-matoid Arthritis because of wide-spread pain. She has shoulder pain, arm pain, elbow pain, wrist, knee and foot pain. She has already seen another alternative doctor who gave her chelation treatments. She was fairly free of pain during this time. Now her pains are back. The chelation also helped against her migraine headaches. She has a water softener. While with the alternative doctor, she had all the mercury taken out of her teeth. I began by explaining that her shoulder and upper arm pain is caused by gallstones in the liver; she can easily wash them out in one evening and be free of shoulder pain the next day. Her hand and foot pain is due to kidney stones and she can dissolve these out in 3 to 4 weeks with our herbal recipe. That leaves the knee pain, which may indeed be rheumatoid arthritis, namely, tooth bacteria invading her knee joints. She also has cramps with her period.

☐ **Protein 24 (HIV) NO**

☒ **Ortho-phospho-tyrosine (Cancer) YES at intestine**

☐ **hCG (Pre-Cancer) NO**

☒ **Fasciolopsis (Parasite) YES at one part of liver**
   Other flukes not tested.

☒ **Isopropyl Alcohol (Solvent) YES high throughout her body**

☒ **Benzene (Solvent) YES**
   Other solvents not tested. Arlette will start on parasite program. She will go off the items on the benzene list as well as shampoo and hair spray and cosmetics that list "Prop."
   Summary: Arlette's appointment came near the end of this series, so her follow-up results got missed. She has worked so hard on her condition, I believe she will be successful.

Susette Ikeda	Breast Cancer and HIV

Susette came with her husband, Mark, for simple arthritis, shoulder pain, and shortness of breath. But she had frequent nausea with fatigue attacks, and her arm pain extended into the armpit. Also, her shortness of breath was accompanied by chest tightness. She placed her hand over the breastbone where the thymus gland is located. These were ominous symptoms. She had already heard her husband's bad news of being HIV positive. I explained to her that HIV is not a sexual disease, although it can be transmitted that way.

☒ **Ortho-phospho-tyrosine (Cancer) YES at side of breast**
(The side under the armpit.) She stated the breast was often painful with striking pain running from under the armpit.

☒ **hCG (Pre-Cancer) YES high everywhere**

☒ **Protein 24 (HIV) YES at thymus and vagina**
Susette had a much worse condition than Mark, with both cancer and the HIV virus.

☒ **Fasciolopsis (Parasite) YES at liver and thymus**

☒ **Fasciolopsis cercaria (Parasite) YES at liver, thymus, blood, saliva**

☐ **Sheep liver fluke (Parasite) NO**
Other flukes not tested.

☒ **Benzene, Isopropyl Alcohol (Solvents) YES high throughout her body**
Other solvents not tested. She will switch off her shampoo and hair spray and use our brands. She will go off the list of benzene polluted products. She will start on parasite killing program. She will avoid eating rare meats.

Summary: Susette's appointment was one of the last to be included in this book so the follow-up was missed.

Ken Stanley	Prostate and Intestinal Cancer

Ken, age 70, came with his wife, without a special reason, but only because his family members were riddled with cancer.

☐ **Protein 24 (HIV) NO**

☒ **Ortho-phospho-tyrosine (Cancer) YES at intestine and prostate**
This was a surprise for him, though.

☒ **hCG (Pre-Cancer) YES everywhere and in blood**

☒ **Fasciolopsis (Parasite) YES high at liver, intestine, prostate**
Note: We don't often see adults in the prostate, even in serious prostate disease.

☒ **Fasciolopsis redia, miracidia, cercaria, eggs (Parasite stages) YES high at liver, prostate, saliva, and semen**

Others not tested. Ken had such high levels of fluke stages in his body fluids that we will sample them for microscope observation.

☒ **Isopropyl Alcohol (Solvent) YES high everywhere**

He has been a heavy cold cereal eater.

☒ **Benzene (Solvent) YES high at thymus, etc.**

Remainder not tested. Ken will start on the parasite program. He will go off propanol containing body products and shampoo and cold cereal. He will go off the benzene list of polluted products.

Summary: Ken's follow-up visit was missed due to the cut-off date for this book. He was serious about his health and probably cured himself.

| 99 | Joshua Kohn | Prostate Cancer |

Joshua's problems began 6 years ago. He is about 45 now. He had mysterious illnesses, one after another, that could not be diagnosed but which went away eventually, on their own. He has kept excellent notes which he brought in and it is evident that he is suffering severe parasitism that may even elude me. (I only have about 120 specimens for testing.)

☐ **Protein 24 (HIV) NO**

☒ **Ortho-phospho-tyrosine (Cancer) YES at prostate**

☒ **hCG (Pre-Cancer) YES high throughout his body**

He has cancer; this did not shock him, considering his history.

☒ **Fasciolopsis (Parasite) YES high at liver and intestine**

☒ **Fasciolopsis redia (Parasite) YES high at saliva, etc.**

Others not tested. We will get a saliva sample for microscope observation. He will start on parasite killing program.

☒ **Isopropyl Alcohol (Solvent) YES high everywhere**

He will go off commercial shampoo and shaving chemicals, also cold cereal.

Two weeks later

☐ **Ortho-phospho-tyrosine, hCG (Cancer) NO**

He is free of cancer and we can direct our attention to his testicular pain problems.

☒ **Styrene (Solvent) YES**

Stop using styrofoam.

☒ **Carbon Tetrachloride (Solvent) YES**

Drinks Magic Springs Natural Drinking Water™ - will go off.

☒ **Xylene (Solvent) YES**

Probably in drinking water. He will switch to his regular faucet water. He may begin on kidney program but continue parasite maintenance program.

Summary: Joshua cleared up his prostate cancer in 2 weeks and is enjoying the new body care products. He does not miss the old polluted ones. He was astonished and dismayed that purchased drinking water may be more polluted, by far, than city water.

Joanne Semak	Intestinal and Cervical Cancer

Elsie is 56 and came in because of an abnormal PAP test. She is scheduled for a colposcopy in 10 days. She would like an alternative.

☐ **Protein 24 (HIV) NO**

☒ **Ortho-phospho-tyrosine (Cancer) YES at intestine, cervix**

☒ **hCG (Pre-Cancer) YES throughout her body**

☒ **Fasciolopsis (Parasite) YES at intestine and liver**

Others not tested. She will start on parasite program.

☒ **Isopropyl Alcohol, Toluene, TCEthylene, Wood alcohol (Solvents) YES**

☐ **Solvents (Remainder) NO**

She will stop using commercial beverages and cold cereal. She will switch off her shampoo and hair spray and use our varieties.

☒ **Mercury, Nickel (Toxic Elements) YES**

She will get metal removed from her mouth as soon as possible.

Summary: Can she accomplish all this and improve the appearance of her cervix in 10 days? Not likely. She needs to postpone sur-

gery for several weeks. Her final results were not ready in time for this book.

Elsa Elizondo   **Not Cancer**

Elsa is 71 years old and came in for urinary tract problems. She is from a midwest state. They have a cat. She has frequent bronchial problems but nobody in the home smokes.

☐ **Protein 24 (HIV) NO**

☐ **Ortho-phospho-tyrosine (Cancer) NO**

☐ **hCG (Pre-Cancer) NO**

There is no cancer, not even pre-cancer in her.

☒ **(Ascaris) Roundworm of cats and dogs, Roundworm of horses (Parasites) YES**

She will treat the cat with our herbal program. She herself will start a kidney program.

Six weeks later

She feels better in many ways. Her energy is up.

☒ **Fasciolopsis (Parasite) YES at intestine**

☒ **Fasciolopsis miracidia (Parasite) YES at intestine, saliva**

☒ **Fasciolopsis redia and eggs (Parasite) YES at intestine, saliva, and blood**

Others not tested. Note how heavily infected with intestinal fluke stages she is. Certainly, kissing would be infectious. But they are not in the liver to cause cancer, nor in the thymus to cause HIV disease.

☒ **Mothballs (Solvent) YES**

Will discard.

☒ **Methylene chloride, Carbon tetrachloride (Solvents) YES**

She will stop using commercial beverages and flavored foods.

☒ **Gasoline (Solvent) YES**

She will be more careful at gas stations.

☐ **Solvents (Remainder) NO**

Note: there is no propanol or benzene, so she is safe from cancer and HIV. But the solvents she has in her are causing her parasite stages to progress and multiply.

☒ **PCB (Toxic Element) YES**

Off detergent.

☒ **Palladium (Toxic Element) YES high**

☒ **Mercury (Toxic Element) YES high**

Others not tested. These could come only from tooth fillings. She is advised to have them all replaced with metal-free plastic. She will start parasite program.

Summary: Elsa's case was included here to show how the stage is often set for cancer without having any serious symptoms. Parasites have learned not to alert us. But a simple increase in consumption of moldy food (contains aflatoxin) such as apple cider vinegar or nuts could cause a propanol build-up in her and then cancer.

---

100 Kim Maddox	Breast Cancer and Near HIV

Kim is a middle age mother of several children. She has had a mole on her breast enlarge and get red and sore. The breast felt full and uncomfortable. It is the same breast where she had many breast infections while nursing babies. The mole is now scaling and flaking.

☒ **Ortho-phospho-tyrosine (Cancer) YES**

☒ **Fasciolopsis (Parasite) YES at liver and intestine**

☒ **Fasciolopsis cercaria, miracidia (Parasite) YES at breast and blood**

She will start on parasite program.

Eight days later

☐ **Ortho-phospho-tyrosine (Cancer) NO**

☐ **Fasciolopsis and all stages (Parasite) NO**

Continue parasite program.

One month later

She is fatigued and feels pressure on her chest.

☒ **Fasciolopsis (Parasite) YES at thymus; NO in liver and elsewhere**

☒ **Fasciolopsis cercaria (Parasite) YES at thymus and edge of breast**

☐ **Ortho-phospho-tyrosine (Cancer) NO**

☐ **Protein 24 (HIV) NO**

☒ **Mycoplasma, CMV (Pathogens) YES**

☒ **Benzene (Solvent) YES**
Uses a toothpaste that contains a special essential oil.

☒ **Isopropyl Alcohol, Acetone (Solvent)s YES**
Note: The adult fluke is not in the liver and there is no cancer, in spite of the presence of isopropanol. The adult fluke and cercaria are in the thymus (one part of it) and yet the HIV virus is not present. Does HIV only come with redia in the thymus? She is advised to stop using essential oil products and go off the entire benzene pollution list as well as shampoo and commercial beverages.

Six days later

☐ **Fasciolopsis and all stages (Parasite) NO**

☒ **Benzene (Solvent) YES**
Still uses products containing the same essential oil.

☐ **Isopropyl Alcohol, Acetone (Solvent) NO**
Note: She is very fond of essential oil products and does not wish to go off them. She sees that she got rid of her cancer the first time without going off them and this proves to her keen mind that she does not absolutely have to go off it.

Seven days later

☐ **Solvents (ALL) NO**
She is off essential oil products.

Summary: Hopefully Kim hasn't ruined her health by having benzene in her thymus for a prolonged time. She just loved her essential oil products and wished the companies making them no harm. Perhaps she stopped in time. She is a conscientious, health-minded, intelligent person.

One week later

She has had a Herpes attack and feels critical of my methods since she feels she should be well by now. She is also losing her hair and has pressure on the chest.

☒ **Fasciolopsis (Parasite) YES at one part of the thymus**

☒ **Fasciolopsis cercaria (Parasite) YES at the same part of the thymus and edge of the breast**

☐ **Fasciolopsis other stages (Parasite) NO**

☐ **Protein 24 (HIV) NO**

☐ **Ortho-phospho-tyrosine (Cancer) NO**

Note: She has the setting for HIV, with adults in the thymus, but does not show the virus. Perhaps it is at its very beginning. Perhaps the redia stage must also be present.

☒ **Benzene (Solvent) YES**

Is using Tom's toothpaste instead of the one with an essential oil; will switch to baking soda.

☒ **Isopropyl Alcohol (Solvent) YES**

☒ **Acetone (Solvent) YES**

She will go back on parasite program and give up all toothpaste and body products this time.

One week later

☐ **Fasciolopsis and all stages (Parasite) NO**

☒ **Benzene, Acetone (Solvents) YES**

Returned to products with essential oils.

☐ **Isopropyl Alcohol (Solvent) NO**

She is accustomed to pure borax shampoo now and likes it.

One week later

☐ **Solvents (ALL) NO**

Including benzene. She has gone off her essential oil products and wants to inform the manufacturer of their benzene pollution. She is justifiably angry about this.

One month later

☒ **PCB (Toxic Element) YES**

Does not like using borax for dishes so went back to detergent but will go back to borax.

One week later

She still has breast pain.

☐ **Fasciolopsis and all stages (Parasite) NO**

☐ **Protein 24 (HIV) NO**

☐ **Ortho-phospho-tyrosine (Cancer) NO**

☒ **PCB (Toxic Element) YES**

Prefers detergent. I reminded her to continue on parasite maintenance program and stay off the entire benzene list.

Final Summary: We need many more persons like Kim who are so shocked that health foods and health products are polluted that it simply is unbelievable. Hopefully, she will turn her anger on the correct culprits after she has accepted the truth.

Lydia Massey	Pancreatic, Intestinal, Uterine Cancer

Lydia is with her husband and needs to be checked for carrier status of the intestinal fluke. Her intelligence is impressive; she includes herself in the health picture of Gerry!

☐ **Protein 24 (HIV) NO**

☒ **Ortho-phospho-tyrosine (Cancer) YES high at pancreas, uterus and intestine!**

She has a high level of cancer in the pancreas and yet was not noticeably ill. However, she has had chronic stomach problems with frequent nausea. She was not too surprised.

☒ **hCG (Pre-Cancer) YES throughout her body**

☒ **Isopropyl Alcohol (Solvent) YES high throughout her body**

☒ **Benzene (Solvent) YES**

☒ **Fasciolopsis (Parasite) YES at liver**

Others not tested. She will start on parasite program. She will go off the benzene list of products and foods. She will go off regular shampoo and use borax. Note: Lydia is in a much more advanced cancerous state than her husband.

| 101 | Shirley Stafford | Liver Cancer and HIV |

Shirley has a healthful lifestyle, without alcohol or nicotine. But she developed a pain over the upper mid-chest (she put her hand right over the thymus gland) and visited her regular doctor. The doctor wanted her to have a mammogram. Her left arm feels heavy. She also has low back pain that runs down her left leg.

☒ Protein 24 (HIV) YES at thymus and vagina

This was almost self-evident, considering the chest pain. My explanations seemed odd to her. She has no known risk factors.

☒ Ortho-phospho-tyrosine (Cancer) YES at liver only

She has cancer of the liver as well.

☒ Fasciolopsis (Parasite) YES at liver and thymus; NO at intestine

☒ Fasciolopsis redia (Parasite) YES

Others not tested. She will start on parasite program.

☒ Benzene (Solvent) YES

Go off all items on the benzene list.

☒ Isopropyl Alcohol (Solvent) YES at one part of the liver only; NO at WBCs!

Note: I could have easily missed the propanol if I had not searched the liver for it. She will go off shampoo and use ours.

Two weeks later

Shirley has not been ill since the last visit. Her arm feels normal now: it had felt heavy before. The pain over her breastbone is gone now.

☐ Protein 24 (HIV) NO

☐ Ortho-phospho-tyrosine (Cancer) NO

☒ Kerosene (Solvent) YES

Be more careful when pouring it.

☐ Solvents (Remainder) NO

☒ **Asbestos (Toxic Element) YES**
Will test home air. Suspect washing machine belt.

☒ **Formaldehyde (Toxic Element) YES**
New recliner chair and foam pillows.

☒ **Mercury (Toxic Element) YES at thymus**

☐ **Toxic Elements (Remainder) NO**
She is advised to replace her metal tooth fillings with metal-free plastic ones. She will do away with new furniture.

Two weeks later
Her low back pain is unimproved. She has brought 2 belts for testing. One of the belts was YES for asbestos. She will start on kidney herbs for low back pain.

Two weeks later
She has scheduled her dental work.

☐ **Protein 24 (HIV) NO**

☐ **Ortho-phospho-tyrosine (Cancer) NO**

☒ **hCG (Pre-Cancer) YES**

☒ **Isopropyl Alcohol (Solvent) YES**
She began using Listerine™; will stop.

☒ **Arsenic (Toxic Element) YES**

☐ **Asbestos (Toxic Element) NO**
The new belt is asbestos free. She will remove pesticide from home.

Summary: It is always a delight to work with a client who can dispose of new furniture or carpets without regrets when health is at stake. Our culture teaches us to value our material things, not our health. Shirley was inspiring to our office with her ease of choosing health before gold crowns and expensive new furniture.

102 Helen Douthet	Cancer and HIV

We have seen Helen in the past five years for painful joints, high blood pressure, and thyroid problems, but was in reasonably good health. After a long absence, she arrived at the office looking very pale and thin. She has just returned from the Mayo Clinic. She said they were unable to diagnose her with anything significant in spite of her

critical condition. She had not made an appointment but was only purchasing vitamins. I coaxed her to take my first test panel.

☒ **Ortho-phospho-tyrosine (Cancer) YES at thymus, bone marrow, liver, intestine and brain!**

☒ **Protein 24 (HIV) YES at thymus, brain, pancreas, blood**
She has widely disseminated disease. How could this be missed by clinical medicine?

☐ **Fasciolopsis adults (Parasite) NO**

☒ **Fasciolopsis miracidia (Parasite) YES at thymus, bone marrow and liver**

☒ **Fasciolopsis redia (Parasite) YES at thymus, bone marrow, and blood**

☒ **Benzene (Solvent) YES**
She will begin parasite program immediately and go off benzene and isopropyl alcohol containing products and return in 2 days for a follow-up. She seemed too ill to do more testing now.

Two days later
She looks exceedingly ill, can barely walk.

☒ **Ortho-phospho-tyrosine (Cancer) YES at thymus, intestine**

☒ **Protein 24 (HIV) YES at thymus and bone marrow**
Notice how both illnesses have shrunk their territory in her body.

☒ **Fasciolopsis miracidia (Parasite) YES**
Continue parasite program.

☒ **Benzene (Solvent) YES high**
The level is much higher than two days ago, she has obviously had a recent high exposure. She has brought some cans, her water, and an air sample to test.

☒ **Benzene (Solvent) YES in Scotchguard™ for fabrics (a spray can), laundry room air (laundry room has an odor), and in her filtered water at sink (purified drinking water)**

☐ **Benzene (Solvent) NO in Carbona™ spot remover, Energine™ cleaning fluid and plain cold tap water**

In view of the possibility that the purified drinking water is contaminated with benzene, she will use purchased drinking water. She does not trust her tap water. She is still an emergency case and needs to follow-up in 3 days.

Three days later

She seems a bit better.

☐ **Protein 24 (HIV) NO**

☐ **Ortho-phospho-tyrosine (Cancer) NO**

☒ **Fasciolopsis redia (Parasite) YES at thymus, bone marrow**

She has had discomfort over her middle abdomen to the point of pain during this week.

☒ **Benzene (Solvent) YES and in WD40™**

Uses on exercise bike - will stop.

Four days later

She is still very ill but feels some improvement. She has partly cleaned the house of chemicals. She has had a "full" feeling on front of neck, still noticeable.

☐ **Protein 24 (HIV) NO**

☐ **Ortho-phospho-tyrosine (Cancer) NO**

She will not eat pork or beef and will not handle meat in the house. She does not eat turkey or chicken because of her sensitivity to Salmonella (gets sick right away).

☐ **Fasciolopsis and all stages (Parasite) NO**

☒ **Benzene (Solvent) YES high**

She is using facial cleanser, a heating pad, shower water, shampoo, polysorbate 80. She will stop until we test each one for benzene.

☒ **Strep pyog, Pseudomon aer, Diplococc pn, Gaffkya (high), Clostridum (high) (Pathogens) YES**

Remainder not tested. Note: all five of these are typically found in teeth. She has a mouth full of metal - mostly gold. She had too many infections (5 out of 6 tests), so I did not continue testing. The implication of AIDS was obvious. She resisted suggestion of dental work. But she will call the dentist regarding cavitations at teeth #1 and #32. I tried to impress on her the need for speedy removal of tooth infections and benzene.

Four days later

Although Helen is not interested in removing the metal from her mouth, she has just returned from seeing the dentist. The dentist found no X-ray evidence of any tooth abscess or cavities, but Helen did have several cavitations cleaned. She is feeling better for the first time.

☒ Benzene, xylene, acetone, wood alcohol, Isopropyl alcohol (Solvents) YES

She will switch to grain alcohol as general cleanser and continue parasite program.

Three days later

She is still getting some low days. She still weighs under 100 pounds but feels she may have gained 1 pound.

☐ Benzene, ether, Isopropyl alcohol (Solvents) NO

☒ Dipetalonema, Echinococcus, E. hist, Echinoporyph, Fishoedrius (Parasites) YES

☒ Pancreatic Fluke (Parasite) YES

Remainder: NO (Box 1). She tested YES for cholesterol crystals and needs to cleanse her liver of gallstones.

Five days later

She is feeling better than 1 week ago, but she still has her ups and downs.

☒ Fishoedrius, Myxosoma (Parasites) YES

☒ Necator (human hookworm) (Parasite) YES high

☒ Moniezia (Parasite) YES high

Tapeworm head, probably escaping from its cyst after solvent action.

☒ Leishmania mex, Taenia sag (Parasites) YES

☐ Parasites (Remainder) NO

☒ Mycoplasma (Pathogen) YES high (systemic)

Probable cause of general aching.

☐ Protein 24 (HIV) NO

☐ Ortho-phospho-tyrosine (Cancer) NO

☒ Fasciolopsis miracidia (Parasite) YES at thymus

☒ Isopropyl Alcohol (Solvent) YES high
Went back to using commercial shampoo.

☐ Benzene (Solvent) NO

☐ Solvents (Remainder) NO
Stay on parasite maintenance program.

Five days later

☒ Benzene (Solvent) YES

☒ Isopropyl Alcohol (Solvent) YES
Using untested body chemicals. Will stop.

Six weeks later

☐ Protein 24 (HIV) NO

☐ Ortho-phospho-tyrosine (Cancer) NO

☒ TCE (Solvent) YES
Off commercial beverages.

☐ Solvents (Remainder) NO
Stay on parasite program.

Six weeks later

She is very much better. She has been on chelation treatment for 1 week. She is on a parasite maintenance program.

☐ Solvents (ALL) NO

☐ Protein 24 (HIV) NO

☐ Ortho-phospho-tyrosine (Cancer) NO

☐ Fasciolopis and all stages (Parasite) NO

☒ Sheep liver fluke (Parasite) YES

☐ Pancreatic fluke (Parasite) NO
She will stay off rare meat.
Summary: Helen had a very close brush with death. Her great dependence on body chemicals of all kinds (lotions, etc.) contributed to

this near tragedy. At one point her weight was 93 pounds, and I feared we had seen her for the last time. If she had followed her friends' advice to hospitalize herself or had returned to the Mayo Clinic, she would not have survived. Although she appeared well at the last visit, her failure to remove dental metal could shipwreck her health in the future.

Gail Lima   Kidney, Bladder Cancer

Gail is a health-minded woman, age 51, who came from Michigan with her husband. She had a long list of problems in spite of eating organic food, very little meat, had no vices and didn't even drink carbonated beverages. She had tinnitus in her left ear, dry skin and lips, tight neck and shoulder so as to give her headaches. Her heart frequently began to pound for no reason. Her knees and wrists were weak and painful. She had low back pain and gas pains and foot pain. She didn't sleep well and felt anxious most of the time. Her energy level and concentration were low. She suffered from panic attacks and depression. She said she had hypoglycemia, chronic fatigue and Candida, 3 modern diseases that suggested parasites and pollution. I will check for tapeworm later.

☒ Ortho-phospho-tyrosine (Cancer) YES at intestine, bladder and kidney

What a surprise and what an unusual place to have cancer (the kidney).

☒ hCG (Pre-Cancer) YES in part of the liver; NO in WBCs

Note: she said she had recently gone to her regular doctor for burning during urination but he looked at her urinalysis and said she was fine. He wanted to arrange an appointment with a psychiatrist for her but she declined. This viewpoint of her doctor's could have been based on her numerous symptoms and health orientation, suggesting hypochondria. Upon checking the urinalysis she brought with her, it showed numerous bacteria, WBCs and cloudiness. She did indeed have a urinary tract infection besides cancer.

☒ Fasciolopsis (Parasite) YES at liver and intestine

☒ Fasciolopsis eggs (Parasite) YES at intestine, blood, bladder, kidney

☒ **Sheep liver fluke metacercaria (Parasite) YES at blood, bladder and kidney**

We will get a urine specimen and search for these.

☐ **Pancreatic fluke (Parasite) NO**

☐ **Human liver fluke (Parasite) NO**

☒ **Mineral oil (Toxic Element) YES**

She uses no lotions or salves however.

☒ **Methyl Ethyl Ketone, Denatured ethyl alcohol, Grain alcohol, Isophorone, TCEthylene, Toluene, Hexane, Regular gasoline, Pentane, Methyl chloride, Carbon tetrachloride (Solvents) YES**

☒ **Isopropyl Alcohol (Solvent) YES at liver and everywhere**

☒ **Benzene (Solvent) YES at thymus**

As each new YES (positive) result was obtained for the solvents, it was more incredible than the last. How could a health-conscious person who drank no carbonated beverages and ate no cold cereal be so toxic with solvents, including the very worst: benzene and carbon tetrachloride? She uses no cosmetics or household cleaners of a toxic kind. When I asked her what she had drunk and eaten the previous day from morning to night, she showed me containers of powders and foil packages of powders. She has been drinking 1½ quarts of a Sunrider product called Nuplus. This seems an unlikely source, but I will analyze it at once. She is also using packets of Vitalite powders. She will go off all beverages except milk, spring water or tap water, fresh squeezed fruit and vegetable juice and single herb teas. She will switch shampoo to borax concentrate. She will start on parasite program.

Six weeks later

☐ **Protein 24 (HIV) NO**

☐ **hCG (Pre-Cancer) NO**

☒ **Ortho-phospho-tyrosine (Cancer) YES at intestine, bladder, kidney**

She still has her cancers. How could a seriously health-conscious person fail to get rid of her cancers in 6 weeks when others get rid of theirs in 6 days?

☒ **Isopropyl Alcohol (Solvent) YES throughout her body!**

448

☒ **Carbon Tetrachloride (Solvent) YES**

☒ **Mothballs (Solvent) YES**

☒ **Cedar Mothballs (Solvent) YES**

Cedar mothballs no doubt have paradichlorobenzene added.

☒ **Mineral oil (Toxic Element) YES**

Uses a commercial lotion. Others not tested due to numerous positives. She is obviously consuming heavily polluted food. She states she has not stopped using her Sunrider supplement powder and other beverage powders because she believes so strongly in them. Upon testing, they were extremely polluted. She will stop using them, although they give her "energy." She also did not switch cosmetics and shampoo to our brands but will do so at once.

BLOOD TEST	Result	Comment
1. Lymphs	very low (13.1%)	bone marrow toxin
2. Potassium	very low (3.8)	adrenals
3. CO2	very high (29)	toxin in the air, we will search house for it
4. Calcium	very low (8.8)	She drinks no milk for fear of toxins in it! She will start on plain yogurt and some milk. 3 cups 2%/day. Also magnesium oxide, 300 mg, 1/day and Vitamin D from Bronsons, 3/day.
5. Phosphate	high (4.5)	dissolving bone. See calcium for recommendations.

☒ **Vanadium(Toxic Element) YES**

Gas leak in her house.

☒ **Arsenic (Toxic Element) YES**

Steam clean carpets. They will tend to these immediately when they get home.

Summary: Gail was extremely disappointed in her health-food powders. She didn't stop using them because she trusted them. Hopefully, she will conquer this life-threatening emotion and get herself well.

Harold Light	Intestinal and Prostate Cancer

Harold is 66 and has always been hard working and active. Now he has shortness of breath, back pain, leg pain, high blood pressure and diabetes. He was put on diabetes medicine 6 months ago, but decided he would rather correct his condition than stay on drugs and eventually need insulin. They have a water softener but live in an apartment complex so they can't disconnect it. They will start getting water for cooking from a different source.

☐ **Protein 24 (HIV) NO**

☒ **Ortho-phospho-tyrosine (Cancer) YES at intestine, prostate, urine**
> He recalls he has had a number of colon polyps removed over the years.

☒ **hCG (Pre-Cancer) YES at intestine, prostate, blood, urine; NO in WBCs**
> Note: again, the WBCs (the immune system) did not show hCG, although it is rather widespread. Is there a problem with his WBCs? Or is it in the nature of hCG not to notify the immune system?

☒ **Fasciolopsis (Parasite) YES at liver, intestine**

☒ **Fasciolopsis eggs (Parasite) YES at liver, intestine, prostate, and blood**
> Others not tested.

☒ **Isopropyl Alcohol (Solvent) YES**

☒ **Benzene (Solvent) YES**
> Others not tested. He will start on parasite killing program and stop using shampoo and shaving chemicals. He will switch to electric shaver. He will go off the benzene list and cold cereal.
>
> *Summary: Harold was showing the typical health deterioration that is considered part of aging. It is actually parasitism and pollution. Pollution with solvents and heavy metals fosters the parasitism. We hope he will stay committed to his purpose to choose a wiser path than drugs and debility.*

---

103 Jerry Thomas	**Bone and Intestinal Cancer**

This 51 year old man came in because of his bone cancer. It started 3 years ago. He began passing blood; he had a tumor on his kidney; the kidney was removed. He has spots on the lungs which were discovered two years ago. He was put on interferon for 9 months; it wasn't working so they took him off again. Then his leg showed cancer 1 year ago, and he had surgery to remove a tumor in his left leg. In May of 1992 he was on chemotherapy, but it didn't help. Another doctor took over at this point. (This is renal cell cancer.) He also has high blood pressure and has been on medication for it for 3 years. There is a water softener in his home; he will turn it off. He uses coffee, tea, chocolate, beer, hard liquor and tobacco.

☐ **Protein 24 (HIV) NO**

☒ **Ortho-phospho-tyrosine (Cancer) YES at intestine and bones; NO at lungs and bronchii**

☒ **hCG (Pre-Cancer) YES everywhere**

☒ **Isopropyl Alcohol (Solvent) YES everywhere**
Off commercial body products and cold cereal.

☐ **Benzene (Solvent) NO**

One week later

☐ **Isopropyl Alcohol (Solvent) NO**

☐ **Ortho-phospho-tyrosine, hCG (Cancer) NO**
His cancer has stopped. We are now focused on healing his lesions.

☒ **Barium (Toxic Element) YES at bones**
He has been spending time in a bus garage; he will avoid it from here on.

☒ **Cadmium (Toxic Element) YES at bones**
The galvanized plumbing is very old. We will test his water.

☒ **Formaldehyde (Toxic Element) YES at bones**
Get rid of foam mattresses.

☒ **PVC, Lutetium (Toxic Elements) YES**
Garage?

☒ **Rubidium, Zirconium (Toxic Elements) YES**

☒ **Holmium (Toxic Element) YES**
Hand cleaner?

☒ **Mercury, Platinum (Toxic Elements) YES**
Tooth fillings.

☐ **Toxic Elements (Remainder) NO**
Summary: Jerry got rid of his cancer in one week, in spite of his addictions. I did not mention them, to increase the chance of his com-

451

ing back to the office and surviving. But he has certainly made a sincere effort in every other way.

Finale

I hope you reach the same conclusions as I did from these case histories:

- **Cancer is simply a side effect** of parasite infestation and solvent accumulation. It is <u>not</u> a permanent, mortal disease.
- **It is amazing how easy** the cancer side effect is to cure— *Fasciolopsis buskii* is one of the first to succumb to the parasite killing herbs—but it often doesn't bring relief, because the problems that started the initial tumor growing haven't been corrected.
- **Cancer blinds us** to our real problems, like seeping dental metal and plastic, toxic body products, hidden pollution in our favorite foods, and toxins in our environment. <u>These</u> destroy our lives.
- **No matter what kind of cancer you have**, a complete program of lifting the burdens on your immune system will miraculously clear it up.
- **Tumors will shrink** if you remove the dozen or so causes that contribute to them. These causes are not mysterious, just more parasites and toxins.

It seems quite clear that ALL cancers are alike, although different organs are picked to be the target. Cancers typically start with tumor formation, due to about a dozen causative factors. These factors cause numerous mutations which are the focus of many current microbiological studies. The tumors turn malignant with the invasion by *Fasciolopsis* and isopropyl alcohol.

How To Test Yourself

This chapter describes how to make and use the electronic device that lets you do the same tests that I did, and that led to the discoveries in this book.

It is natural to be skeptical that you can accumulate isopropyl alcohol from your shampoo, or that there is anything toxic in soft drinks, or you should change your house plumbing, or you should remove your gold crowns. But you can look for toxins in all these items for yourself, and you may luckily find that you do not have them!

It is only from years of experience testing every product clients brought in, or that I sampled from the grocery and drug store, that I make generalizations like "all cold cereals have toxic solvents," or "all meat has parasites." But obviously no one can test them all. Maybe your brand is OK! Or perhaps it is not. Unless you test for yourself you must rigorously follow the advice in this book.

Remember these tests can only say **YES** there is something in this food (or water sample or air sample or pill or potion) that my white blood cells (indicating your immune system) are busy removing. Or **NO** my white blood cells are not working on this[62]. And except for very high amounts, it is hard to say how much of a bad effect the toxin is having. But with repeated testing you can even find that out. Suppose your hair spray tests YES (positive) in your immune system five minutes after using it, but not after twenty minutes. This, you may feel, is an ac-

---

[62] Testing in the white blood cells is the best way I have found to both diagnose and predict illness. You will also be taught how to test any other part of the body.

ceptable level of toxicity. Or you may find it tests YES even though you washed it out of your hair yesterday. That would be a strong indication that you are accumulating at least some of the toxins from your hair spray in your body, and not only must you not use it, you must find a way to reduce your levels! Again, your own tests will be better than my general advice; but without them, you must follow my advice to get well.

All of the results obtained in this book can be duplicated by a person with skills at the high school level. No knowledge of electronics is required.

When possible, we include Radio Shack catalog numbers to describe materials. This is for convenience only. Equivalents are usually available at any electronics store.

A videotape is available that demonstrates how to make and use a Syncrometer™ (see *Sources*).

Leads

If you are new to electronics you will need to know what a *lead* is. A lead is simply a wire used to connect two parts electrically. The method of clipping the lead to the component (part) determines its name. An *alligator clip test lead* uses a small metal clothespin for connecting, while a *mini-hook clip lead* is like a small, spring-loaded crochet hook. The mini-hook is best for attaching to a wire, the alligator clip is best for larger connections like to the test surfaces.

Leads come in many different lengths and are carried by all electronics stores.

The testing device consists of four parts

the test surfaces, probe and handhold, speaker, and circuit. These are connected by leads. The first item to construct is the *test surfaces*.

Test Surfaces

You will need two plates to set test samples on. The plates that hold the samples are intentionally separated from the main circuit because, unless you add shielding, the frequencies on the test plates may interfere with the circuit.

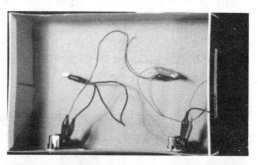

Materials needed:
shoe box
aluminum foil
stiff paper
2 bolts and nuts
nail
4 alligator clip test leads (3 very short, 1 about 24 inches)
2 ordinary light switches.

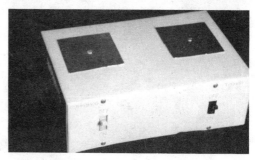

Acceptable:
Cut two 3½ inch squares out of stiff paper such as a cereal box. Cover them with slightly larger squares of aluminum foil, smoothed evenly and

Fig. 82 Test surfaces

tucked snugly under the edges. You have just made yourself a set of open capacitors.

Mount these on the bottom of a shoe box turned upside down. They should be at least two inches apart. Make a hole through each with a small nail, and enlarge with a pencil point until you can fit a small bolt through. Use a washer and a nut to tighten them down. The bolt should be at least one inch long, to make it easy to clip leads to inside the box.

Mount two ordinary light switches on the front side of the shoe box, one in front of each plate. Cut 1 by ½ inch rectangular holes to let the toggle through. Remove the screws that came with the switch, then insert the switch from inside so that OFF is when the toggle is UP (this is the reverse of how most light switches are oriented). Push a pin from the inside through the screw holes, enlarge them, and replace the screws from the outside. If the shoe box is too shallow, flex the "ears" off the switches.

On the shoe box, label the left plate "Substances" and the right plate "Tissues". Label the toggle for each plate with an "OFF" and "ON".

Using a short alligator clip test lead, attach the tissue plate bolt to the tissue switch at one screw terminal. If there are three screw terminals, one will be green for ground–do not use it, use the other two. Attach the other screw terminal on the tissue switch to the substance plate bolt. Attach the substance plate bolt to the substance switch at one screw terminal. Finally attach a long alligator clip test lead to the other substance switch screw terminal. The other end will be attached to the circuit when you build it.

Choose either the "Acceptable" or the "Best" construction technique. You do not have to do both.

Best:

Use a large plastic project box instead of the shoe box. Do not use project boxes with metal lids. If you can not find all plastic boxes, remove the metal top and mount the test plates to the bottom. Use insulating sleeves and solder all connections.

Probe And Handhold

These are what you grasp when testing. The places to attach the probe and handhold are described with the circuit instructions.

Acceptable

For the probe use an empty ball point pen (no ink) with a metal collar by the point. Connect a two or three foot alligator clip test lead to this collar. For the handhold use a cheap metal can opener (the kind that fills your hand) with a second alligator clip test lead attached.

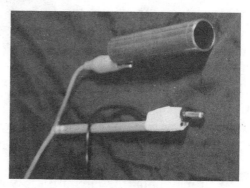

Fig. 83 Handhold and probe

Best

The Archer Precision Mini-Hook Test Lead Set has a banana plug for the probe on one end and a mini-hook on the other end for easy attachment to the circuit. Tape a long, new pencil to the probe; this makes it easier to hold. The best handhold is simply a 4 inch piece of ¾ inch copper pipe (which a hardware store could just saw off for you) connected to the circuit with a three foot alligator clip test lead.

Item discussed	Radio Shack Cat. No.
banana plug probe	Precision Mini-Hook Test Lead Set (contains two, you only need one) 278-1160A

Speaker

Hearing is believing. The sound made when you test substances lets you know if you have a YES (positive) or NO (negative). The better the sound quality the easier it is to hear the difference.

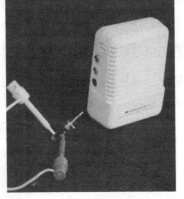

The speaker in the *200 in One Electronic Project Lab*, Cat. No. 28-265 (if you select

Fig. 84 Attaching the speaker

this method of building the circuit) is <u>not</u> satisfactory. However, Cat. No. 28-262 <u>is</u> satisfactory, and no extra speaker is needed.

Acceptable

You may hook the circuit up to your stereo system. Make sure you ask an expert to make the attachment. The leads (wires) you need to do this depend on the terminals your stereo has, but the end of the lead to the circuit should have either alligator clips or mini-hooks for easy attachment. Turn the bass all the way down, and the treble all the way up when you use it. Headsets do not work.

Best

The Archer Mini Amplifier Speaker is inexpensive and small (about the size of a transistor radio), making it easy to take with you. It needs a 9 volt battery. Remove the screw at the center back of the speaker using a Phillips screw driver to gain access to the battery compartment. Also get an 1/8 inch phono jack. Plug the phono jack into the receptacle marked "INPUT", and unscrew the plastic housing on the jack to expose the two posts for attaching wires. Each post should have a small hole in it to attach a mini-grabber lead. If there are no holes use alligator clip leads, but slip a piece of plastic tape between the posts to make sure the alligator clips do not touch each other.

Item discussed	Radio Shack Cat. No.
speaker	Archer Mini Amplifier Speaker 277-1008C
1/8 inch phono jack	Two-conductor Phone Plugs 274-286A (package of 2, you only need 1)
AC/DC adapter (optional)	273-1455C

You are now ready to build the main circuit.

I describe four ways to make a Syncrometer,™ the circuit you can use to test yourself and products:

- **The Easy Way:** buy the *200 in One Electronic Project Lab* by Science Fair, Cat. No. 28-265 or Cat. No. 28-262, at Radio Shack for about $50.00, follow the instructions for connecting *The Electrosonic Human*, then modify the connections as described below
- **The Economical Way:** just buy the parts at Radio Shack for about $35.00, and follow the detailed instructions below (no soldering required)
- **The Rugged Way:** use the parts list, schematic and your electronic expertise
- **The Dermatron Way:** I discovered this method by making some modifications to a commercially available $750.00 ViTel.™ A dermatron is a device invented decades ago to measure <u>body</u> resistance (as opposed to skin resistance which is what lie detectors measure). If you

459

own one you already have the circuit, probe, handhold, speaker and test surfaces. You will just be preparing an additional switch.

Select the most suitable method for your level of experience. You don't have to do all four!

The Easy Way Circuit

Build The Electrosonic Human (in the *200 in One Electronic Project Lab* by Science Fair, Cat. No. 28-265, at Radio Shack). It's easy and fun. If your kit has a different catalog number you may have different connection numbers.

Instead of connecting the probe to terminal T2, just clip it directly to terminal 137, and remove the 137-T2 wire. Similarly, clip the handhold to terminal 76 and remove the 76-26 and 25-T1 wires. This also removes the 4.7K resistor which is not necessary.

Later, when you use the probe to press against your knuckle you may find it painful. In this case try substituting the .005 microfarad capacitor for the .01 microfarad capacitor in the circuit.

If you are using Cat. No. 28-262, you may connect the speaker as described. With Cat. No. 28-265, eliminate the Project Lab speaker by removing 53-173 and 54-174. Connect your speaker instead. Positive (the short post, if using the 1/8 inch phono jack) goes to 53, and negative (long post) goes to 54.

Finally, alligator clip the lead from the test plate shoe box to terminal 50.

Turn the control switch on and keep turning the potentiometer to nearly the maximum. (This reduces the resistance.) Make sure you have good batteries installed. Turn the speaker on. Test the circuit by briefly touching the probe to the handhold. The speaker should produce a sound like popping corn. If it does not, check that your alligator clips are not bending the spring terminals so much that other wires attached there are loose. Finally, turn switches OFF.

The Economical Way Circuit

This is a one hour project, have fun building it!

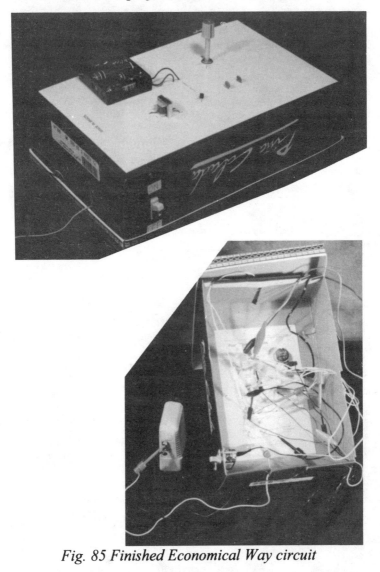

Fig. 85 Finished Economical Way circuit

Materials needed:
shoe box
tape
nail
pointed knife
cheap wire stripper (if needed)
paper clip

Parts List

	Item	Radio Shack Catalog Number
(a)	Ordinary light switch	
(b)	Potentiometer (variable resistor), 50k ohms	271-1716
(c)	Knob to fit the potentiometer	274-428 (package of 2, you only need one, or just wind some masking tape around the shaft in a wad)
(d)	.1 microfarad ceramic disk capacitor	272-1432A
(e)	.0047 microfarad ceramic disk capacitor (.005 will do)	272-130
(f)	MPS2907 PNP silicon transistor or equivalent	276-2023
(g)	Audio output transformer 900 CT: 8 ohm	273-1380
(h)	3 size AA batteries	
(i)	Battery holder for 4 AA's (3 AA battery holder will do)	270-391 has 2 wires coming away from it, one red (for +), one black (for -).
(j)	Microclip test jumpers	278-017 (you need 6 packages of two)

Directions

1. Get a shoe box, save the lid, photocopy the picture in this book and tape it to the bottom (inside) of the box.

Paste This In The Box

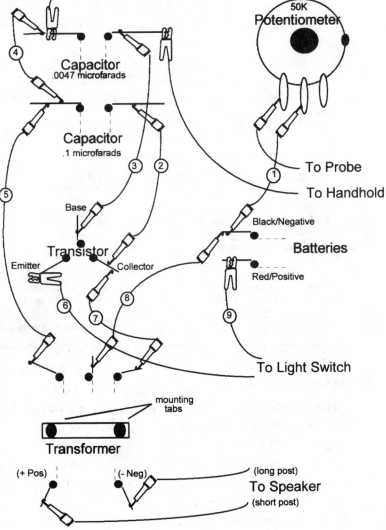

Fig. 86 Parts-layout and connections

464

2.   Mount the light switch (a) just like you did for the test plates on the front of the shoe box. Mount it in the regular way so that ON is UP and label the box clearly. Turn light switch OFF before continuing.

3. Pierce a hole with a large nail or pencil for the shaft of the potentiometer (b), and a smaller hole for the tab on the side of the potentiometer (the tab keeps the potentiometer from rotating when you turn the switch). Remove the nut and washer from the base of the potentiometer shaft, insert the shaft into the hole from the inside of the shoe box. Trim the excess cardboard around the shaft with a knife. Replace the washer, nut, and tighten securely.

4. Attach the knob (c) to the shaft. Use a very small screw driver or pointed knife to tighten.

5. Pierce holes in the box with a pin for the .1 microfarad capacitor (d) and the .0047 microfarad capacitor (e). Push the wires of each capacitor through the holes from the outside. When the ceramic part is almost touching the box, bend the wires inside to keep it in place. The capacitors look very much alike, so be careful not to switch them (open one capacitor package at a time and put the part directly in place, double checking the diagram).

6. Pierce the holes for the transistor (f). Examine the transistor. Hold it in your left hand with the flat side on the left and wires pointing up at you. Notice that the center wire is the "base". Bend the base wire away to the left slightly so you will be able to insert the transistor into the triangle of holes. A diagram on the transistor package tells you that the top wire is the "collector" and the bottom wire is the "emitter". Insert the transistor from the outside of the box so each wire goes where it is supposed to, and bend the wires sideways to secure.

7. Pierce seven holes for the transformer (g). There should be 2 wires on one side and 3 on the other. All wires

should have the ends bared and available for connections. If they are not, strip away ¼ inch of insulation and twist the strands together on each wire to keep them neat (practice using the wire stripper, first, on a different piece of wire). Notice that the transformer has 2 little mounting tabs. Push them through the box and bend them down with a knife or screwdriver on the inside to keep the transformer firmly in place or tape the transformer to the outside of the box. Then thread the 5 wires through their respective holes.

8. Prepare the battery holder (i) by cutting the wires to no more than two inches. Bare the ends of the wires for ¼ inch. You will only use three batteries, so in one of the battery slots, fill the space with a paper clip. Straighten one end of the paper clip. Hook the other end to the spring, and thread the straight part through the hole on the other side. Then bend the straight part down on the outside, out of the way.

9. Next, insert three AA size batteries (h) in the holder (i) (note the plus (+) and minus (-) ends are marked on the holder). Notice that one wire is red (for positive) and one is black (for negative). <u>Don't let the bared ends of the two wires touch.</u> Pierce the holes for the battery wires and insert from the outside. Tape the battery holder to the outside of the box. If your batteries get warm remove them and recheck your connections.

Now to connect everything.

10. Use 9 microclip test jumpers (j) to make the nine connections drawn. Note that connection 6 needs an alligator clip lead to the light switch. Pull on each connection after

you make it, and stuff the extra wire through a slit made in the side of the shoe box with scissors. Make slits wherever you need them. Then clip the lead from your test plate shoe box to the capacitor where shown. Next attach the probe and handhold where shown. Finally attach the speaker where shown. In the picture there are both mini-hook and alligator clips depicted, but it is not important which kind you use, only that you make secure connections.

11. Test the circuit. Turn the speaker on, and the volume half way. Turn the Syncrometer (light switch) ON. Test the circuit by briefly touching the probe to the handhold. The speaker should produce a sound like popping corn (readjust speaker volume to a comfortable level). If you hear nothing, go over each step carefully. Make sure the batteries are fresh. Recheck all connections, especially ones made to stripped wires. Replace the lid and turn the shoe box over so it sits on its lid.

12. Label the potentiometer. Turn the knob almost fully clockwise. Mark the box where the line on the knob points. Grasp the handhold in one hand and press the probe with your thumb. Listen to the pitch. Now turn the knob almost fully counter-clockwise, mark the box, and listen to this pitch. Whichever pitch is higher label MAX (maximum) on the box.

13. You did it! Turn off the speaker and Syncrometer.

After you have used the Syncrometer for a while you may wish to take your device to an electronics shop and ask someone to mount the components in an all plastic box and solder the connections. This would let you travel with it in your suitcase without mashing it into a jumbled mess of wires.

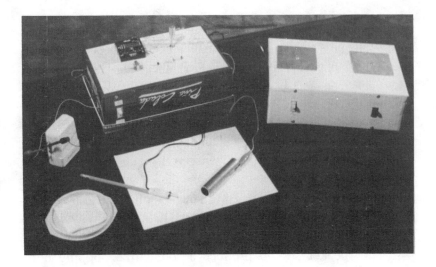

Fig. 87 Economical Way circuit and connections

The Rugged Way Circuit

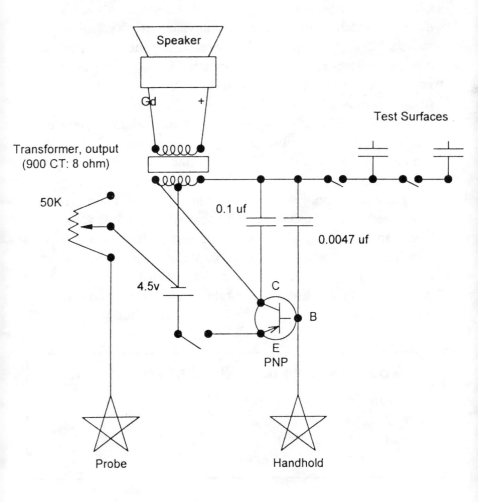

Fig. 88 Schematic

The Dermatron Way

Mount an ordinary light switch in a shoe box as described for The Test Surfaces. This will be called the "tissue switch". Choose one of your test plates as the "substance plate." Your existing switch to that plate is equivalent to the "substance switch." Using an alligator clip, connect the substance plate to one screw terminal on the light switch. Using another alligator clip connect the other screw terminal to your other test surface (the "tissue plate").

You were probably trained to listen for a slight current increase when testing substances. The concept was if the substance was anywhere in the body there would be higher conductance.

You must retrain yourself to listen for something more obvious, *resonance*. Resonance will occur when a substance and a tissue specimen are placed on your test plates that precisely match a body tissue and substance. With the additional information of where the substance has accumulated in the body, you can make much more accurate determinations how problems originate.

You now have the following equipment:

- Electronic circuit with speaker
- Test surfaces
- Probe and handhold
  You are ready to learn to use them.

Troubleshooting

Don't reduce the size of the copper pipes. Keep all wires as short as possible. Use fresh batteries. Don't try to make the Syncrometer all in one box. The test plates are separate for a reason. Keep the lead to the test plate box short, however, and neither it nor the wires to the speaker should pass near other electrical components like the batteries.

Using The Syncrometer

Fill a saucer with cold tap water. Fold a paper towel four times and place it in this dish. It should be entirely wet.

Cut paper strips about 1 inch wide from a piece of white, unfragranced, paper towel. Dampen a paper strip on the towel and wind it around the large metal handhold to completely cover it. The wetness improves conductivity and the paper towel keeps the metal off your skin.

- Turn the Syncrometer and speaker to ON.
- Start with the substance and tissue switches OFF.
- Test the plate connections, if you haven't done so recently. Touch the handhold to the substance plate briefly, then the tissue plate. There should be no crackle from the speaker. Turn the substance switch ON. Touch both plates briefly again. Only the substance plate should crackle. Now turn the tissue switch ON. Both plates should crackle. Turn both plate switches OFF again. Check your connections once a week.

Pick up the handhold, squeeze it free of excess water.

Pick up the probe in the same hand, holding it like a pen, between thumb and forefinger.

Dampen your other hand by making a fist and dunking your knuckles into the wet paper towel in the saucer. You will be using the area on top of the first knuckle of the forefinger or middle finger to learn the technique. Become proficient with both. Immediately after dunking your knuckles dry them on a paper towel folded in quarters and placed beside the saucer. The degree of dampness of your skin affects the resistance in the circuit and is a very important variable that you must learn to keep constant. Make your probe <u>as soon as</u> your knuckles have been dried (within two seconds) since they begin to air dry further immediately.

With the handhold and probe both in one hand press the probe against the knuckle of the other hand, keeping the knuckles tightly bent. Press lightly at first, then harder, taking one second. Count it out as "a thousand and one." Repeat the probe a half second later at the same location. There is an additive effect. The first probe opens your cells' conductance channels. The second probe tests to hear if they are indeed open.; These are considered the two halves of a single complete probe. All of this takes less than three seconds. <u>Don't linger</u> because your body will change and your next probe will be affected.

Subsequent probes are made in exactly the same way. As you develop skill, your probes will become identical. Plan to practice for one to two hours each day. It takes most people at least twelve hours of practice in order to be so consistent with their probes that they can hear the slight difference when the circuit is resonant.

For reference you may wish to use a piano. The starting sound when you touch down on the skin should be F, an octave and a half above middle C. The sound rises to a C as you press to the knuckle bone, then slips back to B, then back up to C-sharp as you complete the second half of your first probe. If you have a multitester you can connect it in series with the handhold or probe: the current should rise to about 50 microamps. If you have a frequency counter the frequency should hit 1000 Hz.

You should reach C-sharp just before the probe becomes painful. Adjust the potentiometer to make this possible. Mark the box STD (standard) at this setting. We will call this the *standard* state.

Two things change the sound of the probe even when your technique is identical:

1. The patch of skin chosen for probing will change its properties. The more it is used, the redder it gets and the higher the sound goes when you probe. Move to a nearby location when the sound is too high to begin with, rather than adjusting the potentiometer.

2. Your body has cycles which make the sound go noticeably higher and lower. If you are getting strangely higher sounds for identical probes, stop and probe every five minutes until you think the sound has gone down to standard. This could take five to twenty minutes. Learn this higher sound so you can avoid testing during this period. Nervousness or excitement raises the sound. Eating may lower it. A method is given in lesson one to determine whether you are in the standard state for testing.

3. You may also find times when it is impossible to reach the necessary sound without pressing so hard it causes pain. You may adjust the potentiometer if that helps. Or wait for your body to return to standard. Remember to set the potentiometer back to STD later. There will be times when the STD pitch is higher than usual (especially in younger persons). Exchanging the .0047 microfarad capacitor for a .01 microfarad capacitor helps fix this.

All tests are momentary.

This means less than one second. It is tempting to hold the probe to your skin and just listen to the sound go up and down, but if you prolong the test you must let your body rest ten minutes, each time, before resuming probe practice!

For our purposes, it is not necessary to locate acupuncture points.

Syncrometer Resonance

The information you are seeking is whether or not there is resonance in the circuit. If there is the test is YES (positive). You hear resonance by comparing the second probe to the first. You are not merely comparing pitch. Resonance is a tone quality in addition to a higher pitch. During resonance a higher pitch is reached faster; it seems to want to go infinitely high. If there is resonance it will be heard as the probe pressure nears maximum, as a rule.

Remember more electricity flows, and the pitch gets higher, as your skin reddens or your body changes cycle. These effects are not resonance.

Resonance is a small extra hum at the high end of the probe. As soon as you hear it, stop probing. Your body needs a short recovery time (10 to 20 seconds) after every resonant probe. The longer the resonant probe, the longer the recovery time to reach the standard level again.

Using musical notes, here is a NO (negative) result: F-C-B-C# (first probe) F-C-B-C# (compare, it is the same sound). Here is a YES (positive) result: F-C-B-C# (first probe) F-D (stop quickly because you heard resonance). (In between the first and second probe a tissue will be switched in per lessons below.)

It is not possible to produce a resonant sound by pressing harder on the skin, although you can make the pitch go higher. To avoid confusion it is important to practice making probes of the same pressure. (Practice getting the F-C-B-C# tune.)

Lesson One

Purpose: To identify the sound of resonance in the circuit.

Materials: Potentized (homeopathic) solutions. Prepare these as follows: find three medium size vitamin bottles, glass or plastic, with non-metal lids. Remove any shreds of paper sticking to the rim. Rinse well with cold tap water. Then rinse again with filtered tap water.

Pour filtered cold tap water into the first bottle to a depth of about ½ inch. Add 50 little grains of table salt. Replace the lid. Make sure the outside is clean. If not, rinse and dry. Now shake hard, holding it snugly in your hand. Count your shakes; shake 120 to 150 times. Use elbow motion so each shake covers about an eight inch distance. Shaken samples <u>are different</u> from unshaken ones, that's why this is so important. When done label the bottle on its side and lid: SALT #1. Wash your hands (without soap).

Next, pour about the same amount of filtered water into the second and third bottles. Open SALT #1 and pour a small amount, like ¼ to ½ of a teaspoon (do not use a spoon) into the second and third bottles. Close all bottles. Now shake the second bottle the same as the first. Clean it and label it SALT #2. Do the same for the third bottle. Label it SALT #2 also and set aside for Lesson Three.

These two solutions have unique properties. SALT #1 <u>always</u> resonates. Use #1 to train your ear. SALT #2 <u>shouldn't</u>

475

resonate. Use #2 to hear when you have returned to your standard state.

Method: Place SALT #2 on the substance plate and SALT #1 on the tissue plate.

1. Turn the Syncrometer and speaker ON.
2. Start with both the substance and tissue switches OFF.
3. Make your first probe (F-C-B-C#).
4. Immediately flip the substance switch ON and repeat the probe. Use only one half second to operate the switch. This is why these switches are mounted "upside down", because it is faster to move the toggle down. The result should be a NO (negative). If the second probe sounds even a little higher you are not at the standard level. Wait a few more seconds and go back to step 2.
5. If the first result was NO, you may immediately flip the tissue switch ON. (Again do this within one half second.) This time the circuit was resonating. Learn to hear the difference between the last two probes.
6. The skin must now be rested When SALT #1 is placed in the circuit there is <u>always</u> resonance whether you hear it or not. Therefore, always take the time to rest the skin.
7. How can you be sure that the skin is rested enough? Any time you want to know whether you have returned to the standard level, you may simply test yourself to SALT #2 (just do steps 2, 3 and 4). While you are learning, let your piano also help you to learn the standard level (starts exactly at F). If you do not rest and you resonate the circuit before returning to the standard level, the results will become aberrant and useless. The briefer you keep the resonant probe, the faster you return to the standard level. Don't exceed one half second when probing SALT #1. Hopefully you will soon hear resonance within that time.
8. This lesson teaches you to first listen to the empty plate, then to SALT #2, then to SALT #1. In later lessons you

simply use two probes, substance and substance-plus-tissue, because we assume you checked for your standard level.

Practice hearing resonance in your circuit every day.

White Blood Cells

Checking for resonance between your white blood cells and a toxin is the single most important test you can make.

Your white blood cells are your immune system's first line of defense. In addition to making antibodies, interferon, interleukins, and other attack chemicals, they also "eat" foreign substances in your body and eliminate them. By simply checking your white blood cells for toxins or intruders you save having to check every other tissue in your body. Because no matter where the foreign substance is, chances are some white blood cells are working on removing it.

It took me two years to find this ideal indicator, but it is not perfect. **Tapeworms are a notable exception.** They can be encysted in a particular tissue which will test positive, while the white blood cells continue to test negative. **Freon is another notable exception.** Also, when bacteria and viruses are in their latent form, they do not show up in the white blood cells. Fortunately, in their active form they show up quite nicely. Again, when toxins or invaders are not plentiful, they may not appear in the white blood cells, although they can be found in a tissue.

Making A White Blood Cell Specimen

Obtain an empty vitamin bottle with a flat plastic lid and a roll of clear tape. The white blood cells are not going into the bottle, they are going <u>on</u> the bottle. The bottle simply makes them easy to handle. Rinse and dry the bottle. Make a second specimen on a clean glass slide if available.

Squeeze an oil gland on your face or body to obtain a ribbon of whitish matter (<u>not</u> mixed with blood). Pick this up with the back of your thumb nail. Spread it in a single, small streak across the lid of the bottle or the center of the glass slide. Stick a strip of clear tape over the streak on the bottle cap so that the ends hang over the edge and you can easily see where the specimen was put (see photo). Wipe the lid beside the tape to make sure no white blood cells are uncovered. Apply a drop of balsam and a cover slip to the slide preparation. Both types of preparation will give you identical results. The bottle type of white blood cell specimen is used by standing it on its lid (upside down). The lid is used because it is flat, whereas the bottom of most bottles is not.

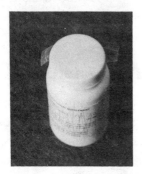

Fig. 89 A White Blood Cell Specimen

Lesson Two

Purpose: To add a white blood cell specimen to the circuit and compare sound.

Method:

1. Turn the Syncrometer and speaker ON.
2. Start with both the substance and tissue switches OFF.
3. Place the white blood cell specimen on the substance plate.
4. Listen to the first probe.

5. Immediately (one half second) turn the substance switch ON and probe again.
6. There should be no difference in sound levels and no resonance.
7. Make sure both plate switches are again OFF.
8. Treat yourself to some junk food. Reserve a piece in a sealed plastic bag.
9. Move your white blood cell specimen to the tissue plate. Place the junk food sample on the substance plate.
10. Listen to the first probe.
11. Immediately (one half second) turn the substance switch ON and probe again. (Remember this should not resonate yet, if you hear any difference you are not at the standard state.)
12. Immediately turn the tissue switch ON and probe a third time. Does this resonate? (If it does, your white blood cells are busy removing the junk food for you.)

Lesson Three

Purpose: To determine your percent accuracy in listening for resonance.

Materials: the SALT #1 and two SALT #2 solutions you made for Lesson One.

Method: move the SALT #1 and SALT #2 labels to the bottom of the bottles so you can not tell which bottle is which.

1. Turn the Syncrometer and speaker ON.
2. Start with both the substance and tissue switches OFF.
3. Mix the bottles up, select one at random, and place it on the substance plate.
4. Make your first probe.

5. Turn the substance switch to ON and make your second probe.
6. Resonance indicates a SALT #1, no resonance indicates SALT #2. Check the bottom. Remember to rest after the SALT #1, whether or not you heard resonance.
7. Repeat steps 3 through 5 a number of times. Work toward getting three out of three correct. Practice every day.

Trouble shooting:

a) If you repeat this experiment and you keep getting the same bottles "wrong", <u>start over</u>. You may have accidentally contaminated or mislabeled the outside of the bottle, or switched bottle caps.
b) If you get different bottles wrong each time, the plates may be contaminated. Wash the outside of the bottles and rinse with filtered water and dry. Wipe the plates very well, too, with filtered water and dry.
c) If all the bottles read the same, your cold tap water is polluted. Change the filter.

Preparing Test Substances

It is possible to prepare dry substances for testing such as a piece of lead or grains of pesticide. They can simply be kept in a plastic bag and placed on the test plate. However, I prefer to place a small amount (the size of a pea) of the substance into a ½ ounce bottle of filtered water. There will be many chemical reactions between the substance and the water to produce a <u>number</u> of test substances all contained in one bottle. This simulates the situation in the body.

Within the body, where salt and water are abundant, similar reactions may occur between elements and water. For example, a strip of pure (99.9% pure) copper placed in filtered water might yield copper hydroxide, cuprous oxide, cupric oxide, copper dioxide, and so forth. These may be similar to some of the reaction products one might expect in the body, coming from a copper IUD, copper bracelet or copper plumbing. Since the electronic properties of elemental copper are not the same as for copper compounds, we would miss many test results if we used only dry elemental copper as a test substance.

Impure Test Substances

It is not necessary to have pure test substances. For instance, a tire balancer made of lead can be easily obtained at an auto service station. Leaded gasoline and lead fishing weights also make good test substances for lead. There is a disadvantage, though, to using impure test substances. You are including the extra impurities in your test. If your lead object also has tin in it, you are also testing for tin. Usually, you can infer the truth by some careful maneuvering. If you have searched your kidneys for leaded gasoline, fishing weights and tire balancers and all 3 are resonant with your kidneys, you may infer that you have lead in your kidneys since the common element in all 3 items is lead. (You will learn how to specify a tissue, such as your kidneys, later.)

Using pure chemicals gives you certainty in your results. You can purchase pure chemicals from chemical supply companies (see *Sources*). Your pharmacy, a child's chemistry set, a paint store, or biological supply company can also supply some.

The biggest repository of all toxic substances is the grocery store and your own home.

You can make test substances out of your hand soap, water softener salt, and laundry detergent by putting a small amount (1/16 tsp.) in a ½ ounce glass bottle and adding about 2 tsp. filtered water. (Or for quick testing just put them dry or wet in a sealed plastic baggie.) Always use a plastic measuring spoon.

Check the items in Toxic Elements (see *The Tests*) to see where they are commonly found. For instance, arsenic is in carpets, stuffed furniture and wallpaper, originating in the pesticide put there. Here are some suggestions for finding sources of toxic products to make your own toxic element test. If the product is a solid, place a small amount in a plastic bag and add a tablespoon of filtered water to get a temporary test product. For permanent use put it in a small amber glass bottle. If the product is a liquid, pour a few <u>drops</u> into a glass bottle and add about 2 tsp. filtered water. Keep all toxic substances in glass bottles for your own safety. Small amber glass dropper bottles can be purchased by the dozen at drug stores (also see *Sources*).

Aflatoxin: scrape the mold off an orange or piece of bread; wash hands afterward.

Acetone: paint supply store or pharmacy.

Arsenic: 1/16 tsp. of arsenate pesticide from a garden shop. A snippet of flypaper.

Aluminum: a piece of aluminum foil (not tin foil) or an aluminum measuring spoon.

Aluminum silicate: a bit of salt that has this free running agent in it.

Asbestos: a small piece of asbestos sheeting, an old furnace gasket, 1/4 inch of a clothes dryer belt that does not say "Made in USA", or a crumb of building material being removed due to its asbestos content (ask a contractor).

Barium: save a few drops from the beverage given clients scheduled for an X-ray. Lipstick that has barium listed in the ingredients.

Benzene: an <u>old</u> can of rubber cement (new supplies do not have it). A tsp. of asphalt crumbs from a driveway.

Benzopyrenes: a piece of toast, hot dog, or flame cooked food. This substance fades in a day, use it while fresh.

Beryllium: a piece of coal; a few drops of "coal oil" or lamp oil.

Bismuth: use a few drops of antacid with bismuth in it.

Bromine: bleached "brominated" flour.

Cadmium: scrape a bit off a galvanized nail, paint from a hobby store.

Cesium: scrape the surface of a clear plastic beverage bottle.

CFC's (Freon): ask an electronics expert for a squirt from an old aerosol can that used Freon as a cleaner. (Squirt into water, outdoors, put the water in a sample bottle.)

Chromate: scrape an old car bumper.

Cobalt: pick out the blue and green crumbs from detergent. A sample of cobalt containing paint should also suffice.

Chlorine: a few drops of pure, old fashioned Clorox.™

Copper: ask your hardware clerk to cut a small fragment off a copper pipe of the purest variety or a ¼ inch of pure copper wire.

Ergot: a teaspoon of rye grains, or rye bread. Add grain alcohol to preserve.

Ether: automotive supply store (engine starting fluid).

Ethyl alcohol (grain alcohol): the purest "drinking" alcohol available. Everclear™ in the United States, Protec™ (potable) in Mexico.

Fiberglass: snip a fragment from insulation.

Fluoride: toothpaste with fluoride.

Formaldehyde: purchase 37% at a pharmacy. Use a few drops only for your sample.

Gasoline: gas station (leaded and unleaded).

Gold: ask a jeweler for a crumb of the purest gold available or use a wedding ring.

Kerosene: gas station.

Lead: wheel balancers from a gas station, weights used on fishing lines, lead solder from electronics shop.

Malonic acid: fresh orange juice.

Mercury: a mercury thermometer (there is no need to break it), piece of amalgam tooth filling.

Methanol: paint supply store (wood alcohol).

Nickel: a nickel plated paper clip, a washed coin.

Patulin (apple mold): cut a sliver of bruised apple that has turned brown, wash and peel first to avoid the benzene in the spray that may be on the peel.

PCB: water from a quarry known to be polluted with it (a builder or electrical worker may know a source).

Platinum: ask a jeweler for a small specimen.

Propyl alcohol: (actually, isopropyl alcohol, not n-propyl alcohol) rubbing alcohol from pharmacy. Use a few drops only, discard the rest. Do not save it.

PVC: glue that lists it in the ingredients (polyvinyl chloride).

Radon: leave a glass jar with an inch of filtered water in it standing open in a basement that tested positive to radon using a kit. After 3 days, close the jar. Pour about 2 tsp. of this water into your specimen bottle.

Silicon: a dab of silicon caulk.

Silver: ask a jeweler for a crumb of very pure silver. Silver solder can be found in electronics shops. Snip the edge of a very old silver coin.

Sorghum mold: 1/8 tsp. sorghum syrup.

Styrene: a chip of styrofoam.

Tantalum: purchase a tantalum drill bit from hardware store.

Tartrazine: (yellow food dye) some yellow jello or orange cheese.

Tin: scrape a tin bucket at a farm supply. Tin solder. Ask a dentist for a piece of pure tin (used to make braces).

Titanium: purchase a titanium drill bit from a hardware store.

Toluene: a tube of glue that lists toluene as an ingredient.

Tungsten: the filament in a burned out light bulb.

Urethane: a piece of plastic foam from new furniture or packaging material.(This will also contain formaldehyde.)

Vanadium: hold a piece of dampened paper towel over a gas stove burner as it is turned on. Cut a bit of this paper into your specimen bottle and add 2 tsp. filtered water.

Xylene: paint store or pharmacy.

Zearalenone: combine leftover crumbs of three kinds of corn chips and three kinds of popcorn.

This list gets you off to a good start. Since few of these specimens are pure, there is a degree of logic that you must apply in most cases. If you are testing for barium in your breast, a positive result would mean that a barium-containing lip stick tests positive and a barium-free lip stick is negative.

A chemistry set for hobbyists is a wonderful addition to your collection of test specimens. Remember, however, the assumptions and errors in such a system. A test for silver using silver chloride might be negative. This does not mean there is no silver present in your body; it only means there is no silver chloride present in the tissue you tested. You are bound to miss some toxins; don't let this discourage you. There is more than enough that you <u>can</u> find.

The most fruitful kind of testing is, probably, the use of household products themselves as test substances. The soaps, colognes, mouthwash, toothpaste, shampoo, cosmetics, breads, dairy products, juices and cereals can all be made into test specimens. Put about 1/8 tsp. of the product in a small glass bottle, add 2 tsp. filtered water and ¼ tsp. grain alcohol to preserve it. If you test positive to these, then you shouldn't use them, even if you can not identify the exact toxin or pathogen.

Finally, there is the error from the filtered water you are using. Test it by tasting it, then searching your white blood cells for it. If you find it there, change the filter and repeat the test. Make a test sample of this water alone.

Lesson Four

Purpose: To determine toxicity of your household products.

Materials: Prepare samples of what you ate at your last meal. Also prepare samples of the soap, shampoo, shaving cream and other products you last put on your body.

Method: Listen for resonance between your white blood cells and the daily foods and products you use.

1. Place your white blood cell specimen on the tissue plate.
2. Place your first sample on the substance plate.
3. Test for resonance.
4. Make two piles. Things that resonate go in the TOXIC pile, things that don't go in the SAFE pile. Don't be surprised if your health brand shampoo "flunks" the test. And if your vitamin C flunks, I hope you write a letter to the manufacturer!

Making Organ Specimens

To test for toxic elements or parasites in a particular organ such as the liver or skin, you will need either a fresh or frozen sample of the organ or a prepared microscope slide of this organ. Meat purchased from a grocery store, fresh or frozen, provides you with a variety of organ specimens. Chicken, turkey, beef or pork organs all give the same results. You may purchase chicken gizzards for a sample of stomach, beef liver for liver, pork brains for brain, beef steak for muscle, sweet breads for thymus, tripe for stomach lining. Other organs may be ordered from a meat packing plant.

Trim the marrow out of a bone slice to get bone marrow. Scrub the bone slice with hot water to free it of marrow to get a bone specimen. Choose a single piece of meat sample, rinse it and place it in a plastic bag. You may freeze it. To make a durable unfrozen sample, cut a small piece, the size of a pea, and place it in an amber glass bottle (½ oz.). Cover with two tsp. filtered water and ¼ tsp. of grain alcohol (pure vodka will do) to preserve it. These need not be refrigerated but if decay starts, make a fresh specimen.

Pork brains from the grocery store may be dissected to give you the different parts of the brain. Chicken livers often have an attached gallbladder or piece of bile duct, giving you that extra organ. Grocery store "lites" provides you with lung tissue. For kidney, snip a piece off pork or beef kidney. Beef liver may supply you with a blood sample, too. Saliva, urine and semen may be your own. Use less than ¼ tsp. of each fluid. Add about 2 tsp. (10 ml) filtered water and a small amount (¼ tsp.) of grain alcohol to preserve them. This dilution of natural fluids is essential to get correct results.

I use ½ oz amber glass bottles with bakelite caps (see *Sources*) to hold specimens. After closing, each bottle is sealed with a Parafilm™ strip to avoid accidental loosening of the cap. However, plastic bags or other containers would suffice.

To make a specimen of skin, use hangnail bits and skin peeled from a callous, not a wart. A few shreds will do. Remember, they must be very close to the test plate when in use; add 2 tsp. filtered water and ¼ tsp. grain alcohol.

Making a Complete Set of Tissue Samples

My original complete set was made from a frozen fish. As it thawed, different organs were cut away and small pieces placed in bottles for preserving in cold tap water and grain alcohol. In this way, organs not available from the grocery store could be obtained. The piece of intestine closest to the anus corresponds to our colon, the part closest to the stomach corresponds to our duodenum. The 2 layers of the stomach and different layers of the eye, the optic nerve and spinal cord were obtained this way.

Another complete set of tissue samples were obtained from a freshly killed steer at a slaughter house. In this way the 4 chambers of the heart were obtained, the lung, trachea, aorta, vein, pancreas, and so forth.

Purchasing a Complete Set of Tissue Samples

Slides of tissues, unstained or stained in a variety of ways for microscope study give identical results to the preparations made by yourself in the ways already described. This fact opens the entire catalog of tissue types for your further study. See "microscope slides and equipment" in *Sources* for places that supply them.

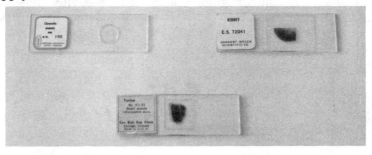

Fig. 90 Some purchased parasite and tissue slides

You now have a set of organ samples, either fresh, frozen, preserved or on slides. You also have a set of test substances, whether chemical compounds, or elements, or products. Your goal is to search in your own organs and body tissues for the substances that may be robbing you of health.

Keeping yourself healthy will soon be an easy, daily routine.

Body Fluid Specimens

The human body emits a wide range of frequencies. Body fluids retain these frequencies and always resonate. To reduce this effect you must dilute all body fluids before using them. Then you will only hear resonance with substances that are actually in the body fluid.

Each of these fluids should be prepared by putting about ¼ tsp. in a ½ oz amber glass bottle. Add about 2 tsp. filtered water and ¼ tsp. grain alcohol for preservation. It is important *not* to shake the specimen, but to mix gently.

Urine. It is desired to have a pure, uninfected urine sample as a tissue specimen. Since this cannot be proved with certainty, obtain several urine samples from different persons whom you believe to be healthy and make several test specimens in order to compare results. Label your specimens Urine A (child), Urine B (woman), Urine C (mine), and so forth.

Semen. A sample from a condom is adequate. Aged specimens (sent by mail, unpreserved and unrefrigerated) work well also. Use one to ten drops or scrape a small amount.

Blood. One to ten drops of blood should be used. A bit of white paper towel for swabbing may be used. Clotted or chemically treated blood is satisfactory. A blood smear on a slide is very convenient.

Milk. Cow's milk is too polluted with parasites and chemicals to be useful. Electronically, a dead specimen is equivalent to a live specimen, so that pasteurization of the milk does not help. A human milk specimen is preferred.

Saliva. Use your own, if you have deparasitized yourself and test negative to various fluke stages. Otherwise find a well friend or child.

You Will Now Be Able to Test in <u>Three</u> Different Ways!

When you test with a substance on one plate and nothing on the other, you are searching your <u>entire body</u> for that substance. Such a test is not very sensitive, but it lets you pick out your worst toxins.

By putting a tissue sample on the other plate you are testing for the substance specifically in that tissue in your body, and this is much more sensitive. The tissue need not be the white blood cells. To find mercury in your kidneys you would use a mercury sample on one plate, and a kidney sample on the other. The technique is the same as when you use white blood cells.

If you put a substance on each plate, a resonating circuit means the two samples have something in common. For example, if you have mercury on one plate and some dental floss on the other, a positive result indicates mercury in the floss.

Lesson Five

Purpose: To watch substances travel through your body.

Materials: Prepare a pint of brown sugar solution (white sugar has isopropyl alcohol pollution) using filtered water. Use about 1 tsp. brown sugar, 1/8 tsp. vitamin C (to detoxify sorghum mold), and a pint of filtered water. Do not shake it; gently mix. Make a sample bottle by pouring about ½ inch into a clean used vitamin bottle. Rinse and dry the outside of the sample bottle. Finally wash your hands with plain water.

Method:

1. Test your skin for the presence of brown sugar, using the newly made sample bottle and your skin specimen. It should not be there (resonate) yet.

2. Prepare a paper applicator by tearing the corner from a white unfragranced paper towel. Fold it to make a wick.

3. Dip the paper wick in the pint of sugar water and apply it to the skin of your inner arm where you can rub freely. Rub it in vigorously for about 10 seconds (otherwise it takes minutes to absorb). Leave the shredded wick on the skin and tape it down with a piece of clear tape about 4 inches long (this increases the time you have to work). Quickly wash your fingers.

4. Place your skin tissue specimen on one plate and the sugar specimen bottle on the other plate.

5. Probe for resonance every 5 seconds. As soon as you hear resonance, implying that the skin has absorbed the sugar solution (which may take a full minute), replace the skin specimen with one of liver and listen for resonance again. There should be none, yet.

6. Alternate between the skin and liver. Soon the skin will be clear and the liver will resonate. Also check the pancreas and muscles to see how quickly sugar arrives there.

7. Check white blood cells and kidneys. It should <u>not</u> appear here (unless it is polluted with a toxin).

8. After five to ten minutes the sugar will be gone from all of these tissues and your experiment is ended. Wash your arm with plain water.

Notice that you have only a few minutes to get all your testing done after the skin has absorbed the test substances.

Lesson Six

Purpose: To verify the isopropyl alcohol and benzene lists.

Method: We will use the Syncrometer to test for a toxin in a product. Assemble the products named in the isopropyl alcohol list (page 45) and benzene list (page 160) ... as many as you can find. Also make sample bottles of benzene and isopropyl alcohol.

1. Place the isopropyl alcohol test substance on one plate and your products, in turn, on the other.
2. Listen to the current with only one of the plates in the circuit. Then listen with both plates in (the test plate switch ON). This method can detect one part per quadrillion in concentration. It is not as sensitive as the skin test (Lesson Five).
3. Repeat, with the benzene test substance.

Even tiny amounts of solvents are toxic! They must not be consumed or be left in our environment.

I have found that too many unsuspected products test positive to <u>benzene</u>. This is such a global tragedy that people must protect themselves by using their own tests. Rather than assurances, regulatory agencies should provide the consumer with cheap and simple tests (dip sticks and papers so we need not lug our Syncrometers around). Even if some test should fail, not all tests would fail to find an important pollutant like benzene. It would come to public attention much faster than the present debacle has.

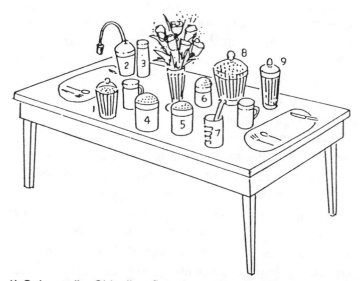

1) *Salmonella*, *Shigella*, aflatoxin, ergot, zearalenone, patulin test sticks; 2) ozonator; 3) Lugol's; 4) vitamin C powder; 5) sodium/ potassium salt; 6) fresh powdered herb spices; 7) food zapper; 8) benzene, isopropyl alcohol, wood alcohol test sticks; 9) heavy metals and lanthanides test sticks.

Fig. 91 Table of the future.

Lesson Seven

Purpose: To test for the presence of aluminum in your brain and your foods.

Materials: An aluminum measuring spoon, a tsp. of free flowing aluminized salt, a square inch of aluminum foil, a package of pork brain from the grocery store, kept frozen. (Other animal sources will do). Or a stained slide of cerebrum, cerebellum or other brain tissue.

Method:

1. Cut a piece of brain tissue (about 1 tsp.) and place in a plastic bag.
2. Place the aluminum samples in separate plastic bags. Add filtered water to each, about 1 tbs. Keep all surfaces and your hands meticulously clean (do not use soap).
3. Place the aluminum sample on one plate and the brain sample on the other plate.
4. Probe for resonance. If the circuit resonates <u>you</u> have aluminum in <u>your</u> brain.
5. If your aluminum specimen actually has cadmium or copper in it, you are <u>also</u> testing for these in your brain. Repeat the aluminum test with other aluminum objects. If they <u>all</u> resonate, you <u>very, very</u> <u>likely</u> have aluminum in your brain. If you can, test yourself to cadmium and copper, separately. If you don't have these in your brain, the aluminum test result is even more likely to be correct.
6. Of course, it would be desirable to have absolute certainty about this. To achieve this, purchase pure aluminum or an Atomic Absorption Standard. These are available from chemical supply companies.

If you do have aluminum in your brain, where is it coming from?

7. Leave your purest aluminum test substance on one plate, and replace the brain sample with these items, testing them one at a time. Remember to rest after each positive result.

- a teaspoon of cottage cheese or yogurt taken from the top of a container of a foil-capped variety
- a piece of cream cheese or butter that was wrapped in foil
- a chip of bar soap or a bit of hand lotion
- a piece of cake or rolls baked in an aluminum pan
- a piece of turkey skin or hot dish that was covered with aluminum foil
- anything baked with baking powder
- a carbonated beverage from an aluminum can

Alternative Lesson:

To test for dental metal in your tissues. Use a piece of amalgam from an old tooth filling. This tests for the rest of the alloys in amalgam fillings as well as mercury. If you can't get a piece of mercury amalgam, use a mercury thermometer (don't break it, just put the bulb on the plate). Choose tissues like kidney, nerves, brain, liver, in addition to white blood cells.

I have never dissected human tissues and subjected them to confirmatory laboratory tests. It seems reasonable that because skin and tongue are directly provable, that other tissues work similarly.

Testing Someone Else

Seat the person comfortably with their hand resting near you. Choose the first knuckle from the middle or first finger just like you do for yourself. Since you are touching this person, you are putting yourself in the circuit with the subject.

To exclude yourself, you need to add inductance to yourself. A coil of about 10 microhenrys, worn next to the skin, works well and is easily made. Obtain insulated wire and wrap 24 turns around a ball point pen (or something about that size), closely spaced. Cut the ends and tape them down securely. Keep it in a plastic bag, even when in your pocket. A commercial inductance of 4.7 microhenrys, worn touching your skin also works well. It can be worn on a string necklace. (Remember to remove the necklace when testing yourself.) The inductance acts as an RF (radio frequency) choke, limiting the alternating current that can flow through you while testing another person.

Test your inductor in this way. Repeat Lesson One with the coil next to your body. No resonance, even to SALT #1, should occur. If it does, make the coil bigger. Remove the inductor when you are not testing others.

Lesson Eight

Purpose: To detect aluminum in the brain of another person.

Materials: same as previous lesson, you wear the inductor.

Method:

1. Place the aluminum sample on one plate and the brain sample on the other plate.
2. Give the other person the handhold. You use the probe. Hold their finger steady in yours.
3. Probe the other person for resonance. The first probe is with only one plate in the circuit. The second is with both plates in the circuit. Resonance implies there is aluminum in the person's brain.

Saliva Testing

This may become your most useful test. The saliva has in it a bit of almost everything toxic that is in you. But it is not the first tissue to carry the HIV virus or a bit of a tapeworm stage. Nevertheless, ortho-phospho-tyrosine, *Salmonella*, mercury in your kidneys, aluminum in the brain all show up in the saliva, too. And saliva can be sent by mail or stored in the refrigerator. It should be frozen for long storage to prevent mold invasion. Or it may have grain alcohol added to preserve it. This test is not as sensitive as having the person present in the circuit, though.

To make a saliva specimen, place a two inch square piece of white, unfragranced paper towel (tear, don't cut) in a light-weight resealable baggie. Hold the open baggie near your mouth. Don't touch the paper towel with your fingers. Drool or spit onto the paper towel until half of it is damp. Zip it shut. Before testing, add enough filtered water to dampen the whole piece of paper.

Lesson Nine

Purpose: To search for shingles or *Herpes*.

Materials: A saliva specimen from the person being tested; they may be thousands of miles away. Also a specimen of the virus as a test substance. This can be obtained from someone else's lesions—one droplet is enough, picked up on a bit of paper towel. The whole thing, towel and all, can be pushed into a glass bottle for preserving. Water and alcohol should be added. It can also be put on a slide, labeled *Herpes, homemade*. A homeopathic preparation of the virus does not give accurate results for this kind of testing, due to the additional frequency imposed on it by potentizing. (However, homeopathic preparations can be used if the potency matches the tissue frequency where it resides. Hopefully, some way of using homeopathic sources will soon be found.)

Method: Place the saliva specimen in its unopened baggie on one plate. You may wish to open it briefly, though, to add enough filtered water to wet all the paper and add ¼ tsp. grain alcohol to sterilize or preserve it.

Place the virus specimen on the other plate and test as usual (like Lesson Six). A positive result means the person has active *Herpes*.

The main disadvantage of saliva testing is that you do not know which tissue has the pathogen or the toxin. You can only conclude that it is present. Usually this is enough information to carry out a corrective program.

Surrogate Testing

Although saliva testing is so easy, it is also possible to use an adult as a surrogate when testing a baby or pet. The pet or baby is held on the lap of the surrogate. A large pet may sit in front of the person. The handhold is held by the surrogate and pressed firmly against the body of the baby or pet. It can be laid flat against the arm, body or leg of a baby and held in place firmly by the whole hand of the adult. The paper covering should be wet. For a pet, the end is held firmly pressed against the skin, such as between the front legs or on the belly. The other hand of the adult is used for testing in the usual way. The adult must wear an inductor for surrogate testing as well as you, the tester.

An ill or bedridden person may be tested without inconvenience or stress. He or she rests their whole hand on the skin of your leg, just above the knee. A wet piece of paper towel, about 4 inches by 4 inches is placed on your leg, to make better contact. You <u>must</u> use an inductor for yourself with this method. You may now proceed to probe on <u>your</u> hand instead of the ill person's.

Lesson Ten

Purpose: To test for cancer.

Materials: Ortho-phospho-tyrosine. Here are three ways to obtain some:

1. Order a pure sample from a chemical company (see *Sources*). Place a few milligrams (it need not be weighed) in a small glass bottle, add 2 tsp. filtered water and ¼ tsp. grain alcohol.

2. All persons with cancer have ortho-phospho-tyrosine in their saliva as well as in the cancerous tissue. Obtain a saliva specimen from a person who has active cancer. Freeze it if you can't prepare it immediately. Keep such specimens well marked in an additional sealed plastic bag. Persons who have recently been treated clinically for cancer are much less likely to have ortho-phospho-tyrosine in the saliva.

3. There is still another way to prepare an ortho-phospho-tyrosine test sample. Common snails from a fish tank or outdoor snails are the natural hosts for *Fasciolopsis buskii* (human intestinal fluke) stages. The stages will produce ortho-phospho-tyrosine when the snails are fed fish food polluted with isopropyl alcohol. Over half the fish food cans I purchased had isopropyl alcohol pollution. Buy several brands of fish food. Test them for isopropyl alcohol and benzene. Obtain some snails, put them in a tank, feed them isopropyl alcohol polluted fish food. (Feed a separate group of snails benzene polluted fish food to obtain samples of HIV.) After two days put each snail in a

zipped plastic bag, and test them individually against someone diagnosed with cancer or their saliva. The snails that the person or saliva tests positive to have ortho-phospho-tyrosine. Put these snails in the freezer to kill them humanely, then crush them and place in a specimen bottle with 50% grain alcohol to preserve. The bottles can be kept sealed and at room temperature.

Similarly, your benzene snails can be tested against someone known to be HIV positive. Saliva does not show the virus in early infections. Any snails that test positive can be used to prepare an HIV test specimen in the same way. The fish food must be tested for both benzene and isopropyl alcohol pollution, and separated appropriately, or you run the risk of making specimens that have both ortho-phospho-tyrosine and HIV.

Method:
1. Test for cancer by placing the test sample you just made (any of the three) on one plate and a white blood cell sample on the other plate.
2. If you resonate with both samples in the circuit you have cancer. Immediately, search for your cancer in your breast, prostate, skin, lungs, colon, and so forth.

As you know by now, you can confirm the cancer by testing yourself to isopropyl alcohol and the human intestinal fluke in the liver. You should eliminate isopropyl alcohol from use and zap all parasites. Keep testing yourself for cancer until it is gone. It should take less than one hour. Also take the herbal parasite program plus Mop Up. Continue to test yourself for isopropyl alcohol and the intestinal fluke in the white blood cells; make sure they are gone. Also test yourself for *Ascaris*, copper, and Freon.

Lesson Eleven

Purpose: To test for HIV.

Materials: Purchase a few milligrams of Protein 24 antigen (a piece of the HIV virus core) or the complete HIV virus on a slide. You may use the vial unopened if only one test specimen is needed. To make more specimens, use about 1 milligram per ½ ounce bottle. Add 2 tsp. filtered water and ¼ tsp. grain alcohol. Or prepare an HIV specimen from snails as described in the previous Lesson.

Method: Search in the thymus (throat sweet breads), vagina and penis for the virus because that is where it will reside almost exclusively for the first year or two. If you don't have those tissue specimens, you could search in urine, blood, saliva, or white blood cells, but only a positive result can be trusted. Also search for the human intestinal fluke and benzene in the thymus. Of course, a positive test in these tissues is very significant. If you are positive, zap parasites immediately. You should test negative in less than an hour. Remove benzene polluted items from your lifestyle. Also test yourself to several varieties of popcorn, brown rice, and corn chips as an indication of zearalenone, which must be eliminated in order to get well. Follow up on yourself every few days to be sure your new found health is continuing. Test yourself for Freon.

Lesson Twelve

Purpose: To test for diseases of all kinds.

Materials: Use slides and cultures of disease organisms. Homemade preparations of strep throat, acute mononucleosis, thrush (*Candida*), chicken pox, *Herpes* 1 and 2, eczema, shingles, warts, measles, yeast, fungus, rashes, colds, sore throats, sinus problems, tobacco virus, and so forth can all be made by

501

swabbing or scraping the affected part. A plastic spoon or bit of paper towel works well. Put a small bit on a slide. Add a drop of balsam and a cover slip. Or put the towel in a bottle, add water and alcohol as described previously. Microscope slides can greatly expand your test set (see *Sources*).

Method: Test yourself for a variety of diseases, using your white blood cell specimen first. Then search in organs like the liver, pancreas, spleen. Notice how many of these common illnesses don't "go away" at all. They are alive and well in some organ. They are merely not making you sick!

Lesson Thirteen

To test for AIDS.

Materials: Benzene sample, slides of tissue samples like thymus, liver, pancreas, penis, and vagina. Also a collection of disease specimens such as the ones used in the previous lesson.

Method: Search in the thymus for benzene. If it is positive throughout the day, <u>you are at risk</u> for developing AIDS, although you may not be ill. Search other tissues for benzene. The more tissues with benzene in them the more serious the situation. Immediately search all your body products and foods for benzene.

Stay off benzene polluted items forever.

Tally up the diseases you tested positive for in Lesson Twelve. Test at least ten. If you had more than half positive you already have AIDS. (50% is my standard, you may set your own; an ideal standard for defining a healthy person should be 0% positive.) Immediately take 900 mg of vitamin B_2.

Lesson Fourteen

Purpose: To test for aflatoxin.

Materials: Do not try to purchase a pure sample of aflatoxin; it is one of the most potent carcinogens known. Having it on hand would constitute unnecessary hazard, even though the bottle would never need to be opened. Simply make specimens of beer, moldy bread, apple cider vinegar, and any kind of peanuts using a very small amount and adding filtered water and grain alcohol as usual.

Method: Test yourself for these. If you have all of them in your white blood cells and the liver then you very, very probably have aflatoxin built up. Next, test your daily foods for their presence in your white blood cells. Those that test positive must be further tested for aflatoxin. Notice the effect of vitamin C on aflatoxin in your liver. Find a time when your liver is positive to aflatoxin (eat a few roasted peanuts from a health food store and wait ten minutes). Take 1 gram vitamin C in a glass of water. Check yourself for aflatoxin every five minutes. Does it clear? If not, take 5 or 10 grams vitamin C. How long does it take?

Lesson Fifteen

Purpose: To test for parasites.

Method: If you test positive to your pet's saliva, you have something in common—a parasite, no doubt. You must search your muscles and liver for these, not saliva or white blood cells, because they are seldom seen in these. Zap yourself for parasites until you no longer test positive to your pets' saliva.

Tapeworms and tapeworm stages can not (and should not) be killed with a regular frequency generator. Each segment, and probably each scolex in a cysticercus has its own frequency and might disperse if your generator misses it. Only <u>zapping</u> kills all and is safe for tapeworms. However, the zapper current does not penetrate and kill an intact cysticercus stage. You must use the Mop Up program.

Be sure to treat your pet on a daily basis with the pet parasite program.

Lesson Sixteen

Purpose: To see how sensitive your measurements can be. (How much of a substance must be present for you to get a positive result?)

Materials: filtered water, salt, glass cup measure, 13 new glass bottles that hold at least ¼ cup, 14 new plastic teaspoons, your skin tissue sample, paper towel.

Method: Some of the best measurement systems available today are immunological (such as an ELISA assay) and can detect as little as 100 fg/ml (femtograms per milliliter). A milliliter is about as big as a pea, and a femtogram is $1/1,000,000,000,000,000$th (10^{-15}) of a gram!

1. Rinse the glass cup measure with filtered water and put one half teaspoon of table salt in it. Fill to one cup, stirring with a plastic spoon. What concentration is this? A teaspoon is about 5 grams, a cup is about 230 ml (milliliters), therefore the starting concentration is about 2½ (2.5) gm per 230 ml, or .01 gm/ml (we will discuss the amount of error later).

2. Label one clean plastic spoon "water" and use it to put nine spoonfuls of filtered water in a clean glass bottle. Use another plastic spoon to transfer one spoonful of the .01 gm/ml salt solution in the cup measure to the glass bottle, stir, then discard the spoon. The glass bottle now

has a 1 in 10 dilution, and its concentration is one tenth the original, or .001 gm/ml.

3. Use the "water" spoon to put nine spoonfuls of filtered water in bottle #2. Use a new spoon to transfer a spoonful of salt solution from bottle #1 to bottle #2 and stir briefly (never shake). Label bottle #2 ".0001 gm/ml".

4. Repeat with remaining bottles. Bottle #13 would therefore be labeled ".000000000000001 gm/ml." This is 10^{-15} gm/ml, or 1 femtogram/ml.

5. Do the skin test with water from bottle #13 as in Lesson Five. If you can detect this, you are one hundred times as sensitive as an ELISA assay (and you should make a bottle #14 and continue if you are curious how good your sensitivity can get). If you can not, try to detect water from bottle #12 (ten times as sensitive as ELISA). Continue until you reach a bottle you can detect.

Calculate the error for your experiment by assuming you could be off by as much as 10% when measuring the salt and water adding up to 20% error in each of the 13 dilutions. This is a total error in bottle #13 of 280%, or at most a factor of 3. So bottle #13 could be anywhere from 0.33 to 3 femtogram/ml. If you can detect water from bottle #13, you are <u>definitely</u> more sensitive then an ELISA, in spite of your crude utensils and inexpensive equipment! Note that the starting error of using 2.5 gm instead of 2.3 gm only adds another 10% error.

If you want to calculate how many salt <u>molecules</u> you can detect, select the concentration at the limit of your detection, and put 2 drops on a square inch of paper towel and rub into your skin. Assume one drop can be absorbed. If you can detect water from bottle #13, you have detected 510,000 molecules (10^{-15} fg/ml divided by 58.5 gm/M multiplied by 6.02×10^{23} molecules/M divided by 20 drops/ml). Water in bottle #12 would therefore have 10 times as many molecules in one drop, and so forth. Even if your error is as much as a factor of 2 (100%), you can still get a good idea of what you can measure.

Atomic absorption standards start at exact concentrations; it is easy to make a more exact dilution series with them. When testing for iridium chloride by this skin test method, I was able to detect 3025 molecules!

Troubleshooting:

Always extend your set until you get a negative result (this should happen by at least bottle #18). If you always "detect" salt, then you <u>shook</u> the bottle!

Never try to reuse a bottle if you spill when pouring into it. Get another new bottle.

Sensitivity of Pollutant-In-Product Testing

Get some slides of *Salmonellas* and *Shigellas* and find some milk that tests positive to at least one. Make a dilution series of the milk up to bottle #14, being careful not to shake the bottles. Start with 2 drops of milk in bottle #1. Use an eye dropper to deliver 2 drops to subsequent bottles. Begin testing at bottle #14, using the slide that tested positive. You will learn to search by frequency later. My sensitivity was routinely around bottle #12, for a variety of pathogens. It was the same for toxic elements starting with standard solutions, about 1000 µg/ml, showing this method is less sensitive than skin testing.

Lesson Seventeen

Purpose: To test for fluke disease.

A small number of intestinal flukes resident in the intestine may not give you any noticeable symptoms. Similarly, sheep liver flukes resident in the liver and pancreatic flukes in the pancreas may not cause noticeable symptoms. Their eggs are shed through the organ ducts to the intestine and out with the bowel movement. They hatch and go through various stages of development outdoors and in other animals. <u>But if you become the total host</u> so that various stages are developing in <u>your</u> organs, you have what I term *fluke disease*. I have found that cancer, HIV, diabetes, endometriosis, Hodgkin's disease, Alzheimer's disease, lupus, MS and "universal allergy syndrome" are examples of fluke disease.

You can test for fluke disease in two ways: electronically <u>and</u> by microscope observation.

Materials: Cultures or slides of flukes and fluke stages from a biological supply company (see *Sources*) including eggs, miracidia, redia, cercaria, metacercaria. Body fluid specimens to help you locate them for observation under a microscope.

Method: Test for fluke stages in your white blood cells first. If you have any fluke stages in your white blood cells you may wish to see them with your own eyes. To do this, you must first locate them. Place your body fluid samples on one plate, your parasite stages on the other plate, and test for as many as you were able to procure, besides adults. After finding a stage electronically, you stand a better chance of finding it physically with a microscope.

Microscopy Lesson

Purpose: To *observe* fluke stages in saliva and urine with a microscope.

Materials:

a. A low power microscope. High power is not needed. A total of 100x magnification is satisfactory for the four common flukes, *Fasciolopsis, sheep liver fluke, human liver fluke* and *pancreatic fluke.*

b. Glass slides and coverslips.

c. A disposable eye dropper.

d. For sanitation purposes (wiping table tops, slides, microscope and your hands) a 50% to 70% alcohol solution (not rubbing alcohol!) is best. Dilute 95% grain alcohol 7 parts alcohol plus 3 parts water. Vodka or 76% grain alcohol can be used undiluted.

e. Formaldehyde, 20%. Formaldehyde 37% is commonly available at pharmacies. Dilute this with equal parts of filtered water to get 18½%, which is close enough to 20%, for the purpose of "fixing" (killing) the specimens. Store in a glass bottle in the garage, away from sunlight. Label. Specimens that are fixed properly do not lose their life-like appearance.

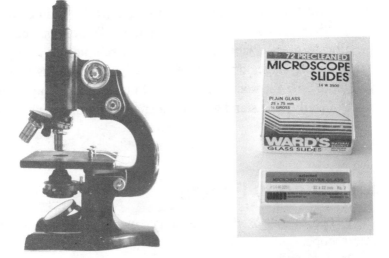

Fig. 92 Microscope, slides and coverslips.

f. Iodine solution. This is only useful for the urine specimens. Lugol's iodine and tincture of iodine are both use-

ful. Ask a pharmacist to prepare *Lugol's Iodine Solution* for you, as follows:
- 44 grams (1½ oz) iodine crystals
- 88 grams (3 oz) potassium iodide crystals

Dissolve both in 1 liter (quart) filtered water. This may take a day of frequent shaking.

Method for saliva:

1. Pour the 20% formaldehyde into a small amber bottle or other receptacle to a depth of about 1/8 inch. Keep tightly closed.
2. The person to be tested is asked to salivate into the bottle so the organisms are immediately "fixed" without undergoing cooling first. The total volume should be about double the original amount of formaldehyde used. Make a mark on the container so the subject knows how much to produce. The resultant concentration of formaldehyde will be about 10%.
3. Shake the bottle a few times. Set it aside for 24 hours to settle (less if testing is urgent).
4. With a dropper, draw up some of the bottom settlings. Put one drop on a slide and apply a coverslip.
5. View under low power of microscope. Compare objects you observe with specimens obtained on slides from biological supply companies.

Note: Persons with HIV and moderate AIDS will show about one to ten parasite stages per slide. It requires several hours of searching. Persons with HIV and severe AIDS show 10 or more fluke stages per slide; this makes the task of finding them much easier. Persons with terminal untreated cancer have many more fluke stages than relatively well persons.

Method for urine:

1. Prepare bottles of formaldehyde fixative ahead of time. Put about ¼ to ½ inch of 20% formaldehyde in each. Keep tightly closed.
2. Add <u>freshly voided</u>[63] urine from cancer or HIV sufferers to the formaldehyde in approximately equal amounts, resulting in a 10% formaldehyde solution. Shake immediately. Let settle several hours. The sediment has a higher number of fluke stages. Cancer victims with cervical or prostate cancer will show higher numbers of stages in urine than other cancer types.
3. Staining the slide is optional. It helps to outline fluke stages slightly. Prepare Lugol's solution as described above.

   Slides may be stained in either of these two ways:
   - Put a drop of "fixed" urine on a slide. Add a drop of 50% Lugol's (dilute 1:1 with filtered water). Apply coverslip.
   - Put a drop of "fixed" urine on a slide. Apply coverslip. Add 1 to 3 drops of 50% Lugol's to edge of coverslip and allow it to seep in.

Note: persons who have been treated for cancer or HIV using any of the known drugs may show only 1 to 2 fluke parasite stages per drop of saliva or urine. For this reason, you may need to search through 20 or more slides to find flukes. Very ill persons may show up to 10 parasites per drop (slide).

Taking Pictures Of What You See

You may be unsure of what you see even if you have the microscope slides of labeled flukes and their stages to study and

---

[63] Urine that has cooled even slightly below body temperature does not show miracidia and redia in their original shapes.

compare. In real life, they vary so much in shape and size that absolute identification is difficult without experience. Unfortunately in a few hours, just as you are getting proficient, your magnificent specimens will be drying out and unfit for observation. To preserve them longer you can seal the edges by painting around the coverslip with fingernail clear enamel. Or dribble hot sealing wax along the edges and then place them in sealed plastic bags (one per bag). Melt sealing wax in a metal jar lid. Make an applicator from a piece of coat hanger wire bent in the shape of a small square to fit around the coverslip and a handle.

Or take photographs. To take pictures of what you see under the microscope you will need a photomicrographic camera, which costs $200.00 and up (see *Sources*). It is easy to use. Remember to label your pictures so you know which slide they came from.

Even photographs do not scientifically prove identity of parasite stages, but it is very good evidence. Proof would require that the saliva or urine sample could be cultured and seen to produce the known parasite stages. Hopefully, this will soon be done.

The Tests

It is tempting to think that the 300+ tests I use are definitive, and by getting rid of the parasites, toxins, solvents, pathogens and fungi we are guaranteed good health. But there are far more of each of these than we will ever have samples of. Fortunately, we think we know the major culprits. If you clean these up, then you can expect most, if not all, of your symptoms to go away.

I see food mold, solvent pollution, metal pollution, and parasitism as being the major threats to our health at this time. Molds prevent the liver from detoxifying solvents. Solvents induce parasites to invade animals and tissues that they have never gotten a foothold in before, causing cancer, HIV/AIDS and a number of other modern diseases. Metal lowers glutathione levels, and with it your immunity to these diseases. These events are totally unsuspected, with virtually no federal research dollars being spent on them compared to the grants for viral and bacterial research. Meanwhile, our beef and poultry supplies are being quietly overrun by parasites, exposing us to new levels of hazard. Even our pets are newly parasitized and can infect us, too!

Although you may think your only goal is to get the human intestinal fluke out of your liver so that ortho-phospho-tyrosine stops being produced, it is just as important to completely clean up your body. This allows you not only to stop the tumors from metastasizing, but to shrink and eliminate them, so that you can become completely well.

Cancer

Although there are no true clinical cancer tests, there are more than two dozen markers.[64] Each can identify a particular cancer with reasonable accuracy. Recently, ortho-phospho-tyrosine has been found to be reliable for many kinds of human malignancies.

The ortho-phospho-tyrosine sample was prepared by dissolving several milligrams in 10 ml filtered water and kept permanently sealed in a ½ ounce amber glass bottle. The hCG sample was similarly prepared.

HIV

There are a variety of antibody tests used clinically, which detect whether you have made antibodies to the HIV virus. Obviously, you must have had the virus at some time in the past in order to make the antibodies. And since nobody ever gets rid of the virus once they have it (unless they de-parasitize), it is a perfectly adequate diagnostic test.

But if you kill the intestinal fluke and its stages, thereby eliminating the virus, you do not stop making the antibodies. For this reason another type of clinical test is needed. Protein 24 (P24) antigen is an actual piece of the HIV virus itself. The P24 test, therefore is testing for the actual virus, not antibodies to it. It is like taking a small piece of elephant skin to the zoo to search for elephants. I selected the clinical P24 test to <u>clinically</u> prove the absence of the HIV virus, because the antibody test would remain positive even after the HIV virus is gone.

---

[64] Stewart Sell, MD, *Diagnostic Uses of Cancer Markers*, The Female Patient, Vol. 9, August 1984.

Another clinical test, PCR-HIV1-RNA (quantitative) also tests for the presence of virus itself. It seeks out the nucleic acid that is specific for the virus. Bear in mind, however, that both the P24 test and PCR tests are still chemical in nature, and are affected by factors which may allow false results to occur. The laboratory test method, of course, tries to take this into account.

My electronic test uses the same P24 antigen, one half milligram dissolved in 3 ml filtered water permanently sealed in a ½ ounce amber glass bottle.

I have also used a slide with lung tissue infected with HIV and got identical results.

Parasites

I test for about 120 different parasites or stages of parasites. (They are divided into Box 1 and Box 2 which you may see referred to in the case histories.) Below is a list of the parasites. They are on slides purchased from biological supply companies. Some are cultures in small vials. Most of them are whole mounts of the adult stage. Some are slides of eggs and other stages.

They are searched for in the white blood cells. This means that encysted forms such as tapeworm cysticercus and Toxoplasma cysts are missed because the immune system is not attacking them. They have to be searched for separately in the tissue suspected (muscles, eyes, etc.).

The importance of testing for a list of parasites is not to cure cancer. *Fasciolopsis buskii*, the human intestinal fluke, has already been identified in my research as the critical cancer parasite. It is the remainder, however, that are undoubtedly contributing to your inability to regain your health. Tracking their demise as you stay on the parasite killing recipe lets you see your progress.

Parasite	Comment
Acanthamoeba culbertsoni	
Acanthocephala	worm
Anaplasma marginale	sporozoa from cows
Ancylostoma braziliense (adult)	hookworm (from dogs and cats)
Ancylostoma caninum	dog hookworm, causes fatigue, anemia, muscle ache
Ancylostoma duodenale male	hookworm
Ascaris eggs	common roundworm of cats and dogs
Ascaris larvae in lung	common roundworm of cats and dogs
Ascaris lumbricoides	common round worm of cats, dogs, humans. Brings with it *Bacteroides fragilis* and *Coxsackie* viruses. Eggs bring *Rhizobium leguminosarum*, *Mycobacterium avium*.
Ascaris megalocephala	roundworm of horse
Babesia bigemina	
Babesia canis smear	sporozoa of dog blood
Balantidium coli cysts	
Balantidium sp. trophozoites parasitic ciliate	
Besnoitia	sporozoa in lung
Blastocystis hominis	yeast in intestine
Capillaria hepatica	roundworm in liver, from rats and cats
Chilomastix cysts	from rats
Chilomastix mesnili (trophozoites)	flagellate in intestine (from rat)
Chilomonas	ciliate
Clonorchis metacercariae	human liver fluke stage
Clonorchis sinensis	human liver fluke adult
Clonorchis sinensis eggs	
Cryptocotyle lingua (adult)	fluke of sea gull
Cryptosporidium parvum	a coccidian, causes diarrhea
Cysticercus fasciolaris	cyst stage of *Taenia taeniaeformis*, tapeworm of pets
Dientamoeba fragilis	a trichomonad, not an amoeba
Dipetalonema perstans	round worm
Diphyllobothrium erinacei (Mansoni) scolex	tapeworm of dogs and cats (head)
Diphyllobothrium latum (scolex)	fish tapeworm (head)
Dipylidium caninum	dog tapeworm
Dipylidium caninum (scolex)	dog tapeworm (head)
Dirofilaria immitis	heartworm of dogs, causes pain over heart, irregular heartbeat in humans
Echinococcus granulosus	small tapeworm (pets)
Echinococcus granulosus (cysts)	tapeworm *cysticercus*, brings *Streptomyces sp.* fungus.
Echinococcus granulosus (eggs)	small tapeworm, stage

Echinococcus multilocularis	tapeworm of pets
Echinoporyphium recurvatum	fluke of poultry
Echinostoma revolutum	flatworm of water foul
Eimeria stiedae	sporozoa of rabbit
Eimeria tenella	sporozoa of large intestine
Endamoeba gingivalis trophozoite	amoeba of gums
Endolimax nana trophozoites, cysts	protozoan
Entamoeba coli cysts	amoeba in small and large intestine
Entamoeba histolytica trophozoites	common amoeba in intestine
Enterobius vermicularis	human pinworm
Eurytrema pancreaticum	common fluke of pancreas (from pigs and cattle), causes diabetes
Fasciola hepatica	sheep liver fluke of mammals, adult
Fasciola hepatica cercariae, eggs, metacercariae, miracidia, rediae	sheep liver fluke stages
Fasciolopsis buskii	human intestinal fluke, adult
Fasciolopsis buskii eggs, miracidia, rediae	human intestinal fluke stages. Brings with it HIV.
Fasciolopsis cercariae	human intestinal fluke stage. Brings with it HIV.
Fischoedrius elongatus	liver fluke of cats
Gastrothylax elongatus	fluke
Giardia lamblia (trophozoites)	common flagellate in intestine
Giardia lamblia cysts	common flagellate in intestine
Gyrodactylus	a fluke
Haemonchus contortus	large stomach roundworm of domestic animals
Haemoproteus	sporozoa, causes bird malaria
Hasstile sig. tricolor (adult)	rabbit fluke
Heterakis	round worm of chickens
Heterophyes heterophyes	fluke of intestine (from crawfish)
Hymenolepis cysticercoides	small tapeworm of pets
Hymenolepis diminuta	small tapeworm of pets
Hypodereum conoideum	fluke of poultry
Iodamoeba butschlii trophozoites and cysts	small amoeba of colon
Leishmania braziliensis	flagellate
Leishmania donovani	infects spleen and liver (from hamsters)
Leishmania mexicana	protozoa
Leishmania tropica	flagellate, infects skin
Leucocytozoon	sporozoa, causes bird malaria
Loa loa	a heart parasite, causes irregular heartbeat
Macracanthorhynchus	spiny headed worm of pig
Metagonimus	fluke of intestine
Metagonimus Yokogawai	a liver fluke
Moniezia (scolex)	large tapeworm of domestic animal (head)

Moniezia expansa	large tapeworm of domestic animals
Monocystis agilis	sporozoa from earth worm
Multiceps serialis	dog tapeworm
Myxosoma	sporozoa from fish gill
Naegleria fowleri	parasite of brain
Necator americanus	human hookworm
Notocotylus quinqeserialis	fluke of intestine (from muskrat)
Onchocerca volvulus	roundworm
Paragonimus Westermanii adult	lung fluke (from pets)
Passalurus ambiguus	rabbit pinworm
Pigeon tapeworm	
Plasmodium cynomolgi	malaria of monkey
Plasmodium falciparum smear	sporozoa of blood, causes malaria
Plasmodium vivax smear	sporozoa of blood, causes benign malaria
Platynosomum fastosum adult	Cat liver fluke
Pneumocystis carinii	sporozoa of the lung from rat
Prosthogonimus macrorchis (eggs)	fluke
Sarcocystis	sporozoa of muscles
Schistosoma haematobium	blood fluke
Schistosoma mansoni	blood fluke of veins
Stephanurus dentalus (ova)	roundworm
Stigeoclonium	
Strongyloides (filariform larva)	human threadworm, causes migraine headache
Taenia pisiformis	tapeworm of cats
Taenia pisiformis (cysticercus)	tapeworm of cats, stage
Taenia saginata (cysticercus)	beef tapeworm, stage
Taenia solium (cysticercus)	pork tapeworm, stage
Taenia solium (scolex)	pork tapeworm
Toxocara (eggs)	roundworm of cats
Toxoplasma (human strain)	sporozoa of mice, cats, etc.; causes eye disease
Trichinella spiralis (muscle)	roundworm, invades muscles, causes myalgia (from pets)
Trichomonas muris	flagellate of rat
Trichomonas vaginalis	protozoa of genital tract
Trichuris sp.	whipworm
Trypanosoma brucei	blood parasite (from rat)
Trypanosoma cruzi	blood flagellate (from mouse)
Trypanosoma equiperdium	causes sleeping sickness
Trypanosoma gambiense	blood flagellate, causes African sleeping sickness (from rat)
Trypanosoma lewisi	blood flagellate of rat
Trypanosoma rhodesiense	blood flagellate, causes sleeping sickness (from rat)
Urocleidus	a fluke

Toxic Elements

I call a substance "toxic" if it can be found in your white blood cells (the immune system). The concept is that if something is found in the white blood cells, it must be harmful to your body or at least useless. Even if the substance isn't harmful, if it preoccupies your immune system, it is a handicap to your body.

Some of the test items, like aluminum silicate, are compounds, not simply elements. Since there are thousands upon thousands of toxic chemicals in our environment and there would be no way of testing them all, my system of using the elements instead of the compounds is a short cut. For this reason, the test is far from perfect. For example, a person may test positive to aluminum silicate but show no aluminum in the white blood cells. So, if I had tested only for aluminum, I would have missed the problem.

Sometimes, toxic elements are present in an organ, but are not present in the white blood cells. For example, there may be mercury stored in the pancreas, but not be showing in the white blood cells at the time I'm testing. I interpret this as reflecting low levels of the toxin. Ideally, a test would search all your organs, but this would be too time-consuming for my technology.

Most of the toxic elements are metals, heavy metals and lanthanides. But some are not; examples are PCBs and formaldehyde.

Some important elements are missing, like iron, zinc and manganese. This is because I never could find them present in the white blood cells, and I finally gave up searching for them.

The most important thing to do after finding the toxic element in your body is to track down the source of it in your environment. Is it in food, air, drugs, vitamins? To test a pill or food, it is put in a plastic bag with filtered water added and tested the same way as the elements. To test the air in a person's

519

home, an open glass jar, containing filtered water, is set out for 3 days in the room to be tested. Fine particles and gas molecules stick to dust in the air and fall into the water. The jar is then used like any other test solution.

Alternatively, a dust sample can be obtained by wiping the kitchen table or counter with a dampened piece of paper towel, two inches by two inches square. It is then placed in a plastic baggie.

Below is a list of the 70 or so toxic elements in the test. Most of them were obtained as Atomic Absorption Standard Solutions and are, therefore, very pure. This prevents mistakes in identifying a toxin. They were stored in ½ ounce brown glass bottles with bakelite caps and permanently sealed with plastic film since testing did not require them to be opened. The exact concentration and the solubility characteristics are not important in this qualitative test. The main sources of these substances in our environment are given beside each item.

Toxic Substance	Sources
Aflatoxin B	beer, bread, apple cider vinegar, moldy fruit, nuts
Aluminum	cookware, deodorant, lotions, soaps
Aluminum silicate	salt, water softener
Antimony	fragrance in lotions, colognes
Arsenic	pesticide, "treated" carpet, wallpaper
Asbestos	clothes dryer belt, hair blower, paint on radiators
Barium	lipstick, bus exhaust
Benzalkonium chloride	toothpaste
3,4 Benzopyrene	flame cooked foods, toast
4,5 Benzopyrene	flame cooked foods, toast
Beryllium	hurricane lamps, gasoline, dentures, kerosene
Bismuth	colognes, lotions, antacids
Bisphenol-A	dental plastic
Boron	
Bromine	bleached "brominated" flour
Cadmium	galvanized water pipes, old tooth fillings
Cerium	tooth fillings
Cesium	clear plastic bottles used for beverages
Chlorine	from Chlorox™ bleach
Chromium	cosmetics, water softener

Cobalt	detergent, blue and green body products
Copper	tooth fillings, water pipes
Dysprosium	paint and varnish
Erbium	packaging for food, pollutant in pills
Europium	tooth fillings
Europium oxide	tooth fillings, catalytic converter
Fiberglass	dust from remodeling or building insulation
Formaldehyde	foam in mattresses and furniture, paneling
Gadolinium	tooth fillings
Gallium	tooth fillings
Germanium	with thallium in tooth fillings (pollutant)
Gold	tooth fillings
Hafnium	hair spray, nail polish, pollutant in pills
Holmium	usually found in presence of PCBs
Indium	tooth fillings
Iridium	tooth fillings
Lanthanum	computer and printing supplies
Lead	solder joints in water pipes
Lithium	printing supplies
Lutetium	paint and varnish
Maleic acid	dental plastic
Maleic Anhydride	dental plastic
Malonic acid	certain plants, dental plastic.
D-malic acid	dental plastic
Mercury	tooth fillings
Methyl Malonic acid	dental plastic
Molybdenum	auto supplies
Neodymium	pollutant in pills
Nickel	tooth fillings, metal glasses frames
Niobium	pollutant in pills, foil packaging for food
Palladium	tooth fillings
Platinum	tooth fillings
Polychlorinated biphenyl PCB	detergent, hair spray, salves
Polyvinyl chloride acetate (PVC)	glues, building supplies, leaking cooling system
Praseodymium	pollutant in pills
Radon	cracks in basement cement, water pipes
Rhenium	spray starch
Rhodium	tooth fillings
Rubidium	tooth fillings
Ruthenium	tooth fillings
Samarium	tooth fillings
Scandium	tooth fillings
Selenium	
Silver	tooth fillings
Sodium fluoride	toothpaste
Strontium	toothpaste, water softener

Tantalum	tooth fillings
Tartrazine	yellow food dye in cheese, jello, etc.
Tellurium	tooth fillings
Terbium	pollutant in pills
Thallium acetate	pollutant in mercury tooth fillings
Thorium nitrate	earth (dust)
Thulium	pollutant in some brands of vitamin C
Tin	toothpaste
Titanium	tooth fillings, body powder
Tungsten	electric water heater, toaster, hair curler
Uranium acetate	earth (dust)
Urethane	plastic teeth and dental resins
Vanadium pentoxide	gas leak in home, dental metal and dental plastic
Ytterbium	pollutant in pills
Yttrium	pollutant in pills
Zirconium	deodorant, toothpaste

Elements like erbium and terbium have only recently come into use. They were formerly called Rare Earth Elements but now are called *Lanthanides*. There are 15 of them: lanthanum cerium, praseodymium, neodymium, samarium, europium, gadolinium, terbium, dysprosium, holmium, erbium, thulium, ytterbium, lutetium, and promethium.

All except promethium are in my test for toxic elements. You can see from the case histories that we have lanthanides in our bodies, widely distributed. They are in our processed foods, in our supplements and medicines, and in our tooth fillings, whether plastic or metal. Is it a good idea for the human species to eat elements that we know nothing about? Several of them absorb UV (ultraviolet) light. Should we be absorbing UV light in this manner when we already have a biological means (riboflavin, vitamin B_2) of doing this that took millions of years to evolve? Some of them have special magnetic properties (gadolinium and samarium). Some of them are phosphors; they give off light when irradiated. A number of them are known to "home in" on cancerous tumors. This is not understood. Why are they in our tablets and capsules? Who is making these polluted products? Evidently, the traditional safeguards against massive pollution don't work. It should be possible to make a test strip that detects Rare Earth Elements as a group, since they have very similar properties. Government agencies should supply them because it is in the public interest to keep society healthy. The public must not rely on reassurances by industry or government that food or body products are pure and safe. People must be able to test them for themselves.

Solvents

This is a list of all the solvents in the test together with the main source of them in our environment. These are chemicals, very pure, obtained from chemical supply companies, unless otherwise stated. Those marked with an asterisk (*) were the subject of a recent book *The Neurotoxicity of Solvents* by Peter Arlien-Soburg, 1992, CRC Press.

Solvent	Source
1,1,1, Trichloro ethane* (TCE)	flavored foods
2, 5-Hexane dione*	flavored foods
2 Butanone* (methyl ethyl ketone)	flavored foods
2 Hexanone* (methyl butyl ketone)	flavored foods
2 Methyl propanol	
2 Propanol (propyl alcohol)	see the isopropyl alcohol list
Acetone	store-bought drinking water, cold cereals, pet food, animal feed
Acetonylacetone (2,5 hexanedione)	flavored foods
Benzene	see the benzene list (page 160)
Butyl nitrite	
Carbon tetrachloride	store-bought drinking water, cold cereals, pet food, animal feeds
Decane	health food cookies and cereals
Denatured alcohol	obtained from pharmacy
Dichloromethane* (methylene chloride)	store-bought orange juice, herb tea blends

Gasoline regular leaded	obtained at gasoline station
Grain alcohol	95% ethyl alcohol obtained at liquor store
Hexanes*	decaffeinated beverages
Isophorone	flavored foods
Kerosene	obtained at gasoline station
Methanol (wood alcohol)	colas, artificial sweeteners, infant formula
Mineral oil	lotions
Mineral spirits	obtained from paint store
Paradiclorobenzene	mothballs
Pentane	decaffeinated beverages
Petroleum ether	in some gasolines
Styrene*	styrofoam dishes
Toluene*	store-bought drinking water, cold cereals
Trichloroethylene* (TCEthylene)	flavored foods
Xylene*	store-bought drinking water, cold cereals

Pathogens

Pathogens are mostly bacteria and viruses, but also may include molds and yeasts. Most of them are on slides, some are preserved cultures, all are purchased from biological supply companies (see *Sources*). They are safe for you to handle.

Bacteria or Virus	Comment
Adenovirus	causes common cold
Alpha streptococcus	respiratory infection
Bacillus anthracis	causes anthrax in cattle
Bacillus cereus	
Bacillus megaterium	soil
Bacterium acnes	causes acne
Bacteroides fragilis	always found with *Ascaris*
Beta streptococcus	causes respiratory infection
Blepharisma	
Bordetella pertussis	"whooping cough"
Borellia burgdorferi	Lyme disease
Campylobacter fetus smear	stomach and vein disease
Campylobacter pyloridis	stomach and vein disease
Candida albicans (pure powder)	common yeast, causes thrush
Capsules of bacteria	
Caulobacter vibrioides	
Central spores (bacillus smear)	

Chlamydia trachomatis	eye disease
Clostridium acetobutylicum	*Clostridium* species inhabit cancerous
Clostridium botulinum	tumors enabling their growth by chang-,
Clostridium perfringens	ing RNA to DNA. Naturally present in
Clostridium septicum (human blood)	colon. Occur in crevices under tooth
Clostridium sporogenes	fillings, dairy products.
Clostridium tetani	
Corynebacterium diptheriae	causes diphtheria
Corynebacterium xerosis	causes stiffness
Coxsackie virus B-1	always found with Bacteroides fragilis
Coxsackie virus B-4	always found with Bacteroides fragilis
Crithidia fasciculata	
Cytomegalovirus (CMV) antigen	
Cytophaga rubra	
Diplococcus pneumoniae	respiratory illness
Eikanella corrodens	
Enterobacter aerogenes	intestinal bacterium
Epstein Barre virus (EBV)	fatigue, found with Strep G[65]
Erwinia carotovora	
Escherichia coli (E. coli)	intestinal bacterium
Gaffkya tetragena	causes respiratory infections
Gardnerella vaginalis	ovarian and genital tract infection
Haemophilus influenzae	bacterial meningitis, infects joints
Hepatitis B antigen	
Herpes simplex 1	causes "cold sores"
Herpes simplex 2	causes genital herpes
Herpes Zoster	"shingles"
Histomonas meleagridis (liver)	
Histoplasma capsulatum	
Human papilloma plantar wart #4	wart
Human papilloma virus #4	wart
Influenza A and B (flu shot)	
Klebsiella pneumoniae	causes pneumonia
Lactobacillus acidophilus	present in tumors and under tooth fillings; can change RNA to DNA,
Lactobacillus casei	
Leptospira interrogans	spirochete, causes arthritis
Measles antigen	
Mumps antigen	
Mycobacterium avium-intracellulare complex	causes lymph node enlargement, found in tumors
Mycobacterium phlei	in dog saliva and in soil
Mycobacterium tuberculosis (infected nodule)	causes tuberculosis

---

[65] Link between EBV, Strep G and Eurytrema made by Paul Grose, 1995.

Mycoplasma	chronic cough
Neisseria gonorrhea	causes gonorrhea
Neisseria sicca	soil
Nocardia asteroides	Parkinson's Disease, heart disease
Proteus mirabilis	urinary tract pathogen
Proteus vulgaris	in oxalate kidney stones
Pseudomonas aeruginosa	found in open wounds
Respiratory syncytial virus	
Rhizobium meliloti	
Rhizobium leguminosarum	forms nitroso compounds, found in tumors
Salmonella enteriditis	intestinal infection, pollutes dairy
Salmonella paratyphi	
Salmonella typhimurium	causes food poisoning, pollutes dairy
Serratia marcescens	occurs in water, soil, milk
Shigella dysenteriae	causes diarrhea, pollutes dairy
Shigella flexneri	depression, pollutes dairy products
Shigella sonnei	
Sphaerotilus natans	
Spirillum serpens	
Staphylococcus aureus	skin bacterium which is common cause of infections, tooth abscesses, heart disease
Staphylococcus epidermidis	infects skin and mucous membranes
Streptococcus lactis	occurs in milk
Streptococcus mitis	lung infection, tooth infection and cavities, abscesses
Streptococcus pneumoniae	pneumonia and inner ear disease
Streptococcus pyogenes	found in abscesses
Streptococcus sp. group G	sore throats, found with Eurytrema
Streptomyces sp.	inhibits RNA and protein formation
Terminal spores bacillus smear	
Tobacco mosaic virus	occurs in tobacco
Treponema pallidum	causes pain over overies
Trichomonas vaginalis	genital tract infection
Troglodytella abrassari	
Veillonella dispar	

Mycotoxins

Mycotoxin	found in	associated with
Aflatoxin	fruit, grains, nuts	cancer
Citrinin		
Citreoviridin		
Cytochalasin B	pasta	mental illness

Ergot	whole grain products, honey, alcoholic beverages	cancer
Griseofulvin		
Kojic acid	coffee, potatoes	diabetes
Ochratoxin		cancer
Patulin	apples and other fruit	cancer
Sorghum	sorghum products	purpura, stroke
Sterigmatocystin	pasta, grains	mental illness
T2-toxin	dried beans	kidney disease, hypertension (high blood pressure)
Zearalenone	chips, popcorn, brown rice	AIDS

Kidney Stones

In this test we search in the kidney for seven kinds of crystals or stones.

Stone	Comment
Cysteine	sulfur containing
Cystine	sulfur containing
Dicalcium phosphate	also causes common arthritis, hardening of arteries, spurs
Monocalcium phosphate	also causes common arthritis, hardening of arteries, spurs
Tri-calcium phosphate	also causes common arthritis, hardening of arteries, spurs
Oxalate	cause of lower back pain 95% of the time
Uric acid	also causes gout and arthritis

Stones begin as tiny crystals, much too tiny to be seen by X-ray. They get deposited in the tiny tubules that make up the kidney, partly blocking the flow of liquid. This leads to "water holding" in your tissues. As more crystals are formed, they begin to deposit in other organs, too, such as joints of feet and hands and the interior of arteries, causing hardening. The usual symptoms are low back pain, pain running down the leg, foot pain, hand pain and gout.

Oxalic acid crystals cause pain in the lower back. Uric acid causes pain in the toes. The phosphates cause pain in the other joints (arthritis). But crystals do not cause pain by themselves. Bacteria find these nutritious deposits, and ultimately, it is they and their refuse that cause pain.

By causing partial blockage, these deposits prevent heavy metals from passing out through the kidneys. Mercury and nickel from tooth fillings are constantly being excreted through the kidney tubules. But as the kidneys get older and the deluge of toxic compounds gets higher, the toxins just attach themselves to the deposits already there. Soon, a pile-up of toxins occurs in the kidney.

The treatment is the same for all persons. It is a combination of herbs and nutritional substances, which, together, can dissolve all the 7 kinds of stones. The recipe is quite long (see Kidney Cleanse, page 591). The reason for this is so the individual kinds of stones don't have to be dissolved separately. This recipe dissolves all the stones in three weeks.

Notice that some very sick or elderly people are told to take half a dose only. Persons with a history of kidney stones, who know they have large stones, are also told to drink half a dose daily. Persons with sensitive stomachs may not tolerate these herbs; they could try killing their parasites first.

It is fair to say that we all develop kidney stones; although they may remain very tiny and cause no pain.

Gallstones

We all have gallstones, so I do not test for this anymore.

Stone	Comment
Cholesterol crystals (encased in bile)	Accumulate in your liver bile ducts.

The Liver Cleanse (page 594) is recommended many times in the Case histories. This will get rid of gallstones, <u>without surgery</u>!

Blood Tests

There are many blood tests that can be performed by a clinical laboratory. In the case histories I do not list all that were done (I typically ordered about 60), but only the ones that I thought significant. Here are some I refer to in the case histories:

Test	Comment
Alk. Phos.	Alkaline phosphatase, bone enzymes. Goes up with bone disease, cancer.
Amylase	An enzyme produced by the pancreas. It should not be in the blood.
Atyp lymphs	Atypical lymphocytes. Misshaped.
Baso	Basophils, a variety of white blood cells. When over 1% is suggestive of cancer.
Blasts	Immature white blood cells, should not be in the blood.
BUN	Blood urea nitrogen. Body waste - controlled by kidneys and liver - too low, due to malonic acid, too high due to bacterial invasion.
Ca125	A cancer marker for ovarian cancer.
Calcium	Too low (below 9.0) if parathyroid problem. Too high (above 10.0) if thyroid problem. May appear normal (9.5), when problem is in both glands.
Chloride	Electrolyte, controlled by adrenal glands.
Cholesterol	High amounts are indicative of blocked bile ducts in the liver, preventing excretion. Low levels reflect liver problems as in cancer.
CO2	Total carbonate. Too low in acid, too high in alkaline conditions.
Creatinine	Body waste derived from our muscles - controlled by kidneys and should be 0.9 to 1.0 mg/dl.

Eos	Eosinophils. Variety of white blood cell; increase with parasitism and allergies. Should be less than 3% of white blood cells.
Estrogen	A major women's hormone. Should not be higher than 100 pg./ml, except in pregnancy.
FBS	Fasting blood sugar (glucose). Blood sugar level measured in the morning in the fasted state. Should not be under 85 mg/DL; controlled by liver, pancreas, adrenals.
Ferritin	A form of iron that is usually high in cancer sufferers
GGT, SGOT, SGPT	Liver enzymes, go up with liver damage.
Hemoglobin	The oxygen carrying part of the red blood cell.
Iron	Should be about 100 mcg/dl, is lowered by copper metal.
LDH	Lactic dehydrogenase, goes up with tumor growth, with muscle stress such as heart stress. Malonic acid elevates.
Lymphs	Lymphocytes. The white cells whose job it is to eat and destroy viruses, and make antibodies. Should be about 25% of white blood cells.
MCV	Mean cell volume (average size of red blood cells). When over 100 suggests pernicious anemia. Corrects itself when *Ascaris* and hookworm are killed.
Monocytes	Rise when you are sick.
Phosphates	Should be less than 4 mg/DL in adults. Higher levels show bone dissolution is occurring. Children should have higher levels.
Platelet count	Goes up with parasitism and minute bleeding. Should be 250 thousand/cu mm. Over 400 thousand/cu mm is extremely high. Causes blood to clot.
Potassium	Should be no less than 4.4 meq/L. An electrolyte
PSA	Prostate specific antigen. A prostate cancer "marker"; it should be less than 4.1 ng/ml.
RBC	Red blood cell count. Below 4.4 million per cubic mm is low. Over 4.7 is due to toxicity from cobalt or vanadium.
Seg	Segmental white blood cells. Those white cells whose job it is to eat and destroy bacteria. Should be about 70% of white blood cells.
Total protein	Blood protein made by the liver; sum of albumin and globulin. Ratio affected by cobalt and vanadium.
Triglycerides	Blood fat, too high with kidney problems, too low in cancer.
Uric acid	Body waste. Too low in glutamine deficiency and in bacterial invasion of organs. Too high in folic acid deficiency.
WBC	White blood cell count. Low levels are below 5,000 per cubic mm.

Building A Zapper

Being able to kill your bacteria and other invaders with electricity becomes much more of a panacea when you can do it all in three 7 minute sessions. No need to single out specific frequencies or to sweep through a range of frequencies one kHz at a time. No matter what frequency it is set at (within reason), it kills large and small invaders: flukes, roundworms, mites, bacteria, viruses and fungi. It kills them all at once, in 7 minutes, even at 5 volts.

How does it work? I suppose that a positive voltage applied anywhere on the body attracts negatively charged things such as bacteria. Perhaps the battery voltage tugs at them, pulling them out of their locations in the cell doorways (called *conductance channels*). But doorways can be negatively charged too. Does the voltage tug at them so they disgorge any bacteria stuck in them? How would the positive voltage act to kill a large parasite like a fluke? None of these questions can be answered yet.

Other fascinating possibilities are that the intermittent positive voltage interferes with electron flow in some key metabolic route, or straightens out the ATP molecule disallowing its breakdown. Such biological questions could be answered by studying the effects of positive frequencies on bacteria in a lab.

The most important question, of course, is whether there is a harmful effect on you. I have seen no effects on blood pressure, mental alertness, or body temperatures. It has never produced pain, although it has often stopped pain instantly. This does not prove its safety. Even knowing that the voltage comes from a small 9 volt battery does not prove safety, although it is reassuring. The clotting of red blood cells, platelet aggregation and functions that depend on surface charges on cells need to be investigated. But not before you can use it. Your safety lies in the short period of exposure that is necessary. Viruses and bacteria disappear in 3 minutes; damaged tapeworm stages, flukes, roundworms in 5; and mites in 7. One need not go beyond this time, although no bad effects have been seen at any length of treatment.

The first seven minute zapping is followed by an intermission, lasting 20 to 30 minutes. During this time, bacteria and viruses are released from the dying parasites and start to invade you instead.

The second seven minute session is intended to kill these newly released viruses and bacteria. If you omit it, you could catch a cold, sore throat or something else immediately. Again, viruses are released from the dying bacteria. The third session kills the last viruses released.

Do Not Zap If You Are Pregnant Or Wearing A Pacemaker.

These situations have not been explored yet. Don't do these experiments yourself. Children as young as 8 months have been zapped with no noticeable ill effects. For them, you should weigh the possible benefits against the unknown risks.

That is all there is to it. Almost all. The zapping current does not reach deep into the eyeball or testicle or bowel contents. It does not reach into your gallstones, or into your living cells where *Herpes* virus lies latent or *Candida* fungus extends its fingers. To reach deeper, the herbal parasite program (page 19) must be added to the zapper treatment.

Killing The Surviving Pathogens

The interior of gallstones may house parasites inaccessible to the zapping. Eliminate this source of reinfection by flushing them out with liver cleanses (page 594). Use ozonated oil in the Liver Cleanse for greater effectiveness.

Although the center of the bowel contents is often unaffected, which lets bowel bacteria like *Shigella, Escherichia coli (E. coli)* and parasite stages survive, sometimes it is nearly all sterilized by zapping. This results in considerable shrinkage of the bowel movement. Eliminate remaining parasites and bacteria with a single dose (2 tsp.) of Black Walnut Hull Tincture, Extra Strength.

The zapper current travels mainly along the intestinal wall where bacteria are scurrying to cross over into your body. Even "good" bacteria are no longer good when they are crossing the wall.

So zapping kills mostly "bad" bacteria. The good news is that perfect bowel habits often result in a few days. Evidently, the good bacteria are benefited by killing the invasive ones. Homemade yogurt and buttermilk (see *Recipes*) are especially good at recolonizing the bowel. But it does not seem wise to culture yourself with special commercial preparations which are often polluted and risk getting parasite stages again when you can become normal so soon anyway. Besides, *acidophilus* bacteria are able to change RNA into DNA and are often found in a growing tumor!

When a large number of parasites, bacteria and viruses are killed, it can leave you fatigued. Try to give yourself a low-stress day after your initial zapping. But there are no significant side effects. I believe this is due to the second and third zapping which mops up bacteria and viruses that would otherwise be able to go on a feeding frenzy with so much dead prey available.

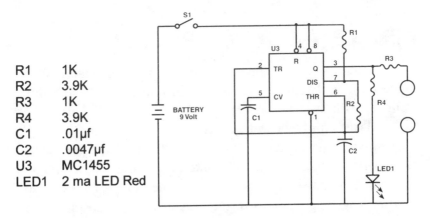

R1   1K
R2   3.9K
R3   1K
R4   3.9K
C1   .01µf
C2   .0047µf
U3   MC1455
LED1   2 ma LED Red

Give this to an electronics person or make it yourself in a shoe box by using the following instructions.

Fig. 93 Zapper schematic.

Remember, too, that newly killed large parasites, like *Ascaris* worms and tapeworm larvae, still house their eggs that remain quite alive, unreachable by zapper current or herbs. Only cysteine and ozonated oil can reach them before they are set free in your body (see the Mop Up program on page 36).

To build your zapper you may take this list of components to any electronics store (Radio Shack part numbers are given for convenience).

Zapper Parts List

Item	Radio Shack Catalog Number
large shoe box	
9 volt battery	
9 volt battery clips	270-325 (set of 5, you need 1)
On-Off toggle switch	275-624A micro mini toggle switch
1 KΩ resistor	271-1321 (set of 5, you need 2)
3.9 KΩ resistor	271-1123 (set of 2, you need 2)
low-current red LED	276-044
.0047 uF capacitor	272-130 (set of 2, you need 1)
.01 uF capacitor	272-1065 (set of 2, you need 1)
555 CMOS timer chip	276-1723 (set of 2, you need 1)
8 pin wire-wrapping socket for the chip	276-1988 (set of 2, you need 1)

short (12") alligator clip leads	any electronics shop, get 6
Microclip test jumpers	278-017 (you need 2 packages of 2)
2 bolts, about 1/8" diameter, 2" long, with 4 nuts and 4 washers	hardware store
2 copper pipes, ¾" diameter, 4" long	hardware store
sharp knife, pin, long-nose pliers	

Hints for absolute novices: Don't let unusual vocabulary deter you. A "lead" is just a piece of wire used to make connections. Label components as you remove them from the package. Practice using the microclips. If the metal ends are L-shaped bend them into a U with the long-nose pliers so they grab better. Chips and chip holders are very fragile. It is wise to purchase an extra of each in case you break the connections.

Assembling The Zapper

1. You will be using the lid of the shoe box to mount the components. Save the box to enclose the finished project.
2. Pierce two holes near the ends of the lid. Enlarge the holes with a pen or pencil until the bolts would fit through. Mount the bolts on the outside about half way through the holes so there is a 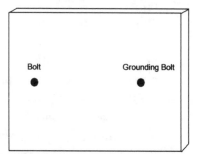 washer and nut holding it in place on both sides. Tighten. Label one hole "grounding bolt" on the inside and outside.
3. Mount the 555 chip in the wire wrap socket. Find the "top end" of the chip by searching the outside surface carefully for a cookie-shaped bite or hole taken out of it. Align the chip with the socket and very gently squeeze the pins of the chip into the socket until they click in place.

4. Make 8 pinholes to fit the wire wrap socket. Enlarge them slightly with a sharp pencil. Mount it on the out-side.

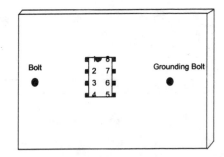

Write in the numbers of the pins (connections) on both the outside and inside, starting with number one to the left of the "cookie bite" as seen from outside. After number 4, cross over to number 5 and continue. Number 8 will be across from number 1.

5. Pierce two holes ½ inch apart very near to pins 5, 6, 7, and 8. They should be less than 1/8 inch away. (Or, one end of each com-ponent can <u>share</u> a hole with the 555 chip.) Mount the .01 uF capacitor near pin 5 on the

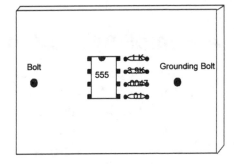

outside. On the inside connect pin 5 to one end of this ca-pacitor by simply twisting them together. Loop the ca-pacitor wire around the pin first; then twist with the long-nose pliers until you have made a tight connection. Bend the other wire from the capacitor flat against the inside of the shoe box lid. Label it .01 on the outside and inside. Mount the .0047 uF capacitor near pin 6. On the inside twist the capacitor wire around the pin. Flatten the wire from the other end and label it .0047. Mount the 3.9 KΩ resistor near pin 7, connecting it on the inside to the pin. Flatten the wire on the other end and label it 3.9. Mount the 1 KΩ resistor and connect it similarly to pin 8 and label it 1K.

6. Pierce two holes ½ inch apart next to pin 3 (again, you can share the hole for pin 3 if you wish), in the direction of the bolt. Mount the other 1 KΩ resistor and la-

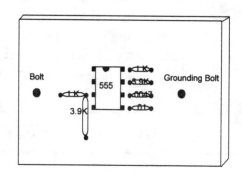

bel inside and outside. Twist the connections together and flatten the remaining wire. This resistor protects the circuit if you should accidentally short the terminals. Mount the 3.9KΩ resistor downward. One end can go in the same hole as the 1K resistor near pin 3. Twist that end around pin 3 which already has the 1K resistor attached to it. Flatten the far end. Label.

7. Next to the 3.9KΩ resistor pierce two holes ¼ inch apart for the LED. Notice that the LED has a positive and negative connection. The longer wire is the anode (positive).

Mount the LED on the outside and bend back the wires, labeling them + and - on the inside.

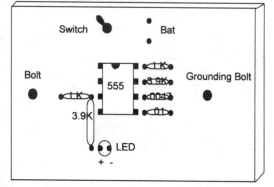

8. Near the top pierce a hole for the toggle switch. Enlarge it until the shaft fits through from the inside. Remove nut and washer from switch before mounting. You may need to trim away some paper

with a serrated knife before replacing washer and nut on the outside. Tighten.

9. Next to the switch pierce two holes for the wires from the battery holder and poke them through. Attach the battery and tape it to the outside.

NOW TO CONNECT EVERYTHING

First, make holes at the corners of the lid with a pencil. Slit each corner to the hole. They will accommodate extra loops of wire that you get from using the clip leads to make connections. After each connection gently tuck away the excess wire.

1. Twist the free ends of the two capacitors (.01 and .0047) together. Connect this to the grounding bolt using an alligator clip.

2. Bend the top ends of pin 2 and pin 6 (which already has a connection) inward towards each other in an L shape. Catch them both

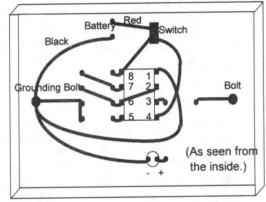

with a alligator clip and attach the other end of the alligator clip to the free end of the 3.9KΩ resistor by pin 7.

3. Using an alligator clip connect pin 7 to the free end of the 1KΩ resistor attached to pin 8.

4. Using two microclips connect pin 8 to one end of the switch, and pin 4 to the same end of the switch. (Put one

hook inside the hole and the other hook around the whole connection. Check to make sure they are securely connected.)

5. Use an alligator clip to connect the free end of the other 1KΩ resistor (by pin 3) to the bolt.

6. Twist the free end of the 3.9KΩ resistor around the plus end of the LED. Connect the minus end of the LED to the grounding bolt using an alligator clip.

7. Connect pin number 1 on the chip to the grounding bolt with an alligator clip.

8. Attach an alligator clip to the outside of one of the bolts. Attach the other end to a handhold (copper pipe). Do the same for the other bolt and handhold.

9. Connect the minus end of the battery (black wire) to the grounding bolt with an alligator clip.

10. Connect the plus end of the battery (red wire) to the free end of the switch using a microclip lead. If the LED lights up you know the switch is ON. If it does not, flip the switch and see if the LED lights. Label the switch clearly. If you cannot get the LED to light in either switch position, you must double-check all of your connections, and make sure you have a fresh battery.

11. Finally replace the lid on the box, loosely, and slip a couple of rubber bands around the box to keep it securely shut.

12. Wrap handholds in one layer of wet paper towel before using. Grasp securely and turn the switch on to zap.[66]

- Optional: measure the frequency of your zapper by connecting an oscilloscope or frequency counter to the hand-

---

[66] I have not detected the copper in the handholds penetrating the skin. Perhaps this is due to the high frequency circuit used. Non-copper handholds are now available from commercial providers.

holds. Any electronics shop can do this. It should read between 20 and 40 kHz.

- Optional: measure the voltage output by connecting it to an oscilloscope. It should be about 7 to 8 volts.
- Optional: measure the current that flows through you when you are getting zapped. You will need a 1 KΩ resistor and oscilloscope. Connect the grounding bolt on the zapper to one end of the resistor. Connect the other end of the resistor to a handhold. (Adding this resistor to the circuit decreases the current slightly, but not significantly.) The other handhold is attached to the other bolt. Connect the scope ground wire to one end of the resistor. Connect the scope probe to the other end of the resistor. Turn the zapper ON and grasp the handholds. Read the voltage on the scope. It will read about 3.5 volts. Calculate current by dividing voltage by resistance. 3.5 volts divided by 1 KΩ is 3.5 ma (milliamperes).

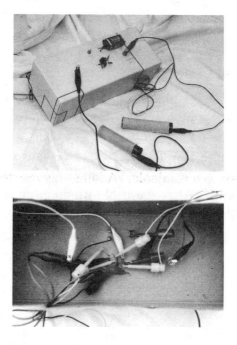

Fig. 94 Finished zapper, outside and inside.

Testing The Zapper

Trying the zapper on an illness to see "if it works" is not useful. Your symptoms may be due to a non-parasite. Or you may reinfect within hours of zapping. The best way to test your device is to find a few invaders that you currently have (see Lesson Twelve, page 501). This gives you a starting point. Then zap yourself. After the triple zapping, none of these invaders should be present.

Recipes

Read old recipe books for the fun and savings of making your own nutritious food. Change the recipes to avoid processed and malonic acid-containing ingredients.

Note: the latest products to fall victim to benzene pollution are **cornstarch** and **baking soda**. You can still use these if they are pure (see *Sources*). Besides this, the new practice of spraying fruits and vegetables with petroleum products to keep them fresh looking has polluted them with benzene. Produce treated this way has an extra glossy appearance and may even be slightly sticky. Carefully avoid such produce. It does not wash off. Peeling is necessary.

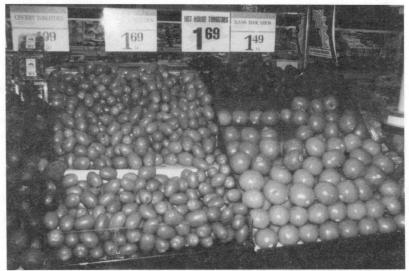

Ask your grocer if the produce they carry has been sprayed for "freshness"; ask the health food store owner, too.

Fig. 95 Glossy fruit and vegetables

Beverage Recipes

Anything made from the malonate-free list (page 117) in your own juicer is fine. Experiment with new combinations to create different flavorful fruit and vegetable juices. Consider the luxury of preparing gourmet juices which satisfy your own individual palate instead of the mass-produced, polluted varieties sold at grocery stores. Remember to wash all fruit, and peel, before juicing. This removes the ever-present pesticides, common fruit mold, and the new food sprays.

Lemonade

1 cup fresh lemon juice, 1 cup honey, 1½ quarts water. Bring honey and water to a boil if you plan to keep it several days. Then add lemon juice and store in the refrigerator. Confectioner's sugar is an optional sweetener.

All honey and maple syrup should have vitamin C added to it as soon as it arrives from the supermarket. This detoxifies mold. Warm it first; then stir in ¼ tsp. per pint.

Green Goodness

head lettuce
grapefruit

Other varieties of lettuce, as well as parsley and spinach, tested positive for benzene. This was also the case for health food store greens, no doubt due to the new practice of spraying for "freshness." If in doubt, ozonate the greens for 20 minutes; then rinse in water with baking soda added. Blend lettuce in juicer or blender to make ¼ cup. Add grapefruit and blend again to make 1 cup. Strain.

Green Drink

cabbage, kale, Swiss chard, turnip greens, or any other broad-leafed edible tops.
grapefruit, lemon, apple, pear, pineapple (strawberries and grapes are too moldy to risk).

Don't use rhubarb or nonedibles! Swiss chard and beet leaves contain a lot of oxalic acid. One leaf of each is enough. Change variety daily.

Blend greens to make ¼ cup. Add fruit to make a total of one cup. Blend together. Strain.

Kill Fertilizer Parasites

Remember to soak all greens and unpeeled vegetables in Lugol's solution for one minute to kill *Ascaris* and tapeworm eggs. They may be present from the manure used for fertilizer and they don't wash off!

Fresh Pineapple Juice

Peel a pineapple. Remove all soft spots. Cut it into cubes. Extract the juice by putting the pineapple through a blender or juicer. There will be very little pulp. Strain the juice and serve it on ice with sprigs of mint. Makes about 1½ cups of juice. Mix the pulp with an equal amount of clover honey and use as topping (kept in freezer) for homemade ice cream, pancakes, or yogurt.

Maple Milk Shake

For each milk shake, blend or shake together: 1 glass of milk and 2 tablespoons maple syrup.

Remember, all dairy products get sterilized.

This includes butter, cream, cheese. If it hasn't been boiled or baked, don't eat it. Add a pinch of salt while boiling. After cooling, it gets baking soda and vitamin C added.

Yankee Drink

Mix together 1 gal. water, 3 cups honey, ½ cup fresh lemon juice or distilled white vinegar, and 1 tsp. ginger.

Hot Vanilla Milk

Add one inch of vanilla bean and one tsp. honey to a glass of milk and bring to a near boil. You may add a pinch of cinnamon or other pure spice. You may even use vanilla extract.

Mark's Lemon-oil Drink

Scrub one lemon; blend it whole, rind, seeds and all. Strain and discard pulp. Add 1 tbs. olive oil and enough honey and water (1½ cup) to make it tasty. Read the label on the lemon-packaging; avoid those that have been sprayed for longer shelf life. Ask your grocer if the information is not by the bin of lemons.

If you are not sure about this, peel the lemon with a sharp knife; you will still get limonene, the active ingredient. Use only one whole lemon a day.

Cream Shake

One egg yolk, one cup of half and half. Honey to sweeten and cinnamon or nutmeg. Blend. Drink only once a day.

Red Milk

One part fresh beet juice (use a juicer) and three parts sterilized half and half milk. Add vitamin C and spice.
Note: Raw beet juice is a liver tonic; start with 1/8 cup only.

C-Milk

Cold milk can absorb a surprising amount of vitamin C powder without curdling or changing its flavor. Try ½ tsp. in a glass of cold milk.

Half And Half

Mix equal parts whipping cream and milk or water.

Buttermilk-C

Stir 1 tsp. vitamin C powder into a glass of milk, more if it won't develop flakes. Add a pinch of salt (pure salt). Additional seasoning may be pepper and herbs or a fenuthyme capsule. Stir and enjoy.

Raw Certified Milk

You may be lucky enough to find this at your health food store. Raw milk has a special factor, lactoferrin. This factor is missing from the liver, spleen and bone marrow in cases of anemia and cancer. One glass of raw milk replenishes it for over a week! Surprisingly, boiling for 10 seconds does not destroy it! Add a pinch of salt before boiling. It is not present in ordinary pasteurized milk.

Moose Elm Drink - also known as Slippery Elm

For very sensitive stomachs when nothing wants to stay down:

1 tbs. moose elm powder
cold (boiled) milk

Start by making a paste as if it were cocoa. Gradually add milk, water or whipping cream to consistency desired. Sweeten with confectioner's sugar or honey. This is very like cocoa; can be drunk hot or cold. Sip one cup a day.

Alginate/Intestinal Healer

For intestines that are sore from surgery, blockage, or inflammation. This beverage is not meant to be digested; it forms a gelatinous ribbon right through the intestine, giving bulk and absorbing toxins along the way. Consume 1 cup a day in tablespoon amounts that you add to soup, stew, pudding, pie, or bouillon.

Bring 2 tsp. sodium alginate powder and 1 pint water to a boil. Stir with wooden spoon handle. Use slow heat – it could take an hour. Add to soup, stew, moose elm beverage, pudding or pie. Consume one to two cups per day.

Food Recipes

Despite the presence of malonic acid, aflatoxins, benzopyrenes, and solvents in many foods, it is possible to have a delicious and <u>safe</u> diet. Many persons need to gain weight, and with the emphasis in today's society on losing weight, consider yourself lucky in this respect. Help yourself to lots of butter, whipping cream, whole milk, avocados, and olive oil. Never throw away the skin or fat in meats. Make your own preserves and baked goods, including breads. Remember, when you are recovering from a major illness it is essential <u>not</u> to diet to lose weight. You must wait two years after you are recovered to try to lose weight.

Daily Foods

Dairy products should contain at least 2% fat to enable you to absorb the calcium in them.

All milk should be sterilized

by boiling it for 10 seconds with a pinch of salt. The salt raises the temperature just enough to kill *Rhizobium leguminosarum*, a dangerous tumor causing bacterium. After cooling, add baking soda, 1/8 tsp. per pint. Follow by the same amount of vitamin C. If it makes mucous, you already have a chronic respiratory infection. Try to clear this up.

Change brands every time you shop to prevent the same pollutants from building up in your body. Choose plastic, not waxed paper containers.

If frying or cooking with fat,[67] use <u>only</u> olive oil, butter or lard (the BHT and BHA preservatives in lard are OK except for seizure sufferers), or chicken fat, or turkey fat simply scooped up from the roaster pan and chilled in the refrigerator. Mix them for added flavor in your dishes. <u>Never use margarine, Crisco, or other hydrogenated fats. Do not cook over flames or grill, even when electric.</u>

---

[67] Earlier I state it is best to be a seafood vegetarian. This is still true. But fat that has been rendered is quite safe.

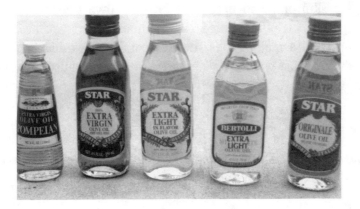

Fig. 96 Olive Oils

Eat lots of **fresh fruits and vegetables.** Wash them off <u>only</u> with cold tap water, not commercial food "wash." Scrub hard with a stiff bristled brush. Then cut away blemishes. Always peel potatoes so you can see the dark spots underneath. Modern dirt is full of chemicals and is toxic to you. Where spraying of fruits, vegetables and greens is permitted, peel everything and don't buy small-leafed greens; they can't be washed free of benzene. Emphasize head lettuce and cabbage.

Be sure to drink plenty of **plain water** from your cold faucet throughout the day, especially if it is difficult for you to drink it with your meals. If you don't like the taste of your own tap water, try to get it from a friend with newer plumbing. Use a glass bottle from a grocery store to transport it (the solvent from a plastic water bottle does not rinse out). Never drink water that has been run through a water softener or copper plumbing or has traveled through a long plastic hose. Don't drink water that has stood in a container for a day. Dump it and rinse the container. To further improve flavor and to dechlorinate attach a small faucet filter made of carbon only. Or buy a filter pitcher (see *Sources*). Don't drink water that has stood in the filter pitcher very long, either.

Regular **table salt** is made of sodium chloride plus impurities, to which a free-running agent is added. Avoid all these by purchasing pure sodium chloride. Keep it free running by adding long grain white rice to it. Sodium chloride is a blood salt. We have a built in sensor that tells us when we have too much in our food. Potassium chloride is a tissue salt. It runs low readily if we have poor adrenal function and don't get enough fruits and vegetables. A blood test always shows both your sodium and potassium levels. It is wise to use a sodium/potassium salt mixture so they stay in balance. A good mixture is: 2 parts sodium chloride and 1 part potassium chloride. A higher proportion of potassium chloride should be approved by your health adviser who will check your blood levels. Another wise rule is to use salt <u>either</u> in cooking <u>or</u> at the table, but not both places. This cuts down on the total consumed.

Because commercial **cold cereals** are very convenient, but have solvents, here are three replacements.

Three Granolas

Granola One
7 cups rolled oats
1 tsp. salt (pure variety)
1 cup wheat germ (fresh, not defatted)
½ cup honey
½ cup sunflower seeds, immaculate quality
½ cup milk with pinch of vitamin C added
½ cup melted butter (already boiled with vitamin C added)
1 cup raisins, rinsed in vitamin C water

Mix dry ingredients together. Mix liquid ingredients and add gradually, while tossing until thoroughly mixed. Place in large ungreased pans and bake in slow (250°) oven. Stir occasionally, baking until brown and dry, usually 1-2 hours. Store in airtight container in freezer.

Granola Two

6 cups rolled oats
½ cup raw wheat germ
1 cup sesame seeds
1 cup sunflower seeds (raw, unsalted)
1 tsp. cinnamon
½ cup melted butter
½ cup honey

Preheat oven to 250°. Toss all ingredients in mixing bowl. Spread thinly on a baking sheet and bake 20-25 minutes. Stir often in order to brown evenly. When golden, remove and let cool. Makes 12 cups.

If you would like to add nuts to your granola recipes, rinse them in cold tap water first, to which vitamin C powder has been added (¼ tsp. per pint). Rub off the skins. This removes aflatoxins and malonate.

Granola Three (Stove Top or Dry Roast)

It is cooked quickly right on top of the stove. The quick, sautéing gives a deep-roasted flavor to the ingredients. The brown sugar melts just a bit, slightly coating each flake.

2 cups raw rolled oats
1/3 cup or more of wheat germ
1/3 cup or more of sesame seeds
1/3 cup or more of sunflower seeds
1/3 cup or more of shredded coconut
¼ cup (packed) brown sugar treated with vitamin C.
¼ tsp. (heaping) salt

1. Use a large, heavy skillet (enamel or glass). Place the oats in the skillet, turn on the heat to medium-low, and stir them constantly for 5 minutes, as they begin to roast.

2. Add wheat germ, sesame seeds, sunflower seeds, and coconut. Keep both the heat and the stirring action constant for ten or more minutes.

3. Sprinkle in brown sugar and salt. Cook for 2-5 more minutes, still stirring. Remove from heat, cool, and store in an airtight container.

Note: this yields about 3½ cups. You can double the amounts, but it is recommended that you make smaller batches more frequently instead, for greater freshness.

Peanut Butter

Use fresh unsalted roasted peanuts—they will be white on the first day they arrive at the health food store from the distributor. (Ask when they will arrive.) Or shell fresh roasted peanuts yourself, throwing away all shriveled or darkened nuts. Grind, adding salt and vitamin C (¼ tsp. per pint) as you

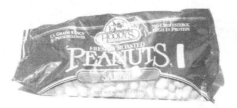

Fig. 97 Light colored, roasted peanuts in the shell had no aflatoxin.

go. Take your own salt shaker with built in vitamin C to the health food store where you grind it. For spreadability, especially for children, mix an equal volume of cold butter, previously boiled, to freshly ground peanut butter. This improves spreadability and digestibility of the hard nut particles. This will probably be the most heavenly peanut butter your mouth has ever experienced.

Spreadable Butter

Bring one quarter pound of butter to a boil in a saucepan. Add a pinch of salt. Count to ten, while it bubbles. Add a pinch of vitamin C. Then add olive oil in equal amount or to suit. Reheat and pour into a butter bowl. Do not save any liquid that separates at the bottom. Refrigerate.

Sweetening and Flavoring

Brown Sugar. Although I am prejudiced against all sugar from a health standpoint, my testing revealed no benzene, isopropyl alcohol, wood alcohol. However it does contain sorghum

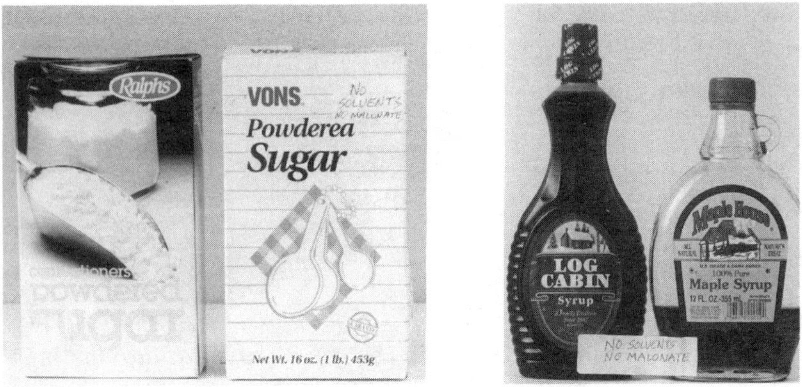

Fig. 98 Safe Sweetening

mold and must be treated with vitamin C to detoxify it. Add ¼ tsp. to a 1 pound package; knead until well mixed.

Confectioner's sugar. This is dextrose or glucose, the same as blood sugar (cane sugar is sucrose). It needs no digestion and can be assimilated much more easily, especially in liver disease. Commercial varieties I tested has no solvents or mold.

Maple syrup. Boil to kill mold spores. Then add vitamin C, ¼ tsp. per pint, to detoxify mycotoxins. Keep refrigerated and use promptly.

Flavoring. Use maple, vanilla (both natural and artificial), and any pure spice. They are free of molds, solvents and malonate.

Honeys. Get at least 4 flavors for variety: linden blossom, orange blossom, plain clover and local or wild flower honey Add vitamin C to newly opened jar to detoxify ergot mold (¼ tsp. per pint). Since jars must be sterilized, purchase your honey in bulk from a health food store.

Jams and jellies. They are not safe unless homemade.

Fruit syrup. Use one package frozen fruit, such as cherries, blueberries or raspberries. Let thaw and measure the amount in cups (it might say on the package). Add an equal amount of clover honey to the fruit. Also add ¼ tsp. vitamin C powder. Mix it all in a quart canning jar and store in the refrigerator. Use this on pancakes, cereal, plain yogurt and homemade ice cream too. Use to make your own flavored beverages in a seltzer maker. If you wish to use fresh fruit, bring it to a boil to sterilize. Use it up in a few days or boil to sterilize it again.

Note for diabetics

Diabetics must not use artificial sweeteners. Nor can they use all the sweeteners listed. Try stevia powder instead.

Preserves

Keep 3 or 4 kinds on hand, such as peach, pineapple, and pear. Peel and chop the fruit. It should not have any bruises. If you use a metal knife, rinse the fruit lightly afterwards. Add just enough water to keep the fruit from sticking as it is cooked (usually a few tablespoons). Then add an equal amount of honey, or to taste and heat again to boiling. Put in sterile jars in refrigerator. Make lemon marmalade the same way, slicing the fruit and peeling thinly. Be sure the lemons were not sprayed! Always add vitamin C powder to a partly used jar to inhibit mold. Never use up partly molded fruit by making preserves out of it. Never use "soft" (actually moldy) bananas to make banana bread. Never make guacamole out of soft (actually moldy) avocados. Throw them out.

Kumquat Marmalade

If you feel starved for "orange" flavor, you will love this recipe.

2½ cups water
2½ quarts whole kumquats, stems removed
2 whole grapefruits
1 lemon
5 or 6 cups powdered sugar
½ tsp. vitamin C

Wash the kumquats, grapefruits, lemon, and put through a food processor until coarsely chopped. Bring the water to a boil, add the fruit, and bring to a boil again. Then cook on low heat, uncovered, about 35 minutes. Stir with wooden spoon occasionally and pick out any seeds that rise to the surface. Stir in sugar according to your taste, again bringing to a boil. Simmer an additional 20 minutes. Stir in vitamin C. Ladle into sterilized glass jars. Cover with plastic lids (see *Sources*).

There are many uses for marmalade besides being good with bread and butter. Try adding to cooked, mashed yams, on homemade ice cream, etc.

C Dressing

½ cup olive oil
¼ cup fresh lemon juice or white distilled vinegar

1 tsp. thyme, fenugreek or both. (Capsules are freshest. The combination is available as Fenuthyme, see *Sources*.)
1 tsp. vitamin C powder
½ tsp. brown sugar

Combine the ingredients in a clean salad dressing bottle. Shake. Refrigerate. The basic recipe is the oil and vinegar in a 2:1 ratio. After mixing these, add any pure spice desired. Or add home made cottage cheese for a creamy texture.

Pasta Pizza Sauce or Red Sauce

Here are two sauces that are excellent on pasta, pizza or salads.

3 red peppers, chopped or in chunks
1 small onion
3 tbs. olive oil
salt to taste
1 cup water
¼ cup white distilled vinegar

Sauce No. 1: Sauté peppers and onion in olive oil for a few minutes. Add generous sprinkling of salt and a cup of water and bring to a boil. Cover pan, lower burner heat and cook for three to five more minutes. Mash (or put into blender) and add vinegar. Blend for a few seconds and add salt (if by taste more is needed). May be kept up to a month in refrigerator if stored in a glass jar with plastic or wooden lid.

Sauce No. 2: Same as Sauce No. 1 except that when a sprinkling of salt is put into pan also add a ½ capsule each of cloves, fenuthyme, and turmeric.

Sour Cream-C

2 cups heavy whipping cream, boiled 10 seconds with a pinch of salt and chilled

¼ tsp. citric acid
¼ tsp. vitamin C powder
1 tsp. fresh onion juice or other seasoning (optional)
   Stir until smooth, refrigerate 2 hours.

Yogurt

Buy a yogurt maker. Be sure to use boiled milk and add vitamin C. When done add fresh blueberries, strawberries, or peaches. Use plain yogurt as starter.

Cottage Cheese "Paneer"

This tastes much better than regular cottage cheese. It's more easily digested, too. Don't throw away the liquid that remains (whey) since it has all the calcium of the milk in it. It is often referred to as "poor-man's beer", drunk ice cold on a hot day.

1/8 tsp. salt
½ gallon milk
juice of 2 lemons

Put milk and salt in saucepan or wok and bring to boil for 10 seconds. Add juice of 1 lemon for each quart of milk. Stir and allow to boil for another few seconds. When curdled, strain through thin cloth (cheesecloth or thin dishtowel) and squeeze all liquid out until desired consistency. Should be very dry if it is to be cut into squares for vegetable dishes, but not too dry if to be used like cottage or cream cheese. Makes 1 cup.

Cottage Cheese "Zuppe"

Drop a carton of cottage cheese into a saucepan and cover with milk or cream. Add 1/8 tsp. baking soda, salt, pepper, garlic and any other herbs. Stir and boil for 20 seconds. When cool, add vitamin C (1/8 tsp. per pint).

Cottage Cheese Cake

This is an excellent way to get more protein into your diet, especially important if you are mostly vegetarian.

1 cup cottage cheese (dry variety)
1 egg
1 tsp. honey or confectioner's sugar
1 tsp. butter
cinnamon

If dry cottage cheese is not available, drain the regular variety. The dryer the cottage cheese the chewier the cheese cake gets. But if you prefer a custard-like consistency, you could use the regular 4% cream cottage cheese without draining; simply blend it for smoothness.

Mix all ingredients and pour into a small glass pie pan with or without a pie shell. Do not use graham crackers or ready-made crust. Sprinkle heavily with cinnamon. Bake at 350° till firm and slightly browned, about 15 to 20 minutes.

Soups

All home made soups are nutritious and safe, provided you use no processed ingredients (like a bouillon cube), or make them in metal pots. Use herbs and pure salt to season. The salt should be added during boiling, not at the end, to raise the boiling temperature and kill more bacteria. Always add a dash of vitamin C or vinegar to draw out calcium from soup bones for you to absorb. Soups are great for the finicky appetite.

Cheese Soup

4 cups home made chicken broth
¾ pound uncolored sharp cheddar cheese, grated or cut up
¼ tsp. vitamin C
1 tsp. freshly grated nutmeg (from whole nutmeg)
1 or 2 potatoes, peeled, cooked and cut into small pieces
1 cup of cream or half and half (unboiled is fine)
salt (pure variety)

Bring all to a boil. After a minute turn the burner to low, cover pan with a lid and cook slowly for at least 20 minutes.

Fish and Seafood recipe

Any kind of fish or seafood is acceptable, provided it is well-cooked. Don't buy food that is already in batter. The simplest way to cook fish is to poach it in milk. It can be taken straight from the freezer, rinsed, and placed in ¼ inch of milk (unboiled is fine) in the frying pan. Add a dash of vitamin C and heat until it is cooked. Turn over and repeat. Throw away the milk. Serve with fresh lemon and herbs.

Baked Apples

Peel and core carefully. Remove all bruises (this is where the mycotoxin, patulin, is). Cut in bite-sized pieces, add a minimum of water and cook or bake minimally. Add a squirt of lemon juice when done. Serve with cinnamon, whipping cream and honey. Make sure you eat the seeds, too.

Ice creams

from the grocery store are loaded with benzene and other solvents. Fortunately there are ice cream makers that do everything (no cranking)! Or try our recipe which uses a blender. Be sure not to add store bought flavors, except vanilla or maple. For lemon flavoring use grated lemon rind. (Buy unsprayed lemons only.)

5 Minute Ice Cream

(Strawberry) Use 2 half pints of heavy whipping cream (boiled, chilled, and vitamin C-ed), 1 package of frozen strawberries (about 10 oz.), and 1/2 cup clover honey. Pour frozen strawberries into blender. Pour whipping cream and honey over them. Blend briefly (about 10 seconds), not long enough to make butter! Pour it all into a large plastic bowl. Cover with a close fitting plastic bag and place in freezer. Prepare it a day ahead. Try using other frozen fruits, such as blueberries and cherries. Keep a few berries out of the blender and stir them in quickly with a non-metal spoon before setting the bowl in the freezer. There are many ice cream recipes to be found in old cook books. Avoid those with processed foods as ingredients. You may add nuts if you rinse them in vitamin C water.

Cookies, cakes and pies

Bake them from scratch, using unprocessed ingredients. Use simple recipes from old cook books.

Seven Day Sample Menu

Because processed foods have many toxins, you must cook as much from scratch as possible. So for convenience sake, keep your meals simple in preparation. You may want to prepare ahead and refrigerate your dressings and toppings. Or you could make a hot soup for dinner, refrigerate, and eat the leftovers for lunch. Don't save leftovers more than two days. Make sure they are covered. Try baking several potatoes at one time, refrigerate and put them in a salad the next night. Variety is the spice of life, so combine the allowed foods in the most creative ways you can imagine. And don't forget herbs and spices; learn to use them from old cook books. When cooking grains, remember to add a bit of salt to raise the boiling temperature.

	Breakfast	Lunch	Dinner
Day 1	Oatmeal and honey with milk, half n' half or whipping cream banana Water Milk ½ cup Green Drink	Fresh ground peanut butter and preserve sandwich Chicken soup Milk Water Lemon Oil Drink	Orange roughy fish Fresh green beans with butter Baked potato with Sour Cream-C topping Pie (homemade) Milk Olive leaf tea (*Sources*)
Day 2	Egg (limit is 2) biscuit Fried potatoes 1 glass milk Green Drink	Chicken sandwich with sour cream dressing Cucumber sliced in vinegar, or avocado Lemon Oil Drink Water Milk	Homemade bean or lentil soup Sardines Dinner roll and butter Salad with homemade dressing Ice cream (homemade) Olive Leaf Tea
Day 3	Wheatena cooked with raisins, salt and milk Banana Green Drink ½ cup milk Water	Tuna sandwich with olive oil Soup Milk Water Olive Leaf Tea	Baked sweet potato with butter and sweetening Fresh spinach w/lemon Bread and butter Chopped, peeled pear or other fruit and whipping cream Cream Shake Water
Day 4	French toast with maple syrup Green Drink Milk Water	Avocado and sour cream sandwich Bread and butter Lemon Oil Drink Water	Lobster or sautéed shrimp Fresh asparagus Potatoes, any style Milk Olive Leaf Tea

Day 5	Cooked cereal
	1 glass milk
	Sliced banana with
	   whipping cream and
	   honey
	1 glass water
	Green Drink
		Cold potato salad with
		   C Dressing
		Soup
		Custard pudding
		Water
		Milk
		Olive Leaf Tea
			1 can sardines or salmon
			   in easy-open can (can
			   openers shed metal)
			Salad of head lettuce,
			   grapefruit, avocado
			   with homemade
			   dressing
			Bread with butter
			Ice-cream or
			Cream Shake
			Water

Day 6	Pancakes
	Banana or chopped
	   fruit with cream
	Milk
	Water
	Green Drink
		Homemade peanut
		   butter sandwich
		Lemon Oil Drink
		Milk
		Water
			Well roasted turkey
			   (dressing must not
			   have celery)
			Mashed potatoes and
			   gravy(save the gravy
			   for next breakfast)
			Cranberry sauce (fresh
			   or canned)
			Salad or coleslaw with C-
			   dressing
			Milk
			Olive Leaf Tea

Day 7	2 Eggs and home-
	   made biscuit with
	   gravy
	Milk
	Fruit juice
	Green Drink
		Salmon sandwich
		   (from flip top can)
		Olive Leaf Tea
		Milk
		Water
			Potatoes au gratin
			Turkey leftovers
			Cob of Corn
			Bread and butter
			Pie (optional)
			Cream Shake

Take most of your supplements with food. Powders can be mixed with a little food and gulped down at the beginning of the meal.

Too Sick To Cook, Too Tired To Eat

Pick three meals from the sample menu that need no cooking and eat them every day, rotating as much as possible.

Recipes for Natural Body Products

You can use just borax (like 20 Mule Team Borax™) for all types of cleaning including your body, laundry, dishes and your house! You don't need all those products you see in commercials for each special task!

Even if you have dry skin, difficult hair or some other unique requirement, just pure borax will satisfy these needs. A part of every skin problem is due to the toxic elements found in the soaps themselves. For instance aluminum is commonly added as a "skin moisturizer". It does this by impregnating the skin and attracting water, giving the illusion of moist skin. In fact you simply have <u>moist aluminum</u> stuck in your skin which your immune system must remove. While borax won't directly heal your skin or complexion, it does replace the agents that are causing damage, so that healing can occur.

Borax Liquid Soap

An empty 1 gallon jug
1/8 cup borax powder
Plastic funnel

Funnel the borax into the jug, fill with <u>hot</u> tap water. Shake a few times. Let settle. In a few minutes you can pour off the clear part into dispenser bottles. This is the soap!

Easier way: use any bottle, pour borax powder to a depth of a ½ inch or so. Add water. Shake. When you have used it down to the undissolved granules, discard them and start over.

Keep a dispenser of borax soap by the kitchen sink, bathroom sink, and shower. It does not contain aluminum as regular detergents and soaps do, and which contribute to Alzheimer's disease. It does not contain PCBs as many commercial and health food varieties do. It does not contain cobalt (the blue or green granules) which causes heart disease and poisons the bone marrow. Commercial detergents and non-soaps are simply not safe. Switch to homemade bar soap and borax for all your tasks! In fact, you could add a tbs. of homemade liquid soap to the borax to make it sudsy. Borax inhibits the bacterial enzyme *urease* and is therefore antibacterial. It may even clear your skin of blemishes and stop your scalp from itching.

For Laundry

Borax (½ cup per load). It is the main ingredient of non-chlorine bleach and has excellent cleaning power without fading colors. It can be combined with homemade soap for extra cleaning power. Your regular laundry soap may contain PCBs, aluminum, cobalt and other chemicals. These get rubbed into your skin constantly as you wear your clothing. For bleaching (only do this occasionally) use original chlorine bleach (not "new improved" or "with special brighteners", and so forth). Don't use chlorine if there is an ill person in the house. For getting out stubborn dirt at collars, rub in homemade bar soap first; for stains, try grain alcohol, vinegar, baking soda (check old recipe books for stain removal tricks).

For Dishes

Don't believe your eyes when you see the commercials where the smiling person pulls a shining dish out of greasy suds. Any dish soap that you use should be safe enough to eat because <u>nothing</u> rinses off clean. Regular dish detergents, <u>including health brands</u>, are now polluted with PCBs. They also contain harmful chemicals like cobalt. Use borax for your dishes. Or use paper plates and plastic (not styrofoam) cups.

In The Dishwasher

Use 2 tsp. borax powder straight or pre-dissolved in water. If you use too much it will leave a film on your dishes. Use vinegar in the rinse cycle to reduce film.

In The Sink

Use a dishpan in the sink. Use ¼ cup borax and add a minimum of water. Also keep a bit of dry borax in a saucer by the sink for scouring. Don't use any soap at all for dishes that aren't greasy and can be washed under the faucet with nothing but running water. Throw away your old sponge or brush or cloth because it may be PCB contaminated. Start each day by sterilizing your sponge (it harbors Salmonella) or with a new one while the used one dries for three full days. Clean greasy pots and pans with a paper towel first. Then use homemade bar soap.

Shampoo

Borax liquid is ready to use as shampoo, too. It does not lather but feels slippery between your fingers (If it is not slippery, the concentration is too low. Check the recipe). It goes right to work removing sweat and soil without stripping your color or natural oils. It inhibits scalp bacteria and stops flaking and itching. Hair gets squeaky clean so quickly (just a few squirts does it) that you might think nothing has happened! You will soon be accustomed to non-lathery soap. Rinse very thoroughly because you should leave your scalp slightly acidic. Take a pint container to the shower with you for rinsing. Put ¼ tsp. citric (not ascorbic) acid crystals (see *Sources*) in it. For long hair use a quart of rinse. Only **citric acid** is strong enough to rinse the borax out, lemon juice and vinegar are not. After shampooing, fill the rinse container with water and pour over your head. Your hair should feel instantly silky. Rinse your whole body, too, since citric acid is also anti-bacterial. All hair shampoo penetrates the eye lids and gets into the eyes although you do not feel it. It is important to use this natural rinse to neutralize the shampoo in your eyes. (Some people have stated that citric acid makes their hair curlier or reddens it. If this is undesirable, use only half as much citric acid.) Citric acid also conditions and gives body and sheen to hair. A single squirt of homemade liquid soap (see *Recipes*) added to borax liquid makes it quite lathery if you need time to adjust to plain borax.

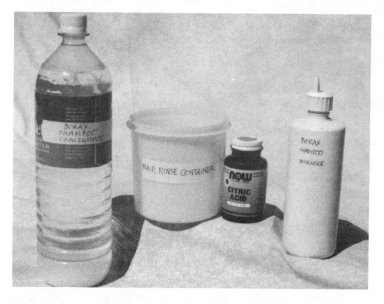

Make a bottle of borax liquid to fill your soap dispensers and shampoo bottle. Use citric acid to rinse and condition
Fig. 99 Borax and citric acid for the shower.

Baking Soda Shampoo

1 tbs. baking soda
1 cup very hot water

Place both in a plastic container and stir with your fingers until dissolved. Scoop it up over your hair by hand; if you pour it, too much runs off.

Hair Spray

I don't have a recipe that holds your hair as well as the bottle of chemicals you can buy at the store. Remarkably, a little lemon juice (not from a bottle) has some holding power and no odor! Buy a 1 cup spray bottle. Squeeze part of a lemon, letting only the clear juice run into the bottle. Fill with water. Keep it in the refrigerator. Make it fresh every week. Spraying with just plain water is nearly as good! For shinier hair, drop a bit of lemon peel into the bottle.

Homemade Soap

A small plastic dishpan, about 10" x 12"
A glass or enamel 2-quart sauce pan
1 can of lye (sodium hydroxide), 12 ounces
3 pounds of lard (BHT and BHA are OK here)
Plastic gloves
Water

1. Pour 3 cups of very cold water (refrigerate water overnight first) into the 2-quart saucepan.
2. Slowly and carefully add the lye, a little bit at a time, stirring it with a wooden or plastic utensil. (Use plastic gloves for this; test them for holes first.) Do not breathe the vapor or lean over the container or have children nearby. Above all <u>use no metal</u>. The mixture will get very hot. In olden days, a sassafras branch was used to stir, imparting a fragrance and insect deterrent for mosquitoes, lice, fleas, ticks.

3. Let cool at least one hour in a safe place. Meanwhile, the unwrapped lard should be warming up to room temperature in the plastic dishpan.
4. Slowly and carefully, pour the lye solution into the dishpan with the lard. The lard will melt. Mix thoroughly, at least 15 minutes, until it looks like thick pudding.
5. Let it set until the next morning; then cut it into bars. It will get harder after a few days. Then package.

If you wish to make soap based on olive oil, use about 48 ounces. It may need to harden for a week.

Liquid Soap

Make chips from your homemade soap cake. Add enough hot water to dissolve. Add citric acid to balance the pH (7 to 8). If you do not, this soap may be too harsh for your skin, while it is excellent for cleaning the sink.

Skin Sanitizer

Make up a 5 to 10% solution of food grade alcohol. Food grade alcohols are grain or cane (ethyl) alcohol. Only the large size Everclear bottle (750 ml or 1 liter) is free of isopropyl or wood alcohol contaminants. Purchase at a liquor store. Next, find a suitable dispenser bottle. Mark it with a pen at about one tenth of the way up from the bottom. Pour 95% grain alcohol (190 proof) to this mark and add water to the top. If using 76% grain alcohol, mark your bottle one tenth of the way up but only add water to the ¾ full mark. Keep shut. You may add a chip of lemon peel for fragrance.

Use this for general sanitizing purposes: bathroom fixtures, knobs, handles, canes, walkers, and for personal cleanliness (but use chlorine bleach for the toilet bowl once a week). Always clean up after a bowel movement with <u>wet</u> toilet paper.

This is not clean enough, though. Follow with a stronger damp paper towel. This is still not clean enough; use a final damp paper towel with skin sanitizer added. After washing hands, sanitize them too, pouring a bit on one palm and put finger tips of the other hand in it, scratch to get under nails, repeat on other hand. Rinse with water. Remember to keep the toilet lid down, while flushing or a spray of *E. coli* will fill the bathroom air, settling on toothbrushes and in water glasses.

Wash your hands if you merely <u>touch</u> the toilet seat.

Do not use this recipe, nor keep any bottles of alcohol in the house of a recovering alcoholic.

Deodorant

Your sweat is odorless. It is the entrenched bacteria feeding on it that make smells. You can never completely rid yourself of these bacteria, although they may temporarily be gone after zapping. The strategy is to control their numbers. Here are several deodorants to try. Find one that works best for you:

Vitamin C water. Mix ¼ tsp. to a pint of water and dab it on.

Citric Acid water. Mix ¼ tsp. to a pint of water and dab it on.

Only a few drops of these acids under each armpit are necessary. If these acids burn the skin, dilute them more. <u>Never</u> apply anything to skin that has just been shaved!

Lemon juice. This acid is not as strong, use what you need.

Cornstarch. Many people need only this. Dab it on.

Use only <u>unpolluted</u> cornstarch (see *Sources*).

Baking soda has been deleted as a deodorant because benzene was found in many boxes (see *Sources* for safe varieties).

Pure alcohol (never rubbing alcohol). The only food grade alcohol is grain or cane (ethyl) alcohol. Dab a bit under each arm and/or on your shirt or blouse. If the alcohol burns, dilute it with water. Be very careful not to leave the bottle where a child or alcoholic person could find it. Pour it into a different bottle!

Pure zinc oxide. You may ask your pharmacist to order this for you. She or he may wish to make it up for you too, but do not let them add anything else to it. It should be about 1 part zinc oxide powder to 3 parts water. It does not dissolve. Just shake it up to use it. After you get it home, you can add cornstarch to it to give it a creamy texture. Heat 3 tsp. cornstarch in 1 cup of water, to boiling, until dissolved and clear. Cool and add some to the zinc oxide mixture (about equal parts). Store unused starch mixture in the refrigerator. Only make up enough for a month. (Yes, this is the same zinc oxide that is used to make the dental cement, ZOE.)

Alcohol and zinc oxide. This is the most powerful deodorant. Apply alcohol first, then the zinc oxide.

Remember that you need to sweat! Sweating excretes toxic substances, especially from the upper body. Don't use deodorant on weekends. Go to the sink and wipe clean the armpits like our grandparents did. These homemade deodorants are not as powerful as the commercial varieties—this is to your advantage.

Brushing Teeth

Buy a new toothbrush. Your old one is soaked with toxins from your old toothpaste. Use food-grade hydrogen peroxide (see *Sources)* if you have only plastic fillings. Dilute it from 35% to 17½% by adding water (equal parts). Store hydrogen peroxide only in polyethylene or the original plastic bottle. Use 4 or 5 drops on your toothbrush. It should fizz nicely as oxygen is produced in your mouth. Your teeth will whiten noticeably in six months.

Before brushing teeth, floss with monofilament fish line (2 or 4 pound). Double it and twist for extra strength. Rinse before use. Or clean up the commercial varieties of floss by soaking in water for a half hour, then drying with a towel. Do not choose waxed or flavored varieties since benzene does not wash off.

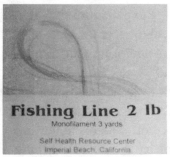

Fishing Line 2 lb
Monofilament 3 yards
Self Health Resource Center
Imperial Beach, California

Fig. 100 Fishing line is a substitute for dental floss

Floss and brush only once a day because even this small trauma invites bacteria and fungus into your blood. If this leaves you uncomfortable, you may use a water pick or simply rub your teeth by hand with a dry cloth towel (paper towels have mercury contamination). Make sure that nothing solid, like powder, is on your toothbrush; it will scour and scratch the enamel. Salt is corrosive—don't use it for brushing metal teeth. Plain water is just as good.

Baking soda is <u>no longer recommended</u> (unless ordered from *Sources*) because it was found to be polluted with benzene.

When battling tooth infection, alternate colloidal silver and white iodine solutions (five drops on brush), and brush twice a day.

For Dentures

Use salt water. It kills all germs and is inexpensive. Salt water plus grain alcohol or food-grade hydrogen peroxide makes a good denture-soak. Rinse well.

Mouthwash

A few drops of food grade hydrogen peroxide added to a little water in a glass should be enough to make your mouth foam and cleanse. Don't use hydrogen peroxide, though, if you have metal fillings, because they react. Don't use regular drug store variety hydrogen peroxide because it contains toxic additives. Health food store varieties contain solvents from the bottling process. (See *Sources* for a good hydrogen peroxide*).* Never purchase hydrogen peroxide in a bottle with a metal cap.

For persons with metal tooth fillings just use plain hot water. A healthy mouth has no odor! You shouldn't need a mouthwash! If you have breath odor, it is probably *Clostridium* growing in the crevice between a tooth filling and the tooth. At least, search for a hidden tooth infection by getting a panoramic X-ray and visiting your dentist.

Contact Lens Solution

A scant cup of cold tap water brought to a boil in glass saucepan. After adding ¼ tsp. pure salt and boiling again, pour into a sterile canning jar. Refrigerate. Freeze some of it.

Lip Soother

For dry, burning lips. Heat 1 level tsp. sodium alginate plus 1 cup water until dissolved. After cooling, pour it into a small bottle to carry in your purse or pocket (refrigerate the remainder). Dab it on whenever needed. If the consistency isn't right for you, add water or boil it down further. You can make a better lip soother by adding some lysine from a crushed tablet, vitamin C powder, and a vitamin E capsule to the alginate mix. If you have a persistent problem with chapped lips, try going off citrus juice.

Foot Powder

Use a mixture of cornstarch and zinc oxide poured into a tall salt shaker with large holes in the lid. Add long rice grains to fight humidity. You may also try arrow root or potato starch. If you don't have zinc oxide use plain cornstarch.

Skin Healer Moisturizer Lotion

1 tsp. sodium alginate
1 cup water

Make the base first by heating these together in a covered, non-metal pan until completely dissolved. Use low heat–it will take over an hour. Use a wooden spoon handle to stir. Set aside. Then make the following mixture:

¼ tsp. vitamin C (ascorbic acid)
¼ tsp. lysine
2 tbs. pure vegetable glycerin
2 vitamin E capsules (400 units or more, each)
1 tsp. olive oil
1 tbs. lemon juice from a lemon or ¼ tsp. citric acid (this is optional)
1 cup water

Heat the water to steaming in a non-metal pan. Add vitamin C and lysine first and then everything else. Pour into a pint jar and shake to mix. Then add the sodium alginate base to the desired thickness (about equal amounts) and shake. Pour some into a small bottle to use as lip soother. Pour some into a larger bottle to dispense on skin. Store remainder in refrigerator. (See *Sources* for sodium alginate and vegetable glycerin. Sodium alginate is also available in capsule form at some health food stores.)

Other Skin Healers

Vitamin C powder (ascorbic acid, not the same as citric acid). Put a large pinch into the palm of your hand. With your other hand pick up a few drops of water from the faucet. Rub hands together until all the powder is dissolved and dispensed. It may sting briefly. Do this at bedtime, especially for cracked, chapped hands. Include lips if they need it.

50% Glycerin. Dilute 100% vegetable glycerin with an equal amount of water. This is useful as an after shave lotion.

Vitamin C liquid. Mix ¼ tsp. vitamin C powder in one pint water (opened capsules will do). This is useful as an after shave lotion and general skin treatment.

Cornstarch. (Unpolluted, see *Sources*.) Use on rashes, fungus, moist or irritated areas and to prevent chafe.

Combining several of these makes them more effective.

Dry skin has several causes: too much water contact, too much soap contact (switch to borax), low body temperature, not enough fat in the diet, or parasites.

Massage Oil

Instead of using ANY oil, which may be benzene polluted, make yourself a cornstarch solution:

    4 tsp. cornstarch
    1 cup water

Boil starch and water until clear, about one minute.

Sunscreen Lotion

Purchase PABA (see *Sources*) in 500 mg tablet form. Dissolve 1 tablet in grain alcohol. Grind the tablet first by putting it in a plastic bag and rolling over it with a glass jar. It will not completely dissolve even if you use a tablespoon of the alcohol. Pour the whole mixture into a 4 ounce bottle of homemade skin softener. Be careful not to get the lotion into your eyes when applying it. A better solution is to wear a hat or stay out of the sun.

Nose Salve

(When the inside of the nose is dry, cracked and bleeding.)

Pour ½ tsp. pure vegetable glycerin into a bottle cap. Add ½ tsp. of water. To apply, use a plastic coffee stirrer or straw. Cut a slit in the end to catch some cotton wool salvaged from a vitamin bottle and twist (cotton swabs, cotton balls and wooden toothpicks are contaminated with mercury, which in turn is polluted with thallium). Dip it into the glycerin mixture and apply inside the nose with a rotating motion. Do each nostril with a new applicator.

Quick Cornstarch Skin Softener

4 tsp. cornstarch
1 cup water

Boil starch and water until clear, about one minute.

Use only <u>unpolluted</u> cornstarch (see *Sources*).

Cornstarch Skin Softener

3 tsp. pure cornstarch
1 cup water
1 tsp. Vitamin C powder (ascorbic acid); or 5 capsules, 1000 mg each

Boil starch and water until clear, about one minute. Add vitamin C and stir until dissolved. Cool. Pour into dispenser bottle. Keep refrigerated when not in use.

After Shaves

Vitamin C. ¼ tsp. vitamin C powder, dissolved in 1 pint water.

Vegetable glycerin. Equal parts glycerin and water or to suit yourself.

Personal Lubricants

Heat these together: 1 level tsp. sodium alginate and 1 cup water in a covered non-metal pan until completely dissolved. Use very low heat and stir with a wooden spoon handle. It takes a fairly long time to get it perfectly smooth. After cooling, pour into a small dispenser bottle. <u>Keep refrigerated</u>.

Or, boil 4 tsp. cornstarch and 1 cup water until completely dissolved in a covered saucepan. Use non-metal dishes and a non-metal stirring spoon. Cool. Pour some into dispenser bottle. Keep refrigerated. This is many person's favorite recipe.

Baby Wipes

Cut paper towels in quarters and stack in a closeable plastic box. Run tap water over them, drain the excess. Add 1 tsp. grain alcohol and/or borax liquid on top. Close. Put a dab of the Quick Cornstarch Softener recipe on top of each wipe as you use it.

People Wipes

¼ tsp. powdered lysine
¼ tsp. vitamin C powder (you may open capsules)
¼ cup vegetable glycerin
1 cup water

Prepare wipes by cutting paper towels in quarters. Use white, unfragranced towels that are strong enough to hold up for this use. Fold each piece in quarters again and stack in a plastic zippered baggy. Pour the fluid mixture over the stack and zip. Store a bag full in the freezer to take on car trips. If you want to keep them a month or more, add 1 tbs. grain alcohol to the recipe.

For bathroom use, dampen a roll of paper towels under the cold tap first. Then pour about ¼ cup of the mixture over the towel roll around the middle. Store in plastic shopping bag or stand in plastic waste basket.

Recipes For Natural Cosmetics

Eye liner and Eyebrow Pencil

Get a pure charcoal pencil (black only) at an art supply store. Try several on yourself (bring a small mirror) in the store to see what hardness suits you. You may need to wet it with water or a vitamin E perle first. Don't put any chemicals on your *eyelids*, since this penetrates into your eye. To check this out for yourself, close your eye tightly and then dab lemon juice on your eyelid. It will soon burn! Everything that is put on skin penetrates. Otherwise the nicotine patch and estrogen patch wouldn't work. Not even soap belongs on your eyelids! Charcoal pencils are cheap. Get yourself half a dozen different kinds so you can do different things.

You could also use a capsule of activated charcoal. Empty it into a saucer. Mix glycerin and water, half and half, and add it to the charcoal powder until you get the consistency you like. Use a brush for eyelashes; use a finger for eyebrows.

Lipstick

Beet root powder (see *Sources*)
100% vegetable glycerin

Combine 1 tsp. vegetable glycerin and 1 tsp. beet root powder in a saucer. Stir until <u>perfectly</u> smooth. Then add ½ tsp. of vitamin E oil. Snip open vitamin E capsules or buy vitamin E oil (see *Sources*). Very thick olive oil can be substituted. Apply liberally with your finger or a lipstick brush. Do not purse or rub your lips together after application. To make the lipstick stay on longer, apply 1 layer of lipstick, then dab some cornstarch over the lips, then apply another layer of lipstick. Store in a small glass or plastic container in the refrigerator, tightly covered in a plastic bag.

Face Powder

Use cornstarch from the original box. You may also try arrow root starch or potato starch. Use your fingers or a tissue to apply because applicators can carry bacteria.

Blush (face powder in a cake form)

Add 50% glycerin to cornstarch in a saucer to make a paste. Slowly add beet root powder to the desired color. To darken it try part of a charcoal capsule. A drop of food grade alcohol will also darken it. To make 50% glycerin, add equal parts of glycerin and water. Try to make the consistency the same as your brand name product, and you can even put it back in your brand name container.

Recipes For Household Products

Floor Cleaner

Use washing soda from the grocery store. You may add borax and boric acid (to deter insects except ants). Use white distilled vinegar in your rinse water for a natural shine and ant repellent. Do not add bleach to this. For the bathroom floor use plain bleach water—follow the label. Never use chlorine bleach if anybody in the home is ill or suffers from depression. Use grain alcohol (1 pint to 3 quarts water) for germ killing action instead of chlorine.

Furniture Duster and Window Cleaner

Mix equal parts white distilled vinegar and water. Put it in a spray bottle.

Furniture Polish

A few drops of olive oil on a dampened cloth. Use filtered water to dampen.

Insect Killer

Boric acid powder (not borax). Throw liberal amounts behind stove, refrigerator, under carpets and in carpets. Since boric acid is white, you must be careful not to mistake it for sugar accidentally. Keep it far away from food and out of children's reach. Buy it at a farm supply or garden store (or see *Sources*). It will not kill ants.

Ant Repellent

Spray 50% white distilled vinegar on counter tops, window sills and shelves and wipe, leaving residue. Start early in spring before they arrive, because it takes a few weeks to rid yourself of them once they are established. If you want immediate action, get some lemons, cut the yellow outer peel off and cover with grain alcohol in a tightly closed jar. Let stand at least one hour. Use 1 part of this concentrate with 9 parts water in a spray bottle. Mix only as much as you will use because the diluted form loses potency. Spray walls, floors, carpets wherever you see them. The lemon solution even leaves a shine on your counters. Use both vinegar and lemon approaches to rid yourself of ants.

To treat the **whole house**, pour vinegar all around your foundation, close to the wall, using one gallon for every five feet. Expect to damage any foliage it touches. Reapply every six months.

Flower and Foliage Spray

Food-grade hydrogen peroxide. See instructions on bottle.

Moth Balls

I found this recipe in an old recipe book. Mix the following and scatter in trunks and bags containing furs and woolens: ½ lb. each rosemary and mint, ¼ lb. each tansy and thyme, 2 tbs. powdered cloves.

Carpet Cleaner

Whether you rent a machine or have a cleaning service, don't use the carpet shampoo they want to sell, even if they "guarantee" that it is all natural and safe. Instead add these to a bucket (about four gallons) of water and use it as the cleaning solution:

Wash water
1/3 cup borax

Rinse water
¼ cup grain alcohol
2 tsp. boric acid
¼ cup white distilled vinegar <u>or</u>
4 tsp. citric acid
1 bottle povidone iodine (optional)

Borax does the cleaning; alcohol disinfects, boric acid leaves a pesticide residue, and the vinegar or citric acid give luster. Povidone iodine kills parasite eggs. If you are just making one pass on your carpet, use the borax, alcohol, boric acid, and iodine. Remember to test everything you use on an unnoticed piece of carpet first.

Health Improvement Recipes

Black Walnut Hull Tincture

This new recipe is four times as strong as the previous one, so it is called **Black Walnut Hull Tincture <u>Extra Strength</u>**.

Your largest enamel or ceramic (not stainless steel, not aluminum) cooking pot, preferably at least 10 quarts
Black walnuts, in the hull, each one still at least 50% green, enough to fill the pot to the top
Grain alcohol, about 50% strength, enough to cover the walnuts
Vitamin C powder, 1 tsp. plus 1 tsp. per quart of tincture
Plastic wrap or cellophane
Glass jars or bottles

The black walnut tree produces large green balls in fall. The walnut is inside, but we will use the whole ball, uncracked, since the active ingredient is in the green outer hull.

Rinse the walnuts carefully, put them in the pot, and cover with the alcohol. Sprinkle on 1 tsp. vitamin C. Seal with plastic wrap and cover tightly. Let sit for three days. Pour into glass jars or bottles, discarding walnuts, and add more vitamin C (1 tsp. per quart). This will keep the color green. If the glass jar has a metal lid, put plastic wrap over the top before screwing on the lid. Potency is strong for several years if unopened, even if it darkens slightly. Refrigerate after opening.

You have just made Extra Strength Black Walnut Hull Tincture. It is stronger than the concentrate made with just a few black walnuts in a quart jar (my earlier recipe), because there are more walnuts per unit liquid. In addition, you will not dilute it before use (although when you take it, it will usually be in water).

When preparing the walnuts, rinse only with cold tap water. You may need to use a brush on areas with dirt. If you are not going to use all of them in this batch, you may freeze them in a resealable plastic bag. Simply refrigerating them does not keep them from turning black and useless. The pot of soaking walnuts should not be refrigerated. Nor does the final tincture need refrigeration until after it is opened.

Exposure to air does cause the tincture to darken and lose potency. To reduce air exposure, fill the pot as much as possible, without touching the plastic wrap, while still keeping a snug fitting lid. Even more importantly, the glass jars or bottles you use to store your tincture should have as little air space as possible, without touching the plastic wrap on top. A large jar should be divided into smaller ones when you are ready to use it. The idea is not to have partial jars, with a lot of air space, sitting for longer than a month or so. To regain some green color, add several tsp. vitamin C, close jar tightly, and let stand 1 day.

There are several ways to make a 50% grain alcohol solution. Some states have Everclear,™ 95% alcohol. Mix this half and half with water. Other states have Everclear,™ that is 76.5% alcohol. Mix this two parts Everclear,™ to one part water. Do not use vodka or the flask-size Everclear; it must be ¾ liter or 1 liter. Smaller bottles have wood alcohol or isopropyl alcohol pollution.

Remember, never use any kind of <u>purchased</u> water to make tincture or you will pollute it yourself.

Black Walnut Hull Tincture (Regular Strength)

This is the potency I used originally. It is included here in case you prefer it or wish to treat a pet. The Extra Strength recipe is four times as potent as the original recipe, so it must be diluted in quarters. (Similarly, if you have a lot of the Regular Strength left and want to use it in place of Extra Strength, simply take four times as much.)

Black Walnut Hull Tincture Extra Strength
Grain Alcohol, about 10%

Mix one part extra strength tincture with three parts of the 10% alcohol. Store in glass containers same as described above.

There are several ways to make a 10% grain alcohol solution. Some states have Everclear,™ 95% alcohol. Mix this one part Everclear to nine parts water. Other states have Everclear that is 76.5% alcohol. Mix this one part Everclear to seven parts water.

Recipe for a small family:
Fill a quart jar with the green balls. Cover with 50% alcohol. Add 1 tsp. vitamin C. Use a plastic bag to cover jar before closing tightly with lid. Let stand on kitchen counter. After 3

days, pour liquid into small glass bottles. Add another ¼ tsp. vitamin C powder to the top of each before closing. The strength of this will be half of the concentrate. So you would need to double the amount taken in the recipe.

Black Walnut Hull Extract (Water Based)

This recipe is intended for alcoholic persons: cover the green balls in the 10 quart (non-metal) pot with cold tap water. Heat to boiling, covered. Turn off heat. When cool, add vitamin C, cover with plastic wrap, and the lid. Let stand for 1 day. It will be darker than the tincture. Do not dilute. Pour into freezable containers. Refrigerate what you will use in two days and freeze the rest. Add vitamin C after thawing or during refrigeration (1 tsp. per quart).

For use: in programs calling for Extra Strength Black Walnut Hull Tincture use four times as much of this water based recipe (8 tsp. instead of 2 tsp. Extra Strength).

Important Note: do not use bottled or purchased water to make this tincture or you could pollute it with isopropyl alcohol!

Quassia recipe

Add 1/8 cup quassia chips to 3 cups water. Simmer 20-30 minutes. Pour off 1/8 cup now and drink it fresh. Refrigerate remainder. Drink 1/8 cup 4 times/day, until a total of ½ cup of chips is consumed. Flavor with spices.

Bowel Program

Bacteria are always at the root of bowel problems, such as pain, bloating and gassiness. They can not be killed by zapping, because the high frequency current does not penetrate the bowel contents.

Although most bowel bacteria are beneficial, the ones that are not, like *Salmonellas*, *Shigellas*, and *Clostridiums* are extremely detrimental because they have the ability to invade the rest of your body and colonize a trauma site or tumorous organ. These same bacteria colonize a cancer tumor and prevent shrinking after the malignancy is stopped.

One reason bowel bacteria are so hard to eradicate is that we are constantly reinfecting ourselves by keeping a reservoir on our hands and under our fingernails.

- So the first thing to do is **improve sanitation**. Use 50% grain alcohol in a spray bottle at the bathroom sink. Sterilize your hands after bathroom use and before meals.
- Second, use **betaine hydrochloride** to kill *Clostridium* (2 tablets 3 times a day).
- Third, use **turmeric** (2 capsules 3 times a day, this is the common spice) which I find helps against *Shigella*, as well as *E. coli*. Expect orange colored stool.
- Fourth, use **fennel** (2 capsule 3 times a day).
- Fifth, use **digestive enzyme tablets** with meals as directed on the bottle. (But only as long as necessary, because these frequently harbor molds.)
- Sixth, use a single 2 tsp. dose of **Black Walnut Hull Tincture Extra Strength**. Add it to a ½ glass of water or fruit juice and sip over a fifteen minute period. Stay seated until any side effect from the alcohol wears off.
- Seventh, <u>if you are constipated</u>, take **Cascara sagrada** (an herb, start with one capsule a day, use up to maxi-

mum on label), **extra magnesium** (300 mg magnesium oxide, 2 or 3 a day), and drink **a cup of hot water** upon rising in the morning. This will begin to regulate your elimination.

- Eighth, take **Lugol's** solution, 6 drops in ½ cup water 4 times a day. This is specifically for *Salmonella*.

It can take all eight to get rid of a bad bacteria problem in a week. Afterward, you must continue to eat only <u>sterile</u> dairy products. Note that the Kidney Cleanse is often effective with bowel problems. Try it also.

You will know you succeeded when your tummy is flat, there is not a single gurgle, and your mood improves!

Enemas

If you should fail to have a bowel movement in a <u>single</u> day it is a serious matter. An ill person cannot afford to fill up further with the ammonia, the toxic amines, and toxic gasses that bowel bacteria produce. Fortunately, enemas are very easy to do. Do an enema before going to bed.

There are several kinds of enema equipment available in pharmacies; most important is NEVER to use anyone else's equipment, no matter how "sterilized" it is guaranteed to be. Get your own. Do not use the equipment used by a professional bowel-cleanser. It is impossible to completely avoid cross-contamination. You must completely avoid it.

A Fleet™ bottle, obtained at your local pharmacy, will do for a starter (other equipment, like shown below, is available, see *Sources*). This is a squeeze bottle with a plastic applicator for insertion. Dump the contents since you are unable to test it for toxins. Refill with warm tap water.

The lubricant can be made in 5 minutes.

4 level tsp. cornstarch
1 cup water

Bring this to a boil and cook for about one minute. Set in the refrigerator to cool quickly. Pour a tsp. or more on top of a plastic bag for convenience in use. The only other lubricants are olive oil and castor oil.

For many of us, the rectum and sigmoid colon have ballooned out into a pocket due to past times of constipation. This is called a *diverticulum*. It is just a few inches from the anus so it is quite accessible by enema.

The diverticulum walls are quite weak due to constant over-stretching. But in just a few weeks of daily cleansing, the pocket will shrink and may even disappear.

Parasites and bad bacteria can escape being killed if they are in the diverticulum. Your entire bowel health can be turned around by killing the invaders of this diverticulum. Two ways of killing rectal parasites are with Lugol's or Black Walnut Tincture enemas.

Lugol's Enema

(Not for persons who are allergic to iodine.) Add 1 tsp. of Lugol's iodine to 1 quart of very warm water; pour into cup-size Fleet™ bottle (giving yourself 4 doses), or enema apparatus. Administer enema slowly and hold internally as long as possible.

Enzyme Enema

Mix a capsule of digestive enzymes with plain enema water. You may also crush a tablet.

Black Walnut Hull Extra Strength Enema

Add 1 to 4 tsp. of Black Walnut Hull Extra Strength to 1 quart of very warm water. Repeat as above.

Do an enema daily for one week to improve bowel function, alternating the above varieties. If you have none of these solutions available, use plain salt water, 1 tsp. per quart. In the absence of salt, use plain water. Remember, you must move your bowels or cleanse at least once a day.

Giving Yourself The Perfect Enema

Any drop you spill and everything you use to do the enema will <u>somehow</u> contaminate your bathroom. Yet you must leave it all perfectly sanitary for your own protection. So follow these instructions carefully.

Spread out a large plastic trash bag on the bathroom floor. Place a plastic grocery bag beside it and a paper plate on it. Set a chair nearby, too. The trash bag is for you to lie on. Lie on your back if you have nobody to help you.

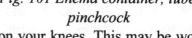

Fig. 101 Enema container, tube, pinchcock

Instructions on commercially available enema bottles advise you to be on your knees. This may be workable for the small squeeze-bottle of ready-made solution you can purchase. It is quite impossible, though, if you are elderly, have painful knees or are simply ill and must try to take in a whole quart from a complex apparatus.

Test the apparatus first, in the bathroom sink to see how it works. Wipe away the grease that comes with it on the applicator; it is sure to be a petroleum product and be tainted with benzene.

Pour a tablespoon of olive oil into the paper plate for the lubricant.

After filling the container with the enema solution, run some through the tubing until the air is out of it and close the pinchcock. Place it on the grocery bag.

Insert the applicator tube as far as you comfortably can. Then lift the container with one hand while opening the valve with the other. The higher you lift it, the faster it runs. Take as much time as you need to run it in. You may wish to set the container on the chair. Very warm liquid is easier to hold. Don't force yourself to hold it all. At any time you may close the valve, withdraw the applicator, and place it on the grocery bag.

Cleaning up the apparatus, the bathroom, and yourself: This topic is seldom discussed, but very important. Notice that some bowel contents have entered the container by reflux action, which is unavoidable. Consider the whole apparatus contaminated. For this reason you must never, never use anybody else's apparatus, no matter how clean it looks.

First, wipe the applicator tube. Then fill the container and run it through the hose into the toilet. Repeat until it appears clean; this is appearance only; you must now sterilize it. Fill it with water and add Lugol's iodine or povidone iodine until intensely red in color. Place the end of the tube in the container to soak. Empty and wipe the outside of the tube with paper. Do not dry the container. Store in a fresh plastic bag. Throw away the trash bag, grocery bag and paper plate. Clean the sink with chlorine bleach. Then wash your hands with skin sanitizer.

If all went well, you may risk taking the next enema on your bed. If not take a shower and stick to the floor location.

Kidney Cleanse

½ cup dried Hydrangea root
½ cup Gravel root
½ cup Marshmallow root
4 bunches of fresh parsley
~~Goldenrod tincture (leave this out of the recipe if you are allergic to it)~~
Ginger capsules
Uva Ursi capsules
Vegetable glycerin
Black Cherry Concentrate, 8 oz
Vitamin B$_6$, 250 mg
Magnesium oxide, 300 mg or ¼ cup Green Drink beverage

Measure ¼ cup of each root and set them to soak, together in 10 cups of cold tap water, using a non-metal container and a non-metal lid (a dinner plate will do). After four hours (or overnight) add 8 oz. black cherry concentrate, heat to boiling and simmer for 20 minutes. Drink ¼ cup as soon as it is cool enough. Pour the rest through a bamboo strainer into a sterile pint jar (glass) and several freezable containers. Refrigerate the glass jar.

Find fresh parsley at a grocery store that does not spray its produce (ask the owner). Boil the fresh parsley, after rinsing, in 1 quart of water for 3 minutes. Drink ¼ cup when cool enough. Refrigerate a pint and freeze 1 pint. Throw away the parsley.

Dose: each morning, pour together ¾ cup of the root mixture and ½ cup parsley water, filling a large mug. Add 20 drops of goldenrod tincture and 1 tbs. of glycerin. Drink this mixture in divided doses throughout the day. Keep cold. <u>Do not drink it all at once</u> or you will get a stomach ache and feel pressure in your bladder. If your stomach is very sensitive, start on half this dose.

Save the roots after the first boiling, storing them in the freezer. After 13 days when your supply runs low, boil the same roots a second time, but add only 6 cups water and simmer only

10 minutes. This will last another 8 days, for a total of three weeks. You may cook the roots a third time if you wish, but the recipe gets less potent. If your problem is severe, only cook them twice.

After three weeks, repeat with fresh herbs. You need to do the Kidney Cleanse for six weeks to get good results, longer for severe problems.

Also take:

- Ginger capsules: one with each meal (3/day).
- Uva Ursi capsules: one with breakfast and two with supper.
- Vitamin B$_6$ (250 mg): one a day.
- Magnesium oxide (300 mg): one a day.

Take these supplements just before your meal to avoid burping.

Some notes on this recipe: this herbal tea, as well as the parsley, can easily spoil. Heat it to boiling every fourth day if it is being stored in the refrigerator; this resterilizes it. If you sterilize it in the morning you may take it to work without refrigerating it (use a glass container).

When you order your herbs, be careful! Herb companies are not the same! These roots should have a strong fragrance. If the ones you buy are barely fragrant, they have lost their active ingredients; switch to a different supplier. Fresh roots can be used. Do not use powder.

- Hydrangea (*Hydrangea arborescens*) is a common flowering bush.
- Gravel root (*Eupatorium purpureum*) is a wild flower.
- Marshmallow root (*Althea officinallis*) is mucilaginous and kills pain.

- Fresh parsley can be bought at a grocery store. Parsley flakes and dried parsley herb do <u>not</u> work.
- Goldenrod herb works as well as the tincture but you may get an allergic reaction from smelling the herb. If you know you are allergic to this, leave this one out of your recipe.
- Ginger from the grocery store works fine; you may put it into capsules for yourself (size 0, 1 or 00).

There are probably dozens of herbs that can dissolve kidney crystals and stones. If you can only find several of those in the recipe, make the recipe anyway; it will just take longer to get results. Remember that vitamin B_6 and magnesium, taken daily, can prevent oxalate stones from forming. But only if you stop drinking regular tea or cocoa. Tea has 15.6 mg oxalic acid per cup[68]. A tall glass of iced tea could give you over 20 mg oxalic acid. Switch to herb teas. Cocoa and chocolate, also, have too much oxalic acid to be used as beverages.

Remember, too, that phosphate crystals are made when you eat too much phosphate. Phosphate levels are high in meats, breads, cereals, pastas, and carbonated drinks. Eat less of these, and increase your milk (2%), fruits and vegetables. Drink at least 2 pints of water a day.

Cleanse your kidneys at least twice a year.

You can dissolve all your kidney stones in 3 weeks, but make new ones in 3 days if you are drinking tea and cocoa and

---

[68] Taken from *Food Values* 14ed by Pennington and Church 1985.

phosphated beverages. None of the beverage recipes in this book are conducive to stone formation.

Liver Herbs

Don't confuse these liver herbs with the next recipe for the Liver Cleanse. This recipe contains herbs traditionally used to help the liver function, while the Liver Cleanse gets gallstones out.

6 parts comfrey root, *Symphytum officinale* (also called nipbone root)
6 parts tanner's oak bark, *Quercus alba* (white oak bark)
3 parts gravel root, *Eupatorium purpureum* (queen of the meadow)
3 parts Jacob's staff, *Verbascum thapsus* (mullein herb)
2 parts licorice root, *Glycyrrhiza glabra*
2 parts wild yam root, *Dioscorea villosa*
2 parts milk thistle herb, *Silybum marianum*
3 parts walnut bark, *Juglans nigra*, (black walnut bark)
3 parts marshmallow root, *Althea officinalis* (white mallow)
1 part lobelia plant, *Lobelia inflata* (bladder pod)
1 part skullcap, *Scutellaria lateriflora* (helmet flower)

Mix all the herbs. Add ½ cup of the mixture to 2 quarts of water. Bring to a boil. Put lid on. Let sit for six hours. Strain and add sweetening such as vegetable glycerin or honey. Drink two cups a day for six to eight weeks. Put the strained herbs in the freezer and use them one more time.

Liver Cleanse

Cleansing the liver of gallstones dramatically improves digestion, which is the basis of your whole health. You can expect your allergies to disappear, too, more with each cleanse you do! Incredibly, it also eliminates shoulder, upper arm, and upper back pain. You have more energy and increased sense of well being.

Cleaning the liver bile ducts is the most powerful procedure that you can do to improve your body's health.

But it <u>should not</u> be done before the parasite program, and for <u>best results</u> should follow the kidney cleanse.

It is the job of the liver to make bile, 1 to 1½ quarts in a day! The liver is full of tubes (*biliary tubing*) that deliver the bile to one large tube (the *common bile duct*). The gallbladder is attached to the common bile duct and acts as a storage reservoir. Eating fat or protein triggers the gallbladder to squeeze itself empty after about twenty minutes, and the stored bile finishes its trip down the common bile duct to the intestine.

<u>For many persons, including children, the biliary tubing is choked with gallstones</u>. Some develop allergies or hives but some have no symptoms. When the gallbladder is scanned or X-rayed nothing is seen. Typically, they are not in the gallbladder. Not only that, most are too small and not calcified, a prerequisite for visibility on X-ray. There are over half a dozen varieties of gallstones, most of which have cholesterol crystals in them. They can be black, red, white, green or tan colored. The green ones get their color from being coated with bile. Notice in the picture how many have imbedded unidentified objects. Are they fluke remains? Notice how many are shaped like corks with longitudinal grooves below the tops. We can visualize the blocked bile ducts from such shapes. Other stones are composites—made of many smaller ones—showing that they regrouped in the bile ducts some time after the last cleanse.

At the very center of each stone is found a clump of bacteria, according to scientists, suggesting a dead bit of parasite might have started the stone forming.

As the stones grow and become more numerous the back pressure on the liver causes it to make less bile. It is also thought to slow the flow of lymphatic fluid. Imagine the situation if your garden hose had marbles in it. Much less water would flow, which in turn would decrease the ability of the hose to squirt out the marbles. <u>With gallstones, much less cholesterol leaves the body, and cholesterol levels may rise.</u>

Gallstones, being porous, can pick up all the bacteria, cysts, viruses and parasites that are passing through the liver. In this way "nests" of infection are formed, forever supplying the body with fresh bacteria and parasite stages. No stomach infection such as ulcers or intestinal bloating can be cured permanently without removing these gallstones from the liver.

For best results, <u>ozonate</u> the olive oil in this recipe to kill any parasite stages that may be released during the cleanse.

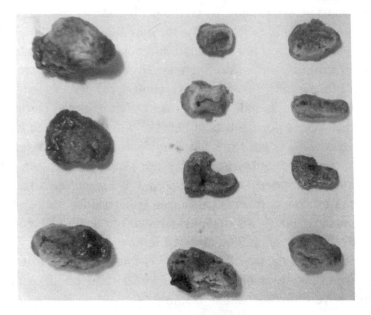

Fig. 102 These are gallstones.

Cleanse your liver twice a year.

Preparation.

- You can't clean a liver with living parasites in it. You won't get many stones, and you will feel quite sick. <u>Zap daily the week before, or get through the first three weeks of the parasite killing program before attempting a liver cleanse.</u> If you are on the maintenance parasite program, you are always ready to do the cleanse.

- Completing the kidney cleanse before cleansing the liver is also <u>highly recommended</u>. You want your kidneys, bladder and urinary tract in top working condition so they can efficiently remove any undesirable substances incidentally absorbed from the intestine as the bile is being excreted.

Ingredients

Epsom salts	4 tablespoons
Olive oil	half cup (light olive oil is easier to get down), and for best results, ozonate it for 20 to 30 minutes, first
Fresh pink grapefruit	1 large or 2 small, enough to squeeze 2/3 to 3/4 cup juice
Ornithine	4 to 8, to be sure you can sleep. Don't skip this or you may have the worst night of your life!
Large plastic straw	To help drink potion.
Pint jar with lid	
Black Walnut Tincture, any strength.	10 to 20 drops, to kill parasites coming from the liver.

Choose a day like Saturday for the cleanse, since you will be able to rest the next day.

Take <u>no</u> medicines, vitamins or pills that you can do without; they could prevent success. Stop the parasite program and kidney herbs, too, the day before.

Eat a <u>no-fat</u> breakfast and lunch such as cooked cereal, fruit, fruit juice, bread and preserves or honey (no butter or milk). This allows the bile to build up and develop pressure in the liver. Higher pressure pushes out more stones.

2:00 PM. <u>Do not eat or drink after 2 o'clock</u>. If you break this rule you could feel quite ill later.

Get your Epsom salts ready. Mix 4 tbs. in 3 cups water and pour this into a jar. This makes four servings, ¾ cup each. Set the jar in the refrigerator to get ice cold (this is for convenience and taste only).

6:00 PM. Drink one serving (¾ cup) of the ice cold Epsom salts. If you did not prepare this ahead of time, mix 1 tbs. in ¾ cup water now. You may add 1/8 tsp. vitamin C powder to improve the taste. You may also drink a few mouthfuls of water afterwards or rinse your mouth.

Get the olive oil (ozonated, if possible) and grapefruit out to warm up.

8:00 PM. Repeat by drinking another ¾ cup of Epsom salts.

You haven't eaten since two o'clock, but you won't feel hungry. Get your bedtime chores done. The timing is critical for success.

9:45 PM. Pour ½ cup (measured) olive oil into the pint jar. Squeeze the grapefruit by hand into the measuring cup. Remove pulp with fork. You should have at least ½ cup, more (up to ¾ cup) is best. You may top it up with lemonade. Add this to the olive oil. Also, add Black Walnut Tincture. Close the jar tightly with the lid and shake hard until watery (only fresh grapefruit juice does this).

Now visit the bathroom one or more times, even if it makes you late for your ten o'clock drink. Don't be more than 15 minutes late. You will get fewer stones.

10:00 PM. Drink the potion you have mixed. Take 4 ornithine capsules with the first sips to make sure you will sleep through the night. Take 8 if you already suffer from insomnia. Drinking through a large plastic straw helps it go down easier. You may use oil and vinegar salad dressing, cinnamon, or brown sugar to chase it down between sips. Take it to your bedside if you want, but drink it standing up. Get it down within 5 minutes (fifteen minutes for very elderly or weak persons).

Lie down immediately. You might fail to get stones out if you don't. The sooner you lie down the more stones you will get out. Be ready for bed ahead of time. Don't clean up the kitchen. As soon as the drink is down walk to your bed and lie down flat on your back with your head up high on the pillow. Try to think about what is happening in the liver. Try to keep perfectly still for at least 20 minutes. You may feel a train of stones traveling along the bile ducts like marbles. There is no pain because the bile duct valves are open (thank you Epsom salts!). **Go to sleep**, you may fail to get stones out if you don't.

Next morning. Upon awakening take your third dose of Epsom salts. If you have indigestion or nausea wait until it is gone before drinking the Epsom salts. You may go back to bed. Don't take this potion before 6:00 am.

2 Hours Later. Take your fourth (the last) dose of Epsom salts. You may go back to bed again.

After 2 More Hours you may eat. Start with fruit juice. Half an hour later eat fruit. One hour later you may eat regular food but keep it light. By supper you should feel recovered.

How well did you do? Expect diarrhea in the morning. Use a flashlight to look for gallstones in the toilet with the bowel movement. Look for the green kind since this is <u>proof</u> that they are genuine gallstones, not food residue. Only bile from the liver is pea green. The bowel movement sinks but gallstones float because of the cholesterol inside. <u>Count them all roughly</u>, whether tan or green. You will need to total 2000 stones before the liver is clean enough to rid you of allergies or bursitis or upper back pains <u>permanently</u>. The first cleanse may rid you of them for a few days, but as the stones from the rear travel forward, they give you the same symptoms again. You may repeat cleanses at two week intervals. Never cleanse when you are ill.

Sometimes the bile ducts are full of cholesterol crystals that did not form into round stones. They appear as a "chaff" floating on top of the toilet bowl water. It may be tan colored, harboring millions of tiny white crystals. Cleansing this chaff is just as important as purging stones.

How safe is the liver cleanse? It is very safe. My opinion is based on over 500 cases, including many persons in their seventies and eighties. None went to the hospital; none even reported pain. However it can make you feel quite ill for one or two days afterwards, although in every one of these cases the maintenance parasite program had been neglected. This is why the instructions direct you to complete the parasite and kidney cleanse programs first.

CONGRATULATIONS

You have taken out your gallstones <u>without surgery</u>! I like to think I have perfected this recipe, but I certainly can not take credit for its origin. It was invented hundreds, if not thousands, of years ago, THANK YOU, HERBALISTS!

This procedure contradicts many modern medical viewpoints. Gallstones are thought to be formed in the gallbladder, not the liver. They are thought to be few, not thousands. They are not linked to pains other than gallbladder attacks. It is easy to understand why this is thought: by the time you have acute pain attacks, some stones <u>are</u> in the gallbladder, <u>are</u> big enough and sufficiently calcified to see on X-ray, and <u>have</u> caused inflammation there. When the gallbladder is removed the acute attacks are gone, but the bursitis and other pains and digestive problems remain.

The truth is self-evident. People who have had their gall-bladder surgically removed still get plenty of green, bile-coated stones, and anyone who cares to dissect their stones can see that the concentric circles and crystals of cholesterol match textbook pictures of "gallstones" exactly.

Lugol's Iodine Solution

It is too dangerous to buy a commercially prepared solution. It is certain to be polluted with isopropyl alcohol or wood alcohol. Make it yourself or ask your pharmacist to make (not order) it for you. The recipe to make 1 liter (quart) is:

44 gm (1½ ounces) iodine, granular
88 gm (3 ounces) potassium iodide, granular

Dissolve the potassium iodide in about a pint of the water. Then add the iodine crystals and wait till it is all dissolved. This could take a few hours with frequent shaking. Fill to the liter mark (quart) with water. Keep out of sight and reach of children. Do not use if allergic to iodine. Be careful to avoid bottled water for preparation.

White Iodine

88 gm potassium iodide, granular

Add potassium iodide to one quart or one liter cold tap water. Potassium iodide dissolves well in water and stays clear; for this reason it is called "white iodine." Label clearly and keep out of reach of children. Do not use if allergic to iodine.

Vitamin D Drops

1 gram cholecalciferol (see *Sources*)
10 cups olive oil

Mix in a non-metal container. It may take a day of standing to dissolve fully. Refrigerate. Ten <u>drops</u> contain 40,000 IU. Use within a year. This is enough for 250 people, each getting 10 cc. (2 tsp.). The dosage for adults during dental work or with bone disease is: one drop (no more, no less) daily, placed on tongue or on bread, for <u>3 weeks only</u>. After 21 days use 2 drops a week <u>only</u>. You can get too much of this.

Sources

This list was accurate as this book went to press. <u>Only the vitamin sources listed here were found to be pollution-free, and only the herb sources listed here were found to be potent</u>, although there may be other good sources that have not been tested. The author has a financial interest in New Century Press and family members in the Self Health Resource Center. Other than that, she has no financial interest in, influence on, or other connection with any company listed.

Note to readers outside the USA:

Sources listed are typically companies within the United States because they are the most familiar to me. You may be tempted to try a more convenient manufacturer in your own country and hope for the best. <u>I must advise against this</u>! In my experience, an uninformed manufacturer <u>most likely</u> has a polluted product! Your health is worth the extra effort to obtain the products that make you well. One bad product can keep you from reaching that goal. This chapter will be updated as I become aware of acceptable sources outside the United States. Best of all is to learn to test products yourself.

When ordering chemicals for internal use, always specify a <u>food</u> grade.

Item	Source (These are manufacturers. Ask for a distributor near you.)
Amber bottles, ½ ounce	Drug store, Continental Glass & Plastic, Inc. (large quantities)
Arginine	Spectrum Chemical Co., Seltzer Chemicals, Inc.
Aspartic acid	EDOM Labs, a crushed tablet will do.

Baking soda (sodium bicarbonate)	Spectrum Chemical Co.
Beet root	San Francisco Herb & Natural Food Co.
Belts for clothes dryer	Three that tested negative to asbestos are: Maytag™ 3-12959 Poly-V belt, Whirlpool™ FSP 341241 Belt-Drum Dr. (replaces 660996), and Bando™ V-Belt A-65. Bando American makes other belts, some of which might be the right size for your dryer. Call for a dealer near you, make sure it says "Made In America", not all do.
Betaine hydrochloride	General Nutrition Corporation
Biotin	Spectrum Chemical Co.
Black cherry concentrate	Health food store
Black Walnut Hull Tincture	Self Health Resource Center, Nature's Meadow, New Action Products
Borax, pure	Grocery store
Boric acid, pure	Now Foods, health food store, pharmacy
Calcium	Spectrum Chemical Co.
Cascara sagrada	Natures Way, health food store
CFH capsules	see Fenuthyme
Charcoal capsules	Health food store or drug store.
Chemical Supply Companies	Sigma-Aldrich Chemical Co., Spectrum Chemical Co., ICN Biomedicals, Inc. (research chemicals only, including genistein), Boehringer Mannheim Biochemicals (research only)
Cholecalciferol	Spectrum Chemical Co.
Citric acid	Now Foods or health food store
Cloves	San Francisco Herb & Natural Food Co. (ASK for fresh)
Coenzyme Q10	Spectrum Chemical Co., Seltzer Chemicals, Inc.
Colloidal silver maker	SOTA Instruments Inc.
Cornstarch	Spectrum Chemical Co., Lady Lee brand in the grocery store, Argo brand (25 lb. sack only) from CPC International, Inc.

Cysteine	Spectrum Chemical Co.
Denture making	New Century Press has current information
Electronic parts	A Radio Shack near you.
Electronic pest deterrant	New Tech Inovations
Empty gelatine capsules size 00	Health food store
Enema equipment	Medical Devices International
Epoxy coating	F. W. Dempsey Construction Co.
Fenuthyme	Natures Way
Filters, pure charcoal	Pure Water Products (pitchers), Seagull Distribution Co. (faucet, shower, whole house)
Folic acid	Spectrum Chemical Co.
Germanium	Jarrow Formulas, Inc.
Ginger capsules	Now Foods
Glutamine	Spectrum Chemical Co.
Glutathione	Spectrum Chemical Co., Seltzer Chemicals, Inc.
Glycine	Spectrum Chemical Co.
Goldenrod tincture	Dragon River Herbals, Blessed Herbs
Grain alcohol	Liquor store, get only 750 ml or 1 liter
Grains and legumes from India	Bazaar of India Imports
Gravel root (herb)	San Francisco Herb & Natural Food Co.
Hydrangea (herb)	San Francisco Herb & Natural Food Co.
Hydrogen peroxide 35% (food grade)	New Horizons Trust
Iodine, pure	Spectrum Chemical Co.
L-glutamic acid powder (This is not glutamine.)	Spectrum Chemical Co., or crush tablets from Schiff Bio-Food Products
L-lysine powder	Spectrum Chemical Co.
Lecithin	Spectrum Chemical Co.
Lugol's iodine	For slide staining (not internal use) from Spectrum Chemical Co., and farm animal supply store. For internal use must be made from scratch.
Magnesium oxide	Spectrum Chemical Co.
Marshmallow root (herb)	San Francisco Herb & Natural Food Co.

Methionine	Spectrum Chemical Co.
Microscope slides and equipment	Carolina Biological Supply Company, Ward's Natural Science, Inc., Southern Biological Supply Company, Fisher-EMD
Microscopes	Carolina Biological Supply Company, Ward's Natural Science, Inc., Edmund Scientific Co.
Niacinamide	Spectrum Chemical Co.
Olive leaf tea	San Francisco Herb & Natural Food Co.
Ornithine	Spectrum Chemical Co., Seltzer Chemicals, Inc.
Ortho-phospho-tyrosine	Sigma-Aldrich Chemical Co.
Ozonator	Phase II Enterprises
P24 antigen sample	Bachem Fine Chemicals Inc.
PABA (para amino benzoic acid)	Bronson Pharmaceuticals
Pantothenic acid	Spectrum Chemical Co.
Peroxy	See Hydrogen peroxide.
Photo-micrographic camera and film	Ward's Natural Science, Inc.
Plastic lids for Ball's mason jars	Alltrista Corporation
Potassium iodide, pure	Spectrum Chemical Co.
Salt (sodium chloride), pure	Spectrum Chemical Co., get USP grade
Soap, homemade	Sacred River Soap
Sodium alginate	Spectrum Chemical Co. or health food store
Stevia powder	Now Foods
Syncrometer	Self Health Resource Center
Syncrometer video	Self Health Resource Center
Taurine	Spectrum Chemical Co.
Thioctic acid	Spectrum Chemical Co.
Tooth Truth	New Century Press
Urinary phenol test	National Medical Services, for the test, have your doctor specify "chronic benzene exposure"
Uva Ursi	Natures Way or health food store
Vegetable glycerine	Starwest (5 gallon buckets only) or health food store

Vitamin B$_1$	Spectrum Chemical Co.
Vitamin B$_2$ (riboflavin)	Spectrum Chemical Co., Nutrition Headquarters
Vitamin B$_6$	Spectrum Chemical Co., EDOM Labs, Seltzer Chemicals, Inc.
Vitamin B$_{12}$	Spectrum Chemical Co.
Vitamin C (ascorbic acid)	Hoffman-LaRoche (all other sources I tested had either toxic selenium, yttrium, or thulium pollution!)
Vitamin D	See cholecalciferol
Vitamin E capsules	Bronson Pharmaceuticals
Vitamin E Oil	Spectrum Chemical Co.
Water filter pitchers	See filters.
Wormwood capsules	Self Health Resource Center, Kroeger Herb Products, New Action Products
Wormwood seed	R. H. Shumway
Zinc oxide	Spectrum Chemical Co.

Alltrista Corporation
PO Box 2729
Muncie, IN 47307-0729

Bachem Fine Chemicals Inc.
3132 Kashiwa St.
Torrance, CA 90505
(310) 539-4171

Bando American Inc.
1149 West Bryn Mawr
Itasca, IL 60143
(800) 829-6612
(708) 773-6600

Bazaar of India Imports
1810 University Ave.
Berkeley, CA 94703
(800) 261-7662

Blessed Herbs
109 Barre Plaines Rd.
Oakham, MA 01068
(508) 882-3839

Boehringer Mannheim
Biochemicals
9115 Hague Rd.
P.O. Box 50414
Indianapolis, IN 46250
(800) 262-1640
(317) 849-9350

Bronson Pharmaceuticals
Div. of Jones Medical Industry
1945 Craig Road
P.O. Box 46903
St. Louis, MO 63146-6903
(800) 235-3200 retail
(800) 525-8466 wholesale

Carolina Biological Supply Co.
2700 York Rd.
Burlington, NC 27215
(800) 334-5551
(919) 584-0381

Continental Glass & Plastic Inc
841 West Cermak Rd.
Chicago, IL 60608-4582
(312) 666-2050

CPC International Inc.
Englewood Cliffs, NJ 07632-9976

Dragon River Herbals
PO Box 74
Ojo Caliente, NM 87549
(800) 813-2118
(505) 583-2118

Edmund Scientific Co.
101 E. Gloucester Pike
Barrington, NJ 08007
(856) 573-6250

EDOM Labs, Inc.
860 Grand Boulevard
P.O. Box 780
Deer Park, NY 11729
(516) 586-2266
(800) 723-3366

Fisher Scientific EMD
485 S. Frontage Rd.
Burr Ridge, IL 60521
(800) 955-1177

F. W. Dempsey Construction
4228 East 2nd Street
Long Beach, CA 90803
(562) 433-5520

Hoffman-LaRoche
340 Kingsland St.
Nutley, NJ 07110-1199
(800) 892-6510
(201) 235-5000

General Nutrition Corporation
Pittsburgh, PA 15222

ICN Pharmaceuticals, Inc.
Biomedical Division
3300 Hyland Ave.
Costa Mesa, CA 92626
(714) 545-0113
(800) 854-0530

Jarrow Formulas, Inc.
1824 S. Robertson Blvd.
Los Angeles, CA 90035-4317
(800) 726-0886
(310) 204-6936

Kroeger Herb Products
805 Walnut St.
Boulder, CO 80302
(800) 225-8787
(303) 443-0261
(for retail call:)
Hanna's Herb Shop
5684 Valmont Rd.
Boulder, CO 80301
(800) 206-6722

Medical Devices International
3849 Swanson Ct.
Gurnee, IL 60031
(708) 336-6611

National Medical Services
3701 Relsh Road
Willow Grove, PA 19090
(215) 657-4900

Nature's Way
10 Mountain Springs Pkwy
Springville, UT 84663
(800) 962-8873
(801) 489-1500

New Action Products
P.O. Box 540
Orchard Park, NY 14127
(800) 455-6459
(716) 662-8000
New Action Products CANADA
PO Box 141
Grimsby, Ont. Canada
(800) 541-3799
(716) 873-3738

New Century Press
1055 Bay Blvd., Suite C
Chula Vista, CA 91911
(800) 519-2465
(619) 476-7400

New Horizons Trust
53166 St. Rt. 681
Reedsville, OH 45772
(800) 755-6360
(614) 378-6366

New Tech Inovations
4715-92nd Avenue
Edmonton, AB T6B2V4
CANADA

Now Foods
395 Glen Ellen Road
Glen Ellen, IL 60108
(630) 545-9098

Nutrition Headquarters, Inc.
Carbondale, IL 62901

Superior Health Products
13549 Ventura Blvd.
Sherman Oaks, CA 91423
(800) 700-1543 (818)986-9456

Pure Water Products
10332 Park View Ave.
Westminster, CA 92683
(800) 478-7987

R. H. Shumway
P.O. Box 1
Graniteville, SC 29829
(803) 663-9771

San Francisco Herb & Natural
Food Co.
1010 46th St.
Emeryville, CA 94608
(800) 227-2830 wholesale
(510) 601-0700 retail

Sacred River Soap Co.
4342 Elenda Street
Culver City, CA 90230
(310) 204-4807

Seagull Distribution Co.
3372 Baltimore St.
San Diego, CA 92117
(858) 483-0264

Schiff Bio-Food Products
Moonachie, NJ 07074

Self Health Resource Center
1055 Bay Blvd., #A
Chula Vista, CA 91911
(800) 873-1663
(619) 409-9500 (USA)
(780) 475-2403 (Canada)

Seltzer Chemicals, Inc.
5927 Geiger Ct.
Carlsbad, CA 92008-7305
(760) 438-0089

Sigma-Aldrich Chemical Co.
3500 Dekalb Street
St. Louis, MO 63118
(314) 771-5765
(800) 325-5832

SOTA Instruments Inc.
PO Box 866
Point Roberts, WA 98281-0866
(Canada) PO Box 26161
Central Postal Station
Richmond, BC V6Y 3V3
(800) 224-0242

Southern Biological Supply Co.
P.O. Box 368
McKenzie, TN 38201
(800) 748-8735
(901) 352-3337

Spectrum Chemical Co.
14422 South San Pedro Street
Gardena, CA 90248
(800) 772-8786
(310) 516-8000

Starwest Botanicals, Inc
11253 Trade Center Dr.
Rancho Cordova, CA 95742
(916) 638-8100
(888) 273-4372

Ward's Natural Science, Inc.
5100 West Henrietta Road
Rochester, NY 14586
(716) 359-2502
(800) 962-2660

Hope For The Future

Human society has searched for the cause of cancer for **100 years**, and *failed*, <u>even though</u>:
- the mission was entrusted to our best researchers in the academic, medical and industrial sectors
- they had private contracts, a monopoly
- there was incredible funding

Because the true cause could have been found by an ordinary person of reasonable intelligence with a High School education and moderate funds, <u>if only legally permitted</u>, I recommend that society withdraw the trust, advantages and resources given to the above institutions and lay open the enterprise of advancement in health issues to the non-professional person who shows dedication to the task.

It should be legal for a lay person to offer to the public any form of non-invasive health analysis, from astrology to magnetics to radionics to homeopathy to using the device described in this book, provided qualifications, methods and fees are disclosed in advance.

We must have FREEDOM to select health solutions for our physical welfare, the same as we have freedom to select religious solutions for our spiritual welfare. Freedom of religion was hard won. Many sincere and intelligent persons opposed it and still oppose it today, because they feel it is not moral to allow people to choose the "wrong" spiritual path. Similarly, the government passes laws to "protect" you from choosing the "wrong" (non-professional) health path. But those laws prevented us from finding the cure to cancer (unless you count "five year survival" as a cure). I recommend repealing these

611

laws. Religious freedom changed the religious structure on earth profoundly; freedom to select health solutions could have a similar impact.

The only reason I publish and <u>do not patent</u> the new technology described in this book is to make *Self Health* possible. Self Health means freedom in health matters—freedom to consult about illness not only with medical doctors (MD's), but with resources that are illegal now, like health advisors, researchers, technicians, and other physicians. It means freedom to select and order your own tests and get the results.

If your ankle is swollen and painful after a fall, and you go to the emergency room, you can not order an X-ray of it although the need is obvious. A doctor must make the order (and you pay the additional doctor's fee). Then you are not allowed to look at it (only doctors can diagnose). And just try to get a copy of your medical records; your doctor will instead insist on mailing them to your next doctor (because you might misinterpret them). The story is the same for blood, urine and hormone tests. Lay people can understand a great deal of this information, and learn even more on their own, if they were only encouraged instead of prohibited.

Because Self Health, by its very concept, undermines the existence of the medical profession as we know it, those espousing Self Health, hopefully soon to be the majority of persons, need to be protected from the legal wrath of medical institutions as they try to retain total control.

Index

D

Mop Up Program - 36